CONTENTS

3 Axis I Disorders Usually First Diagnosed in Infancy, Childhood, or Adolescence: Attention-Deficit and Disruptive Behavior Disorders 23

5 "Adult" Disorders That May Begin in Childhood or Adolescence 103

Child and Adolescent

Psychiatry

Third Edition

CONCISE
GUIDES

Robert E. Hales, M.D.
Series Editor

CONCISE GUIDE TO
Child and Adolescent Psychiatry

Third Edition

Mina K. Dulcan, M.D.

D. Richard Martini, M.D.

MaryBeth Lake, M.D.

Washington, DC
London, England

Copyright © 2003 American Psychiatric Publishing, Inc.
ALL RIGHTS RESERVED

Diagnostic criteria included in this book are reprinted, with permission, from *Diagnostic and Statistical Manual of Mental Disorders,* 4th Edition, Text Revision. Copyright © 2000, American Psychiatric Association.

Manufactured in the United States of America on acid-free paper
07 06 05 04 03   5 4 3 2 1
Third Edition

American Psychiatric Publishing, Inc.
1000 Wilson Boulevard
Arlington, VA 22209-3901
www.appi.org

Typeset in Adobe's Times and Helvetica

Library of Congress Cataloging-in-Publication Data
Dulcan, Mina K.
   Concise guide to child and adolescent psychiatry / Mina K. Dulcan, D. Richard Martini, MaryBeth Lake.—3rd ed.
      p. ; cm. — (Concise guides)
   Includes bibliographical references and index.
   ISBN 1-58562-074-2 (alk. paper)
   1. Child psychiatry—Handbooks, manuals, etc. 2. Adolescent psychiatry—Handbooks, manuals, etc. I. Martini, D. Richard. II. Lake, MaryBeth, 1966– III. Title. IV. Concise guides (American Psychiatric Publishing)
   [DNLM: 1. Adolescent Psychiatry—methods—Handbooks. 2. Child Psychiatry—methods—Handbooks. 3. Mental Disorders—Adolescence—Handbooks. 4. Mental Disorders—Child—Handbooks. WS 39 D881c 2003]
RJ499.3.D84 2003
618.92′ 89—dc21   2002043677

British Library Cataloguing in Publication Data
A CIP record is available from the British Library.

8 Psychopharmacology 259

LIST OF TABLES

4 Other Axis I Disorders Usually First Diagnosed in Infancy, Childhood, or Adolescence

5 "Adult" Disorders That May Begin in Childhood or Adolescence

6 Developmental Disorders

7 Special Clinical Circumstances

8 Psychopharmacology

9 Psychosocial Treatments

ABOUT THE AUTHORS

Mina K. Dulcan, M.D.

Margaret C. Osterman Professor of Child Psychiatry; Head, Department of Child and Adolescent Psychiatry, Children's Memorial Hospital; Director, Warren Wright Adolescent Program, Northwestern Memorial Hospital; Professor of Psychiatry and Behavioral Sciences and Pediatrics; Chief, Child and Adolescent Psychiatry, Northwestern University, Feinberg School of Medicine, Chicago, Illinois

MaryBeth Lake, M.D.

Director of Training in Child and Adolescent Psychiatry, Department of Child and Adolescent Psychiatry, Children's Memorial Hospital; Assistant Professor of Psychiatry and Behavioral Sciences, Northwestern University, Feinberg School of Medicine, Chicago, Illinois

D. Richard Martini, M.D.

Director, Consultation Liaison, Intake, and Emergency Services, Department of Child and Adolescent Psychiatry, Children's Memorial Hospital; Associate Professor of Psychiatry and Behavioral Sciences and Pediatrics, Northwestern University, Feinberg School of Medicine, Chicago, Illinois

INTRODUCTION

to the Concise Guides Series

The Concise Guides Series from American Psychiatric Publishing, Inc., provides, in an accessible format, practical information for psychiatrists, psychiatry residents, and medical students working in a variety of treatment settings, such as inpatient psychiatry units, outpatient clinics, consultation-liaison services, and private office settings. The Concise Guides are meant to complement the more detailed information to be found in lengthier psychiatry texts.

The Concise Guides address topics of special concern to psychiatrists in clinical practice. The books in this series contain a detailed table of contents, along with an index, tables, figures, and other charts for easy access. The books are designed to fit into a lab coat pocket or jacket pocket, which makes them a convenient source of information. References have been limited to those most relevant to the material presented.

Robert E. Hales, M.D., M.B.A.
Series Editor, Concise Guides

PREFACE TO THE THIRD EDITION

Since the publication in 1999 of the second edition of the *Concise Guide to Child and Adolescent Psychiatry*, the pace of research on the diagnosis and treatment of emotional and behavioral problems in children and adolescents has accelerated. The Surgeon General's Conference on Children's Mental Health: Developing a National Action Agenda, held in 2000, highlighted the mental health needs of youth and their families and focused on the priority of developing, disseminating, and implementing scientifically proven prevention and treatment services. The full report is available at http://www.surgeongeneral.gov/cmh/default.htm.

New data most relevant to clinical practice have been distilled for this third edition, and each section of the book has been updated. The American Psychiatric Association has graciously permitted the reprinting of tables of diagnostic criteria from DSM-IV. Where relevant, updated information in the text of the *Diagnostic and Statistical Manual of Mental Disorders*, Fourth Edition, Text Revision (DSM-IV-TR) (American Psychiatric Association 2000) has been incorporated into this book.

■ ACKNOWLEDGMENT

Jean Stiman, who loves books, again provided enthusiastic support and assistance without which this book could not have been completed.

INTRODUCTION

The *Concise Guide to Child and Adolescent Psychiatry,* Third Edition, was written for the novice in child and adolescent psychiatry who has some knowledge of adult psychiatry. This book offers an introduction to mental health care in children and adolescents and should be used in conjunction with clinical supervision. In the interest of brevity, complex theoretical notions, new research, and areas of controversy have been simplified. Each section on a disorder or clinical situation includes a listing of relevant treatment methods. Treatment techniques are described in Chapters 8 and 9. Each chapter has additional reading for those who wish more detail. General textbooks in child and adolescent psychiatry are listed at the end of Chapter 2. The American Academy of Child and Adolescent Psychiatry has published practice parameters—clinical guidelines that are valuable distillations of the scientific literature and the wisdom of experienced clinicians—in the *Journal of the American Academy of Child and Adolescent Psychiatry.* Each is listed in the relevant chapter of this book.

Throughout this book, *children* refers to both prepubertal children and adolescents, unless otherwise specified. *Parent* is used for the child's primary adult caregiver(s), whoever that may be.

■ CHANGE IN CHILDREN AND ADOLESCENTS

The primary "work" of children is to grow and change in multiple dimensions. Rigid descriptions of mental disorders and psychiatric symptoms do not capture the liveliness and energy of children as they develop and cope with internal and external difficulties. A child's tendency to change is a therapeutic ally. As clinicians, we work with the natural dynamics of the interaction between our interventions and the developmental processes.

All disorders in childhood can exert lasting effects far beyond the boundaries of the primary psychiatric disorder. Developmental complications are often cumulative and may disrupt a wide range of functions. Social, cognitive, and psychological development, and even physical growth (Pine et al. 1996) may be impaired. Progressive learning delays, school failure, low self-esteem, demoralization, impaired relationships with family members, and rejection or neglect by peers are common complications of childhood-onset disorders. Prompt intervention can reduce these developmental consequences.

Regardless of the etiology of the primary disorder, biological, cognitive, psychodynamic, familial, social, economic, and cultural factors are critical in determining the course of illness. The effects of early developmental deficits may be compensated for or exacerbated by later opportunities or barriers. The family or social environment can amplify strengths or aggravate weaknesses. The adult outcome of a childhood disorder in a specific patient is a result of the interaction between therapeutic forces and risk and protective factors. The ultimate prognosis may depend more on the ability of the child and family to learn to cope with the illness than on the severity of the disorder. Resilient individuals may even turn childhood symptoms such as excessive sensitivity (separation anxiety disorder), unrelenting stubbornness (oppositional defiant disorder), or uncontrolled activity and enthusiasm (attention-deficit/hyperactivity disorder) into strengths in adulthood. Compensatory abilities and an enhancing environment can result in achievement and adaptation far above that predicted from early deficits.

■ OVERVIEW OF DIAGNOSIS

Use of DSM-IV-TR for Children and Adolescents

"Adult" psychiatric disorders in DSM-IV-TR (American Psychiatric Association 2000) can begin during childhood. Any Axis I diagnosis can be used for a child if the criteria are met. Some disorders have slightly adapted criteria for children. The DSM-IV-TR "disorders usually first diagnosed in infancy, childhood, or adolescence" include diagnoses that typically begin in childhood. Some behavior patterns are normal at certain developmental stages but become pathological if they persist (becoming, for example, separation anxiety disorder, functional enuresis, functional encopresis, or oppositional defiant disorder). Most Axis I disorders, however, are not "normal" at any age. The only Axis II disorder in the childhood section of DSM-IV-TR is mental retardation. Pervasive developmental disorders (including autistic disorder) and specific developmental disorders (learning, motor skills, and communication disorders) are on Axis I. In this book, key DSM-IV-TR criteria for each disorder are highlighted. For full details, refer to DSM-IV-TR (American Psychiatric Association 2000).

DSM-IV-TR contains a variety of clinical circumstances, classified as "V codes" or "other conditions that may be a focus of clinical attention," that are not psychiatric diagnoses but may prompt assessment and treatment. Any of these codes may be used for children's conditions, but some are especially common in clinical settings. The most prevalent conditions are listed in Table 1–1, and many are discussed in Chapter 7, "Special Clinical Circumstances." Although some clinicians are tempted to use V codes to avoid "labeling" a child, these categories should be used only if the child's symptoms do not meet the criteria for another DSM-IV-TR disorder.

All DSM-IV-TR diagnoses (except for tic disorders) require evidence that the symptoms are causing impairment in social, academic, or occupational functioning.

Medical conditions are listed on Axis III. The full range of medical problems, from a fever or earache to a brain tumor, may be signaled first by behavioral or emotional symptoms or declining school performance. Children with chronic medical disorders or physical disabilities are at increased risk for psychiatric disorders (see Chapter 7).

Axis IV is used for reporting psychosocial and environmental problems relevant to diagnosis, treatment, and prognosis. Stressors with unique effects during development include parental absence or

TABLE 1–1.	**DSM-IV-TR conditions especially relevant to children and adolescents that may be a focus of clinical attention**

Relational problem related to a mental disorder or general medical condition

Parent–child relational problem

Sibling relational problem

Physical abuse of child

Sexual abuse of child

Neglect of child

Noncompliance with treatment

Child or adolescent antisocial behavior

Borderline intellectual functioning (coded on Axis II) (IQ 71–84)

Bereavement

Academic problem

Identity problem

Source. American Psychiatric Association 2000.

neglect, physical and sexual abuse, psychiatric disorder in a caregiver, and puberty. On Axis V, the clinician uses the Global Assessment of Functioning Scale (GAF) to rate the lowest level of functioning for the past week. The Children's Global Assessment Scale (Shaffer et al. 1983) may be used to supplement the GAF.

Comorbidity

Psychiatric disorders typically occur in combinations. This is true not only in young people treated in the most intensive settings, such as inpatient units and residential treatment facilities, but also in outpatients. Comorbidity is common even in community epidemiological surveys, although less so than in children who have been referred for clinical services. Combinations of disorders may be unexpected, such as a youth with impulsive hyperactivity or aggressive conduct problems who also suffers from depression or anxiety. Rating scales are a useful supplement to the diagnostic process, to avoid overly narrow focus on the presenting problem.

■ OVERVIEW OF TREATMENT

Until recently, psychiatric treatment in children was more an art than a science. Treatment methods were applied regardless of diagnosis and reflected the training and beliefs of the therapist rather than the characteristics of the patient. Newer trends include consideration of biological factors, multimodal treatment approaches, multidisciplinary teams, and use of evidence-based interventions. With improvements in diagnostic criteria and evaluation techniques and the design and rigorous testing of therapy models and medications for specific disorders, treatment selection is increasingly scientific.

In contrast to treatment in adults, a child is typically brought to the clinical setting by someone else. Although the child is identified as "the patient," each case has at least two clients: a parent or guardian and the child, whose needs and desires may conflict. In addition, treatment often involves other family members; teachers and school counselors; government agencies, such as child protective services or the juvenile court; community organizations; and financial providers, such as welfare, Medicaid, and insurance companies. Because children depend on adults for their basic needs and have little autonomy in choosing caregivers, residence, schools, or activities, the clinician must work in partnership with the parents and other support systems to reestablish developmental progress and maximize adaptive outcome.

■ REFERENCES

American Psychiatric Association: Diagnostic and Statistical Manual of Mental Disorders, 4th Edition. Washington, DC, American Psychiatric Association, 1994

American Psychiatric Association: Diagnostic and Statistical Manual of Mental Disorders, 4th Edition, Text Revision. Washington, DC, American Psychiatric Association, 2000

Pine DS, Cohen P, Brook J: Emotional problems during youth as predictors of stature during early adulthood: results from a prospective epidemiologic study. Pediatrics 97:856–863, 1996

Shaffer D, Gould MS, Brasic J, et al: A Children's Global Assessment Scale (CGAS). Arch Gen Psychiatry 40:1228–1231, 1983

■ ADDITIONAL READING

Rapoport JL, Ismond DR: DSM-IV Training Guide for Diagnosis of Childhood Disorders. New York, Brunner/Mazel, 1996

2

EVALUATION AND TREATMENT PLANNING

■ EVALUATION

A comprehensive evaluation includes obtaining a biopsychosocial history; performing a mental status examination; ordering any additional tests; and obtaining records (with parental permission) from the child's school, pediatrician, and agencies such as child protective services or the juvenile court. The clinician should request reports of all prior psychiatric, psychological, developmental, and medical evaluation and treatment. Assessment should continue throughout the course of treatment as the child, parents, and situation change. When the presenting problems are urgent or narrowly circumscribed, treatment may be initiated after a focused evaluation with more complete assessment as time permits.

Before the evaluation, the clinician should tell the parents how long the evaluation will take, what it will cost, and what they can expect at the end. The clinician should advise parents on how to prepare the child for the first visit. Some parents invite the child out for an ice-cream cone but bring him or her to the child psychiatry clinic instead. Needless to say, this does not enhance the child's cooperation, although it does provide the clinician with useful data about the parents.

In conducting an evaluation, the clinician must constantly be mindful of the patient's developmental level, which determines whether a behavior (e.g., temper tantrums, separation anxiety) is pathological. Developmental stage influences the nature of symptoms, expectable reactions to stressors, ability to communicate and to understand concepts, and capacity to participate in different types of treatment.

The structure of an evaluation is determined by the child's age, the nature of the presenting problems, and practical factors. It is often useful to begin by meeting briefly with the child and parents together, to clarify and understand each person's views of the presenting problems and the goals of the evaluation and to develop an initial impression of family interaction. For children younger than 6 years, it may be convenient to obtain the entire history from the parents before seeing the child. Older children, especially adolescents, should be involved early in the evaluation process. Adolescents are often concerned about confidentiality and should be told that what they say will be shared only with their permission, unless they are at risk for physical harm, such as from suicide, homicide, substance abuse, high-risk sexual behavior, or running away. Clinicians are legally mandated to report suspected physical or sexual abuse to child protection authorities.

Use of Multiple Informants

No single informant or technique can give a full description of a child. Children, teachers, parents, other relatives, community members, and clinicians each have their own point of view and opportunities for observation. Lack of agreement in the reports of parents and teachers, or between two parents, often results from genuine variations in the behavior of children in different settings and with different people. Ideally, both parents should be interviewed, even if they are not living together, because their cooperation will enhance the likelihood of successful treatment. Each parent has a unique perspective on the child's development and environment. A telephone interview may be substituted if a parent lives far away.

History From Parents

The elements of a complete history from the parents or caregivers are outlined in Table 2–1. The construction of a time line, including

---

TABLE 2–1.   **Outline of biopsychosocial history**

Chief symptom and reasons for referral

History of present illness

Development of the symptoms

Attitudes of child and parents toward the symptoms

Effects of the symptoms on the child and family

Stressors

Prior psychological or psychiatric evaluations

Prior treatment

Psychotherapy: type, frequency, duration, effects

Medication: exact doses, schedule, beneficial and adverse effects

Environmental changes and effects

Current developmental status

Habits

Motor abilities and activity level

Attention

Speech and language

Academic performance

Relationships with peers

Risk-taking behaviors

Sexual development and behavior

Hobbies, activities, athletic interests and skills

Relationships with family members and other significant adults

Review of behavioral and psychological symptoms

Medical review of systems

Past history

Psychiatric

Medical

Neurological

Developmental history

Pregnancy and delivery

Neonatal period, infancy, early childhood

Temperament

Milestones

Motor

Cognitive

Speech and language

Social

TABLE 2–1.   **Outline of biopsychosocial history** *(continued)*

Developmental history *(continued)*
   School history
   Traumatic events
Psychosocial and psychiatric history of each parent
Developmental history of the couple/family life cycle
Family medical history
Current family circumstances, concerns, liabilities, resources

symptoms, major life events, and changes in the family and environment, can help organize a complex history.

An important element in the developmental history is the child's *temperament,* or "style" of behavior. Children can be rated on each of the nine dimensions listed in Table 2–2. The *goodness of fit* between the child's temperament and the parents' temperament, expectations, and child-rearing skills significantly affects developmental course and outcome. In addition, certain trait clusters (Table 2–3) have predictive value. Both *difficult* and *slow-to-warm-up* children are at risk for emotional and behavior problems, whereas *easy* children are relatively protected.

TABLE 2–2.   **Dimensions of temperament**

1. Activity level
2. Rhythmicity (regularity and predictability of biological functions)
3. Approach to or withdrawal from novel stimuli
4. Adaptability to environmental change
5. Intensity of reaction
6. Threshold of responsiveness (intensity of stimulation required to evoke a response)
7. Quality of mood (positive, neutral, or negative)
8. Distractibility
9. Attention span and persistence

Source.   Adapted from Thomas A, Chess S: *Temperament in Clinical Practice.* New York, Guilford, 1986.

TABLE 2–3. **Temperament clusters**

Easy
  Positive mood
  Regular biological rhythms
  Adaptable
  Low intensity of reactions
  Positive approach to novelty

Difficult
  Negative mood
  Irregular biological rhythms
  Slow to adapt
  Intense reactions
  Negative response to novelty

Slow to warm up
  Gradual adaptation after repeated contact
  Mild intensity of reactions
  Negative response to novelty

Source.   Adapted from Thomas A, Chess S: *Temperament in Clinical Practice.* New York, Guilford, 1986.

Patient Interview

During the patient interview, the child provides his or her view of the medical history and current symptoms, strengths, and concerns and the clinician makes observations. Children and adolescents often report their anxiety and depression, clandestine conduct problems, and drug use more accurately than their parents do. Parents typically report history, observable behavior problems, and family background more accurately than the child does. The details of the interview vary with developmental stage. The content of the mental status examination is outlined in Table 2–4.

The therapist should begin the patient interview by informally discussing nonthreatening topics before focusing on the presenting symptoms. For patients who are not very verbal, an opportunity to draw (with pencils, crayons, or washable markers) can help them feel comfortable enough to engage in conversation. Young children

---

TABLE 2–4.   **Mental status examination**

Physical appearance and grooming
Interactions with clinician
Understanding of the purpose of the interview
Motor activity level and coordination
Tics, stereotypies, mannerisms
Mood and affect
Anxiety
Obsessions or compulsions
Attention, persistence, frustration tolerance
Impulsivity
Oppositionality
Verbal or physical aggression
Speech and language
Hallucinations, delusions, thought disorder
Clinical estimate of intelligence
Judgment and insight

---

initially may want the parent to be present and may be more comfortable with play materials (e.g., dollhouse, stuffed animals, blocks, clay) than with a formal interview. Some clinicians previously believed that asking children direct questions about their symptoms was harmful, but research has disproved this theory. Clinicians must ask children direct questions (using wording that is adapted to the child's developmental level) to understand their emotional states.

Family Evaluation

Each person living with the patient, as well as noncustodial parents, grandparents, and siblings who are no longer living at home, may be crucial to understanding family dynamics, including unexpected sources of emotional support and areas of conflict. Meeting simultaneously with all significant family members to collect information and to observe interactions is often useful. Families with young children may benefit from the use of role playing, family drawings,

TABLE 2–5. **Family developmental tasks**

Forming a "marital coalition" to meet the needs of the adults for intimacy, sexuality, and emotional support

Establishing a "parental coalition" to form flexible relationships with children and present a consistent disciplinary front

Emphasizing nurturance, enculturation, and emancipation of children

Coping with crises

Source. Adapted from Fleck S: "A General Systems Approach to Severe Family Pathology." *American Journal of Psychiatry* 133:669–673, 1973.

or puppet play. The clinician may ask the family to complete a task during the session in order to assess family interactions. A family tree or genogram helps the clinician to organize data on family members and their relationships.

Regardless of a family's structure, the well-being of the child requires that certain tasks be accomplished (Table 2–5). Well-functioning families respond resiliently to stress, communicate effectively, assign roles that suit the needs and abilities of each family member, respond appropriately to emotions, solve problems both within and outside the boundaries of the family, and find effective and humane ways to control the behavior of family members.

Tasks of the initial session of a family assessment include the following:

- Ascertaining family members' views of the problem
- Beginning to establish a relationship with each family member to facilitate the treatment alliance
- Gathering data by observation and with questions
- Making test interventions and assessing their effects
- Proposing a provisional plan for the next steps

Mental health care for young people is unlikely to succeed without considering their parents' needs. Parents struggling with their own untreated psychiatric disorders may be unable to meet the child's emotional and physical needs, and there may be a "contagious" effect on the child. The clinician's most important contribution may be to arrange for the parent to receive psychiatric assessment and pharmacological and/or psychotherapeutic treatment. The clinician may need to use both empathy and judicious persuasion to induce the parent to assume a "patient" role.

Standardized Evaluation Instruments

Selected parent, teacher, and self-report behavior checklists, questionnaires, and rating scales supplement the clinical evaluation by providing a systematic review of behaviors and psychiatric symptoms. Scores may be compared with those obtained from large community-based samples or groups of clinically referred children. Ratings may also be done at intervals to measure progress. The most commonly used broad-spectrum package consists of the Child Behavior Checklist (CBCL) parent rating form, the Teacher Report Form (TRF), and the Youth Self-Report (YSR) Form (Achenbach System of Empirically Based Assessment; http://www.aseba.org). More specific instruments are available for one or more diagnoses. Structured and semistructured diagnostic interview protocols (Table 2–6) are more commonly used in research but often have clinical usefulness.

TABLE 2–6.   **Examples of standardized diagnostic assessment interviews**

Structured diagnostic interview
  Diagnostic Interview Schedule for Children (DISC)
Semistructured diagnostic interviews
  Diagnostic Interview for Children and Adolescents (DICA)
  Schedule for Affective Disorders and Schizophrenia for School-Aged
    Children and Adolescents (Kiddie-SADS)

Note.   For references and more detail, see *Journal of the American Academy of Child and Adolescent Psychiatry,* Special Section: Diagnostic Interviews, 39:1, January 2000.

Medical Evaluation

A standard evaluation includes a medical history and physical examination (within the past 6 months or more recently if the onset of problems is acute) to identify any medical causes of symptoms or coexisting medical disorders. Neurological consultation or testing (e.g., electroencephalogram, brain scan) generally is indicated only if focal signs or symptoms are present or if the history suggests seizures, regression in cognitive or physical functioning, or sequelae of brain injury. Laboratory tests may be obtained, especially if pharmacological treatment is anticipated. Urine testing for drugs and, in female adolescents, a pregnancy test are often indicated.

School Assessment

School reports are almost always useful. Attention, learning, quality and quantity of homework and classwork, behavior in class and on the playground, and social relationships are sensitive indicators of the presence of psychiatric symptoms and of developmental status. After obtaining parental consent, the clinician may talk with the teacher or school counselor, obtain school records (educational testing, behavior, grades, and attendance), arrange for teachers to complete standardized checklists, and perhaps even visit the school to observe the youngster.

Psychological Testing

Standardized tests administered by a clinical psychologist can assess intellectual potential, cognitive skills, and fund of knowledge (Table 2–7). Individually administered tests provide a more accurate evaluation than those given to entire classrooms of children. Tests have been criticized because of cultural influences on performance, unresponsiveness to "creative" responses, the dangers of using a rigid construct of intelligence that masks individual strengths, the use of test results to exclude children from mainstream education, and potential insults to developing self-esteem. Despite these concerns, IQ tests provide a global assessment that has clinical

TABLE 2–7. Individually administered tests of intellectual capacity and learning

Intelligence

Kaufman Assessment Battery for Children (K-ABC)	Ages 2.5 through 12.5 years
	Less dependent than Wechsler Intelligence Scales or Stanford-Binet Intelligence Scale on schooling and culturally based information
	IQ portion emphasizes problem-solving style and ability to process information
	Achievement Scale also included
Kaufman Adolescent and Adult Intelligence Test (KAIT)	Ages 11 through 85 years
	Distinguishes between learned information and capacity to solve novel problems
Kaufman Brief Intelligence Test (K-BIT)	Screening test to estimate IQ
Leiter International Performance Scale—Revised	Ages 2 through 20 years
	Nonverbal test for use with children who are hearing impaired or autistic or who do not speak English
Peabody Picture Vocabulary Test—Revised (PPVT-R)	Age 2.5 years through adulthood
	Brief test of receptive vocabulary abilities; often used as a screening test to estimate verbal IQ
Stanford-Binet Intelligence Scale, Fourth Edition	Age 2 years through adulthood
	Heavily language based
	15 subtests grouped into verbal reasoning, short-term memory, quantitative reasoning, abstract/visual reasoning

TABLE 2-7. **Individually administered tests of intellectual capacity and learning** *(continued)*

Wechsler Preschool and Primary Scale of Intelligence—Third Edition (WPPSI-III)	Ages 2.6 through 7.3 years 12 subtests grouped into verbal and performance scales
Wechsler Intelligence Scale for Children—Third Edition (WISC-III)	Ages 6 through 16 years 13 subtests grouped into verbal and performance scales
Wechsler Adult Intelligence Scale—Third Edition (WAIS-III)	Age 16 years through adulthood 11 subtests grouped into verbal and performance scales
Academic achievement	
Kaufman Test of Educational Achievement (K-TEA)	Ages 6 through 18 years Screening test for achievement in reading, math, and spelling
Wechsler Individual Achievement Tests, Second Edition (WIAT-II)	Ages 5 through 19 years Grades kindergarten through 12 Parallels Wechsler IQ tests Screener version measures skills in reading, math reasoning, and spelling Comprehensive Battery adds listening comprehension and written and oral expression
Wide Range Achievement Test, Third Edition (WRAT-3)	Age 5 years through adulthood Brief screen for assessing skills in word recognition, spelling, and written arithmetic computation
Woodcock-Johnson Psychoeducational Battery—Revised (WJ-R)	Age 2 years through adulthood Comprehensive test that assesses cognitive ability: memory, processing, comprehension, and reasoning; and achievement: reading, writing, and math skills

TABLE 2–7.   Individually administered tests of intellectual capacity and learning *(continued)*

Adaptive behavior (required to diagnose mental retardation)

Vineland Adaptive Behavior Scales

Age birth through 19 years

Semistructured interview with parent

Adaptive Behavior Composite Score includes Communication, Daily Living Skills, Socialization, and Motor Skills (up to age 5 years)

Basic Survey, Expanded, and Screener versions available

Classroom Edition—brief written form for teachers to complete predictive value, particularly when combined with an evaluation of adaptive behavior. Projective tests such as the Children's Apperception Test (CAT) or the Rorschach Inkblot Technique are not generally useful in making diagnostic or treatment decisions. The most commonly used test for assessing infants (ages birth to 3 years) is the Bayley Scales of Infant Development, Second Edition. It has three subsections: Mental Scale, Motor Scale, and Behavior Rating Scale.

■ TREATMENT PLANNING

Treatment plans are based on both psychiatric diagnosis and identified target symptoms. The strengths and vulnerabilities of the patient and the resources and liabilities of the family are critical factors in treatment planning. The social environment, including school, neighborhood, and social support networks, strongly influences choice of treatment strategy. The practical realities of the quality and availability of community resources, and the family's ability to pay for or to attend treatment sessions, often compel the clinician to modify an "ideal" or comprehensive plan. Realistic and efficient selection and sequencing of treatment modalities are central to effective decision making. Clinical judgments regarding anticipated treatment effectiveness, efficiency, and risk–benefit ratio may lead to selection of a single form of treatment or multimodal therapies. Interventions may be administered simultaneously or sequentially, as the child or family requires or is able to make use of additional treatment.

Parental motivation or ability to carry out the treatment plan may strongly influence treatment decisions. For example, unusual strengths of a family may avert hospitalization of a psychotic or suicidal child, or limitations may prevent implementation of family therapy or maintenance of the child living at home. For children from disrupted homes or abusive or neglectful environments, the first priority may not be psychiatric care, but social services, such as a safe and stable home, food, supervision, and medical care. In complex cases, a case manager who coordinates the involvement of various agencies and services (sometimes called "wraparound") may be able to maintain a child in the community, which results in a better outcome at a lower overall cost.

Each of a child's symptoms may appear to call for a different intervention. In setting priorities, factors to consider include the following:

- Risk of physical harm to the child or to others
- Symptoms that will likely increase in severity and chronicity if not treated rapidly (e.g., school avoidance)
- Patient and family motivation and resistance
- Symptoms or family members that are most accessible to treatment
- Problems that are most urgent to the patient or family

Treatment planning is an ongoing process. Continual reassessment is necessary as the effects of interventions are seen and as additional information about the child and family comes to light.

■ FEEDBACK

The clinician's findings and recommendations are typically presented to both the parents and the child. The clinician decides whether to meet with them together or separately, and in what order. Depending on the ability of each to listen or understand, parents and child are educated about the nature of the child's and the family's strengths, psychiatric liabilities or disorders, and the expected course and possible complications of the disorder. The clinician should answer questions about etiology at the level that scientific knowledge allows, while assiduously avoiding blaming or being judgmental. Parents and many children already feel guilty about real or perceived failures, and the empathic clinician is cautious to ameliorate these feelings.

Parents, and usually the child, should help determine which treatment strategy to follow. The clinician describes recommended and alternative interventions in terms of the process (duration, costs) and the anticipated benefits and risks. A successful feedback conference helps the family to understand their strengths and weaknesses, respect their child's abilities and the difficulties he or she faces, sense the interplay of multiple etiological factors, realize the implications of the child's diagnosis and prognosis, ponder the practicalities involved, acknowledge hopes and fears, and integrate the recommendations with the rest of their lives. Even the best treatment has little chance of success without the cooperation of the family and the child (to the extent possible for developmental stage and psychopathology). The treatment plan should be consistent with the family's resources. Finding areas in which improvement may be quickly attained builds the family's confidence in themselves and in the therapeutic process.

■ ADDITIONAL READING

American Academy of Child and Adolescent Psychiatry: Practice parameters for the psychiatric assessment of children and adolescents. J Am Acad Child Adolesc Psychiatry 34:1386–1402, 1995

American Academy of Child and Adolescent Psychiatry: Practice parameters for the psychiatric assessment of infants and toddlers (0–36 months). J Am Acad Child Adolesc Psychiatry 36 (suppl):21S–36S, 1997

Cepeda C: Concise Guide to the Psychiatric Interview of Children and Adolescents. Washington, DC, American Psychiatric Press, 2000

Halperin JM, McKay KE: Psychological testing for child and adolescent psychiatrists: a review of the past 10 years. J Am Acad Child Adolesc Psychiatry 37:575–584, 1998

Lewis M (ed): Child and Adolescent Psychiatry: A Comprehensive Textbook, 3rd Edition. Philadelphia, PA, Lippincott, Williams & Wilkins, 2002

McGoldrick M, Gerson R, Shellenberger S: Genograms: Assessment and Intervention, 2nd Edition. New York, WW Norton, 1999

Wiener JM, Dulcan MK (eds): Textbook of Child and Adolescent Psychiatry, 3rd Edition. Washington, DC, American Psychiatric Press, 2003

3

AXIS I DISORDERS USUALLY FIRST DIAGNOSED IN INFANCY, CHILDHOOD, OR ADOLESCENCE

Attention-Deficit and Disruptive Behavior Disorders

DSM-IV-TR (American Psychiatric Association 2000) organizes those disorders that typically begin before adulthood into a separate section. Mental retardation (coded on Axis II) and the learning, motor skills, and communication disorders are presumed to be present at birth and to become manifest as expectations for competence increase with age. They are covered in Chapter 6, along with the pervasive developmental disorders. Reactive attachment disorder, rumination disorder, and pica characteristically begin during infancy. Attention-deficit/hyperactivity disorder (ADHD) and oppositional defiant disorder (ODD) most often appear in early childhood, whereas conduct disorder (CD) and tic disorders develop in middle childhood through adolescence. Enuresis and encopresis are diagnosed in early childhood when developmentally appropriate stages of toilet training are not achieved. Separation anxiety disorder and selective mutism become apparent when age-appropriate independent social behavior is impaired. This chapter covers attention-deficit and disruptive behavior disorders. The remaining diagnoses in this section of DSM-IV-TR are covered in Chapter 4.

In DSM-IV-TR, disruptive behavior disorder includes CD and ODD. Unlike ADHD, these disorders are characterized by willful disobedience. CD and ODD often present concurrently with ADHD, however. All three of these conditions are sometimes called externalizing disorders, emphasizing the prominence of externally directed behaviors. Parents and teachers are generally more distressed than the child, who often denies symptoms, blames others for problems, and is reluctant to undergo treatment. These syndromes are characterized by the chronicity and severity of clusters of problem behaviors that differentiate them from the mild behavior problems that are highly prevalent in typical children.

■ ATTENTION-DEFICIT/HYPERACTIVITY DISORDER

Clinical Description

The syndrome of hyperactivity, impulsivity, and inattention was previously labeled "minimal brain damage," "minimal brain dysfunction," "hyperkinetic syndrome," or "hyperactivity."

DSM-IV-TR defines three subtypes of ADHD: combined type (meeting criteria for both inattention and hyperactivity–impulsivity), predominantly inattentive type, and predominantly hyperactive–impulsive type (Table 3–1). The predominantly inattentive type is similar, but not identical, to the DSM-III (American Psychiatric Association 1980) category of attention-deficit disorder without hyperactivity. Children with the predominantly inattentive subtype tend to be described as "daydreamers" or "spacey," more often have comorbid anxiety and depression, are more likely to be neglected by peers, have fewer conduct and behavior problems, and present less frequently to psychiatric settings than do those with the combined type. The predominantly hyperactive–impulsive group consists largely of very young children for whom the inattention criteria are not yet developmentally appropriate.

Clinical skill, familiarity with normal development, and rigorous application of the diagnostic criteria are needed to diagnose

TABLE 3–1.　**DSM-IV-TR diagnostic criteria for attention-deficit/hyperactivity disorder**

A.　Either (1) or (2):

(1)　six (or more) of the following symptoms of **inattention** have persisted for at least 6 months to a degree that is maladaptive and inconsistent with developmental level:

Inattention

(a)　often fails to give close attention to details or makes careless mistakes in schoolwork, work, or other activities

(b)　often has difficulty sustaining attention in tasks or play activities

(c)　often does not seem to listen when spoken to directly

(d)　often does not follow through on instructions and fails to finish schoolwork, chores, or duties in the workplace (not due to oppositional behavior or failure to understand instructions)

(e)　often has difficulty organizing tasks and activities

(f)　often avoids, dislikes, or is reluctant to engage in tasks that require sustained mental effort (such as schoolwork or homework)

(g)　often loses things necessary for tasks or activities (e.g., toys, school assignments, pencils, books, or tools)

(h)　is often easily distracted by extraneous stimuli

(i)　is often forgetful in daily activities

(2)　six (or more) of the following symptoms of **hyperactivity–impulsivity** have persisted for at least 6 months to a degree that is maladaptive and inconsistent with developmental level:

Hyperactivity

(a)　often fidgets with hands or feet or squirms in seat

(b)　often leaves seat in classroom or in other situations in which remaining seated is expected

(c)　often runs about or climbs excessively in situations in which it is inappropriate (in adolescents or adults, may be limited to subjective feelings of restlessness)

(d)　often has difficulty playing or engaging in leisure activities quietly

(e)　is often "on the go" or often acts as if "driven by a motor"

(f)　often talks excessively

TABLE 3–1. **DSM-IV-TR diagnostic criteria for attention-deficit/hyperactivity disorder *(continued)***

Impulsivity

(g) often blurts out answers before questions have been completed

(h) often has difficulty awaiting turn

(i) often interrupts or intrudes on others (e.g., butts into conversations or games)

B. Some hyperactive-impulsive or inattentive symptoms that caused impairment were present before age 7 years.

C. Some impairment from the symptoms is present in two or more settings (e.g., at school [or work] and at home).

D. There must be clear evidence of clinically significant impairment in social, academic, or occupational functioning.

E. The symptoms do not occur exclusively during the course of a pervasive developmental disorder, schizophrenia, or other psychotic disorder and are not better accounted for by another mental disorder (e.g., mood disorder, anxiety disorder, dissociative disorder, or a personality disorder).

Code based on type:

> **314.01   Attention-deficit/hyperactivity disorder, combined type:**   if both criteria A1 and A2 are met for the past 6 months
> **314.00   Attention-deficit/hyperactivity disorder, predominantly inattentive type:**   if criterion A1 is met but criterion A2 is not met for the past 6 months
> **314.01   Attention-deficit/hyperactivity disorder, predominantly hyperactive-impulsive type:**   if criterion A2 is met but criterion A1 is not met for the past 6 months

Coding note: For individuals (especially adolescents and adults) who currently have symptoms that no longer meet full criteria, "in partial remission" should be specified.

ADHD, because inattention, impulsivity, and overactivity are common in children, especially boys. Children with ADHD may appear quite different to observers in different environments. Teachers expect more extended concentration and physical stillness than do parents. When the child is in a highly structured or novel setting, is engaged in a stimulating activity (e.g., a computer game), or is alone with an interested adult, symptoms may not be apparent at all, except in the most severe cases of ADHD. Symptoms typically worsen in situations that are unstructured, boring, and minimally supervised or that require sustained attention or mental effort. Problems, therefore, are often far more apparent to the teacher in a busy classroom than to the clinician in a quiet office. The clinical waiting area may provide a more realistic sample of behavior. Core deficits in ADHD include impairment relative to expected developmental level in learning and following rules (e.g., how to solve academic problems or how to behave in school and with friends) and difficulty in inhibiting impulsive responses to internal wishes or needs or to external attractions or provocations (Barkley 1998).

Many children with ADHD have high levels of motor activity in a variety of settings. When children are expected to be highly active (e.g., on the playground), children with and without ADHD have similar activity levels. In the classroom, however, restlessness, fidgeting, and walking or running around without permission cause problems. The child with ADHD often energetically explores new places and things. On entering a room, the child may immediately begin to touch and climb. He or she may inadvertently break things or hurt him- or herself or others.

Children with ADHD have great difficulty with motivation, sustained attention, organization, and completion when tasks are difficult, complex, long, or boring. These youngsters are unusually prone to seek immediate gratification. Resulting school problems include delayed learning, poor study skills, incomplete homework and tests with careless mistakes, and disruptive behavior. These problems may lead to erratic or failing grades, special class placement, suspension, expulsion, or dropping out.

Peers perceive children with ADHD as immature and irritating and often avoid or neglect them because of their low frustration tolerance; difficulty following rules; and intrusive, bossy, and socially inappropriate behavior. Peers learn quickly that it is easy to tease children with ADHD or to set them up to get into trouble with adults.

Epidemiology

Prevalence estimates of ADHD vary, due to differences in diagnostic criteria, samples, and assessment methods. DSM-IV-TR cites a rate of 3%–7% in school-age children. Community surveys have found ADHD in as many as 17% of boys and 8% of girls of elementary school age and 11% of boys and 6% of girls in adolescence. A rigorous record-based birth cohort community study found a cumulative incidence by age 19 of 7.5% for definite ADHD (Barbaresi et al. 2002). ADHD is present in 30%–50% of child psychiatric outpatients and 40%–70% of child psychiatric inpatients, often in combination with other psychiatric disorders. In elementary school–age children, the boy-to-girl ratio is typically 9 to 1 in clinical settings but in community surveys is 2–3 to 1. Girls are more likely to have the predominantly inattentive type than the combined type, and, compared with boys, are less likely to have comorbid disruptive behavior disorders and more likely to have comorbid anxiety and depression. Although in most ways, boys and girls with ADHD are similar in symptoms, impairment, and response to treatment, girls with ADHD are less likely to be identified or receive treatment than are boys with the disorder.

ADHD has been found to exist in all countries where studies have been done. Greater reported prevalence in the United States appears to result from differing diagnostic practices and cultural expectations. Because all children in the United States are expected to attend school until age 18 years, academic and behavior problems are often detected in youth who, in other countries, would no longer be in school.

Comorbidity

ADHD commonly occurs in association with other psychiatric disorders, particularly ODD and CD. As many as 50% of clinically referred children with ADHD also have CD, and many others have ODD; therefore, much of the ADHD literature is actually about the combination of ADHD plus ODD or CD. In clinical settings, approximately one-third of patients with ADHD also have a mood and/or anxiety disorder. Although ADHD is very common in youth with Tourette's disorder, relatively few children with ADHD also have Tourette's. The presence of ADHD not uncommonly complicates the clinical course of mental retardation and specific learning disorders. In adolescents, comorbid substance abuse is seen.

Etiology

ADHD is a heterogeneous syndrome, and various factors contribute to etiology. The common feature is relative dysfunction in the prefrontal cortex, which controls many "executive functions" such as planning, organization, and impulse control. One subgroup may have a predominantly genetic etiology, whereas in another, ADHD may be the result of biological environmental insults. Although school and home environment can influence the severity of ADHD symptoms, child-rearing practices do not cause ADHD. A wide variety of biological findings reflect possible etiologies. Neurochemical studies of ADHD suggest that multiple neurotransmitter systems are involved, including norepinephrine and dopamine. Anatomic imaging studies have found that, as a group, children with ADHD show differences relative to control subjects in brain areas associated with executive functioning: smaller frontal lobe volume, different symmetry of the caudate nucleus, and smaller volume of the cerebellar vermis. Imaging findings are not specific enough to be useful in the diagnosis of ADHD, only in ruling in or out a suspected focal brain finding. Functional magnetic resonance imaging (fMRI) research offers promise in understanding the underlying brain mechanisms of attention and impulse control.

Genetics

The genetic contribution to the etiology of ADHD is substantial. In addition, children with ADHD without conduct problems are likely to have relatives with learning problems. Children with both ADHD and CD are more likely to have relatives with CD, adult antisocial behavior or personality, and substance abuse. Mood disorders are common in families with ADHD. The hereditary component of ADHD is probably polygenic, rather than a single-gene defect. The specific mechanism of genetic transmission in ADHD has not been identified.

Medical Factors

Children with identifiable medical or neurological causes represent a small proportion of the ADHD population, and many children with medical risk factors do not have ADHD (Table 3–2).

Nonlocalizing neurological "soft signs" (e.g., clumsiness, left–right confusion, perceptual–motor dyscoordination, dysgraphia) are common in children with ADHD, but 15% of children without ADHD have as many as five soft signs, and children with anxiety disorders also have these signs. The presence or absence of soft signs is not helpful in diagnosis but may have implications for treatment and prognosis.

TABLE 3–2.	Medical contributions to attention-deficit/ hyperactivity disorder
Prenatal	Young mother
	Poor maternal health
	Maternal use of cigarettes, alcohol, or drugs
Birth complications	Bleeding
	Hypoxia
	Toxemia
	Prolonged labor
Perinatal	Low birth weight
	Postmaturity
Infancy	Malnutrition
Toxicity	Lead poisoning
Genetic disorders	Fragile X syndrome
	Glucose-6-phosphate dehydrogenase deficiency
	Generalized resistance to thyroid hormone
	Phenylketonuria
Brain injury	Trauma
	Infection

Course and Prognosis

Mothers of some youngsters with ADHD (especially those meeting hyperactive–impulsive criteria) recall excessive intrauterine kicking or report, "When he began to walk, he ran." Although ADHD can be diagnosed by age 3 years, considerable overlap with normal high activity level, impulsivity, limited frustration tolerance, and short attention span is found before age 5 years. Diagnosis is often delayed until elementary school, where expectations for physical stillness, prolonged attention, and conformity to social norms are greater and there is greater comparison to peers. Verbally skilled, nonoppositional children who do not have learning disabilities and who are not severely hyperactive may not be given a diagnosis until they experience the greater academic demands for organization and concentrated effort in middle school or high school, or even college or graduate school.

ADHD is not a benign or self-limited childhood disorder; it has a chronic or even lifelong course. As children mature, physical hyperactivity typically decreases. However, in adolescence, most continue to be symptomatic. As many as 30%–50% of clinically diagnosed hyperactive children continue to have the diagnosis of ADHD in adulthood, and other young adults have some symptoms of ADHD with impaired functioning. Secondary effects include low self-esteem and significantly compromised social skills. These individuals have more school failure, car accidents, changes in residence, court appearances, felony convictions, suicide attempts, and problems with relationships than do young adults without ADHD. Children with ADHD are at increased risk for substance abuse or delinquency as adolescents only if they also had CD in childhood. "Pure" ADHD may increase the risk for substance abuse disorders in adulthood, however (Biederman et al. 1997). Comorbid ADHD and CD in childhood also predict antisocial behavior and antisocial personality disorder in adolescence and adulthood. The absence of significant conduct problems or defiant, aggressive behavior toward adults in childhood predicts a better prognosis for ADHD. Childhood comorbid anxiety or mood disorders tend to persist (Biederman et al. 1996).

Parental responses to children with ADHD can aggravate or improve the course of the child's illness. Observation studies indicate that mothers tend to have more controlling, directive, structure-setting, and negative responses to their children with ADHD than control mothers have to their children (Tallmadge and Barkley 1983). Although parents had been blamed for being anxious and intrusive and reinforcing the child's problem behavior, when the ADHD child's behavior is improved by stimulant medication, the parents immediately become more positive and less controlling (Tallmadge and Barkley 1983). Much of the parent–child conflict appears to be caused by comorbid ODD rather than by the ADHD per se. Children with ADHD are often more compliant with their fathers' requests than with their mothers'. Living with a child who has ADHD, especially one who also has CD or ODD, can push parents and siblings beyond the point at which they can cope adaptively with the stress. Given the strong genetic contribution to ADHD, it is not uncommon for one or both parents to be struggling to master their own inattention and impulsivity. ADHD provides an example of how an early-onset disorder, often with a genetic or neurological etiology, can be modified by life experiences and developmental processes, including educational programming; neighborhood supports; individual compensatory strengths such as easy temperament, engaging personality, athletic abilities, and intelligence; and family emotional, social, and financial resources.

Evaluation

Children and adolescents with ADHD commonly do not admit to symptoms of hyperactivity, inattention, and impulsivity. The patient interview is useful, nonetheless, for the clinician to observe the child's behavior and to identify any comorbid psychiatric disorders. The parent interview is crucial for both ADHD diagnosis and more comprehensive assessment. Key parts of the history include obstetrical history (e.g., maternal substance use, prenatal or perinatal injury), medical history (e.g., seizures, thyroid disorder, head trauma, tics, medication use), screening questions for sleep disorders, traumatic events (including neglect or abuse), family residence (e.g., lead exposure from paint or exhaust fumes), family psychiatric history, family medical history (e.g., thyroid disorder), and any factors that may increase the risk of medication abuse by the child, siblings, or parents. Special emphasis is placed on school reports of grades, learning, and behavior (including behavior on the school bus and in the cafeteria). Normed parent and teacher rating scales are key— either general ones like the Child Behavior Checklist (CBCL) and the Teacher Report Form (TRF) (see Chapter 2) or DSM-IV-TR–based symptom ratings such as the SNAP-IV (rating form and scoring instructions available at http://adhd.net).

The physical examination should include possible signs of physical anomalies, thyroid disorder, or chronic illness, as well as baseline findings relevant to subsequent medication treatment such as height and weight, tics, and cardiac status. Neurological examination or tests (e.g., electroencephalogram [EEG] or brain scan) are indicated only in the presence of focal neurological signs or clinical suggestions of a seizure disorder or a decline in neurological functioning. Acuity of vision and hearing should be tested. Laboratory measurement of thyroid function or blood lead level (and possibly free erythrocyte protoporphyrin) is indicated only if suggested by history or physical examination. A baseline electrocardiogram (ECG) is indicated if treatment with a tricyclic antidepressant (TCA) is being considered. An ECG is optional prior to treatment with clonidine.

Psychological testing is useful to assess intellectual ability, academic achievement, and possible specific learning disorders. Although observations during testing may provide data on attention, distractibility, impulsivity, ability to stay seated, and frustration tolerance, a normal performance on individual testing does not preclude the diagnosis of ADHD. Neuropsychological evaluation may be requested to evaluate specific deficits suggested by history, physical examination, or routine psychological testing. Speech and language evaluation may be needed.

ADHD is a clinical diagnosis made on the basis of interviews and standardized parent and teacher behavior rating scales. EEG, brain imaging, laboratory tests, psychological tests, and computerized tests of vigilance are not diagnostic for ADHD.

Differential Diagnosis

Because the usual long-term course of ADHD is gradual improvement, sustained worsening behavior (apart from periods of environmental stress) suggests the emergence of a different psychiatric disorder. A positive treatment response to stimulant medication does not confirm a diagnosis of ADHD or eliminate another diagnosis. Clinical expertise is necessary to differentiate ADHD from normal high activity level. Problems of recent onset and brief duration may represent an adjustment disorder. For a diagnosis of ADHD, some symptoms causing impairment must have been present before age 7 years, and criteria must have been met for at least the past 6 months. Various physical problems (medical disorders, sleep disorders, or lack of adequate sleep or nutrition) can interfere with attention. Hyper- or hypothyroidism, as well as the effects of certain medications (theophylline, carbamazepine, benzodiazepines, or phenobarbital) and the abuse of drugs, can mimic ADHD. In addition, situational anxiety, child abuse or neglect, posttraumatic stress disorder, or understimulation in school can present with inattention, hyperactivity, or impulsivity. CD and ODD are characterized by deliberate or provocative noncompliance, as distinguished from the impulsive or inattentive failure to comply seen in ADHD, although these disorders often occur with ADHD. Depression or anxiety may present with deficits in attention. Anxious children may appear fidgety and restless, but they can verbalize worries or fears. Symptoms of anxiety are most apparent in new situations, whereas ADHD typically worsens with increased familiarity. Mania or bipolar mixed state may take uncharacteristic forms in prepubertal children and should be considered, especially in patients with a family history of bipolar disorder. Mood disorders are generally more episodic than ADHD and have prominent symptoms of sadness or hypomania.

Accurate differential diagnosis is particularly crucial to rule out psychosis, because stimulant treatment can exacerbate psychotic symptoms and disorganization. Children with ADHD do not have hallucinations, delusions, or formal thought disorder. However, distractibility and excessive talking may resemble "loose" thought patterns, and impulsivity may lead to potentially dangerous behavior and a lack of awareness of the environment that may be confused with poor reality testing. Children with pervasive developmental disorder (PDD) often show hyperactivity, inattention, and impulsivity, but a diagnosis in the PDD category (including autistic disorder) preempts a diagnosis of ADHD. Children with undiagnosed mental retardation or learning disorders are often mistakenly referred for stimulant treatment because of inattention, distractibility, and inability to follow directions in school.

Monitoring Treatment

Treatment outcome is best evaluated by the reports of caregivers in various settings. Regular reports on behavior and academic progress from teachers and other observers are useful. Brief rating scales completed by teachers weekly during dose titration and at intervals thereafter are an efficient means of gathering school-related information. The items on the Child Attention Problems (CAP) Rating Scale (Barkley 1990) are similar to many of the DSM-IV-TR symptoms of ADHD (Table 3–3). Scoring of inattention and overactivity is based on a large normative sample (Table 3–4).

The IOWA Conners Teacher Rating Scale covers both ADHD symptoms and defiance or oppositional behavior (Loney and Milich 1982; Pelham et al. 1989). Some investigators and clinicians use computerized laboratory tests of attention, vigilance, and impulsivity, such as the Continuous Performance Test (CPT), to assess medication effect. Because these tests measure a limited domain of performance in an artificial environment, they should not be substituted for clinical judgment based on the reports of observers in different settings. Observations and productivity and accuracy on timed samples of reading or math problems are far more ecologically valid.

TABLE 3–3.   **Child Attention Problems (CAP) Rating Scale**

Child's name: _____   Child's age:_____
Today's date: _____   Child's sex: Male ❏
                                                Female ❏

Filled out by: _____

Below is a list of items that describes pupils. For each item that describes
the pupil now or within the past week, check whether the item is Not true,
Somewhat or sometimes true, or Very or often true. Please check all items
as well as you can, even if some do not seem to apply to this pupil.

	Not true	Somewhat or sometimes true	Very or often true
1. Fails to finish things he/she starts	❏	❏	❏
2. Can't concentrate, can't pay attention for long	❏	❏	❏
3. Can't sit still, restless, or hyperactive	❏	❏	❏
4. Fidgets	❏	❏	❏
5. Daydreams or gets lost in his/her thoughts	❏	❏	❏
6. Impulsive or acts without thinking	❏	❏	❏
7. Difficulty following directions	❏	❏	❏
8. Talks out of turn	❏	❏	❏
9. Messy work	❏	❏	❏
10. Inattentive, easily distracted	❏	❏	❏
11. Talks too much	❏	❏	❏
12. Fails to carry out assigned tasks	❏	❏	❏

Please feel free to write any comments about the pupil's work or behavior
in the last week.

Source.   Reprinted with permission from Craig Edelbrock, Ph.D., 1967. (In the
public domain; may be reproduced but not changed or sold.) Available on the Internet at http://www.dbpeds.org/pdf/cap.pdf.

TABLE 3–4. **Child Attention Problems (CAP) Rating Scale scoring**

Each of the 12 items is scored 0, 1, or 2.

Total score: Sum of the scores on all items

Subscores:

    Inattention: Sum of scores on items 1, 2, 5, 7, 9, 10, and 12

    Overactivity: Sum of scores on items 3, 4, 6, 8, and 11

Scores recommended as the upper limit of the normal range (93rd percentile):

	Boys		**Girls**	
Age (years)	6–11	12–16	6–11	12–16
Inattention	9	9	8	7
Overactivity	6	7	5	4
Total score	15	16	12	11

Source.   Personal communication, Craig Edelbrock, Ph.D., 1986. Scoring form available on the Internet at http://www.dbpeds.org/pdf/capscore.pdf.

Treatment

The cornerstones of treatment are education about the disorder, appropriate school and class placement and academic remediation (if necessary), and medication treatment. Mild cases of ADHD may respond to parent education, behavior modification, and school consultation alone, especially in young children. If medication and environmental modification do not lead to sufficiently improved behavior, academic performance, and social adjustment, or if comorbid psychiatric conditions are present, then additional treatments should be considered, based on the specific problems of the child and family.

Parent Education

Education of parents regarding the nature of the disorder and its management is key to the treatment of ADHD. Efficient parent education methods include parent groups in the clinical setting, books (see Appendix), and referral to a support group such as CHADD (Children and Adults With Attention-Deficit/Hyperactivity Disorder) (see Appendix). Parents are taught to manage the child's environment by providing consistent routines and structure, reducing excessive stimulation, and averting predictable opportunity for misbehavior. At home, parents are advised to establish specific spaces for homework, remove easily damaged furnishings, closely monitor peer activities, and avoid taking the child to supermarkets and shopping malls. Parents can be coached on how best to work with the school to meet their child's needs.

School-Related Interventions

Special education is not always required but is useful for many ADHD patients. The clinician may assess the need for special services after the child is receiving the maximum benefit from medication. The parent (and the clinician, with parental permission) should inform school officials about the child's vulnerabilities and strengths. Regular reports from the teacher on behavior and academic performance are essential for best outcome. An Individualized Education Program (IEP) can be developed with the school to ensure that the child will receive needed services.

Useful and practical adaptations by teachers include consistent classroom structure and routines, seating the child near the teacher and away from disruptive peers or distractions, dividing assignments into small segments, reducing the quantity of repetitive classwork or homework, and communicating consistently with parents. A notebook for documenting assignment and completion of homework that is carried daily between teacher and parent can be effective. The Daily Report Card (see Chapter 9) targets specific behaviors, and can be completed by the teacher with consequences provided by the parent. Closely supervised recess, physical education, bus, and cafeteria arrangements are sometimes needed. If these modifications are not sufficient, a small and perhaps self-contained classroom or resource room with a high teacher-to-student ratio, one-to-one tutoring, or remediation of specific learning disorders can be beneficial.

Academic transitions require careful planning. The move from elementary school, with smaller classes and fewer teachers, to middle school and then to high school is often very difficult for youngsters with ADHD. The decrease in structure and supervision along with the increased expectations for autonomous functioning and organization may result in dramatic exacerbation of academic and behavior problems.

Pharmacotherapy

Medication is the primary treatment for the core symptoms of ADHD. The vast majority of children with ADHD have a positive response to one or more drugs. Unfortunately, despite more than 50 years of research, specific predictors of response to one or all psychostimulants have not been demonstrated. Dosage titration requires individual tailoring to optimize behavior and learning in different settings throughout the day. Drug treatment may continue for years, with periodic dosage adjustments needed. A few patients no longer need treatment by adolescence, but many individuals require medication through adolescence and even into adulthood.

The psychostimulants methylphenidate and amphetamine are the oldest and most established pharmacological agents in child psychiatry; their short-term clinical effectiveness and safety have been confirmed in more than 100 double-blind studies. The specific medications and their use are covered in Chapter 8. Prevalence of medication prescription varies widely among communities. Overall, the number of elementary school–age children taking methylphenidate is the same as conservative estimates of the prevalence of ADHD (3%–5%). Medications appear to be underutilized in some areas, however, especially when schools and parents have difficulty accessing diagnostic and treatment resources. In some practices, stimulants may be prescribed too freely, with insufficient evaluation and follow-up.

Other drugs (see Chapter 8), such as atomoxetine, a norepinephrine reuptake inhibitor, antidepressants (bupropion or TCAs), or α-adrenergic agents (clonidine or guanfacine), can be considered if stimulants are only partially effective or produce unacceptable side effects or if the child or family is at high risk for abuse of the stimulant medication. Other medications may also be indicated to treat comorbid aggression, anxiety, or depression.

Psychotherapeutic Interventions

Behavior modification can improve academic achievement, reduce specifically targeted behavior problems, and decrease symptoms that are not helped by stimulants. Both punishment (time-out and response cost) and contingent rewards are required, and consistent, intensive, and prolonged (months to years) treatment may be needed. Response cost is the removal of points, rewards, or privileges following misbehavior as specified in a behavior modification plan. Parents and teachers must learn the specific techniques and be willing to invest the time and energy to implement them. Stimulants and behavior modification at home and at school may have separate and additive effects on motor behavior, attention and learning, and social functioning. Generalization and maintenance of improvement is unfortunately limited. Children may need to be taught social skills before behavior modification or medication can improve peer relationships. In a highly structured program (often not feasible to implement or maintain, however), the behavior of children with ADHD can be nearly normalized, but 30%–60% will improve further with the addition of a low dose of stimulant medication.

Cognitive-behavior therapy, in which children learn social and academic problem-solving strategies, monitor their own performance, remind themselves of rules, and praise themselves for accomplishments, generally is not effective in reducing ADHD symptoms, most likely because the child rarely uses the learned skills unless he or she is specifically cued by an adult. Individual psychotherapy may be useful to address comorbid disorders or sequelae of trauma. Family psychotherapy may reduce the conflict that results from raising a child with ADHD or may address primary marital dysfunction. Group therapy provides a setting where social skills deficits can be observed and remediated.

Unestablished Treatments

Dietary treatments remain popular with some families despite the minimal evidence of efficacy and the difficulty complying with special diets. Research on the Feingold diet (which omits salicylates and food dyes) is inconclusive, but elimination of food dyes might be helpful for a subgroup (5%) of children with ADHD, particularly those younger than 6 years. Double-blind studies do not confirm parents' reports of acute effects of food dyes. Even for those children whose condition improves with a restricted diet, stimulants are a more potent treatment than diet. Despite anecdotal reports, there is no scientific evidence that sugar, food allergies, herbal remedies, yeast, trace minerals, or megavitamins influence the etiology or treatment of ADHD. Systemic reactions (irritability, fatigue) due to a variety of allergies or deficiencies or excesses in food intake may affect behavior and attention in some children. Some nonprofessionals have recommended caffeine as a more "natural" treatment of hyperactivity, but studies have found significant side effects and no evidence of efficacy.

Other unproven treatments that have enthusiastic advocates (often with financial interests) include anti–*Candida albicans* medication, neurotherapy (biofeedback training of brain waves), sensory integrative training, optometric vision training, chiropractic manipulation, metronome therapy, herbal regimens, homeopathy, massage, and acupuncture.

■ CONDUCT DISORDER

Clinical Description

Children and adolescents with CD repeatedly violate important societal rules or the personal rights of others (Table 3–5). The division of youths with CD into subgroups has been controversial. Previous diagnostic criteria identified two groups: 1) those who were socialized (i.e., had friends) and whose delinquent behavior occurred in the context of gangs or peer groups and 2) those who were socially

TABLE 3–5. **DSM-IV-TR diagnostic criteria for conduct disorder**

A. A repetitive and persistent pattern of behavior in which the basic rights of others or major age-appropriate societal norms or rules are violated, as manifested by the presence of three (or more) of the following criteria in the past 12 months, with at least one criterion present in the past 6 months:

Aggression to people and animals
(1) often bullies, threatens, or intimidates others
(2) often initiates physical fights
(3) has used a weapon that can cause serious physical harm to others (e.g., a bat, brick, broken bottle, knife, gun)
(4) has been physically cruel to people
(5) has been physically cruel to animals
(6) has stolen while confronting a victim (e.g., mugging, purse snatching, extortion, armed robbery)
(7) has forced someone into sexual activity

Destruction of property
(8) has deliberately engaged in fire setting with the intention of causing serious damage
(9) has deliberately destroyed others' property (other than by fire setting)

Deceitfulness or theft
(10) has broken into someone else's house, building, or car
(11) often lies to obtain goods or favors or to avoid obligations (i.e., "cons" others)
(12) has stolen items of nontrivial value without confronting a victim (e.g., shoplifting, but without breaking and entering; forgery)

Serious violations of rules
(13) often stays out at night despite parental prohibitions, beginning before age 13 years
(14) has run away from home overnight at least twice while living in parental or parental surrogate home (or once without returning for a lengthy period)
(15) is often truant from school, beginning before age 13 years

B. The disturbance in behavior causes clinically significant impairment in social, academic, or occupational functioning.

TABLE 3–5.	**DSM-IV-TR diagnostic criteria for conduct disorder** *(continued)*

C. If the individual is age 18 years or older, criteria are not met for antisocial personality disorder.

Code based on age at onset:

> **312.81 Conduct disorder, childhood-onset type:** onset of at least one criterion characteristic of conduct disorder prior to age 10 years
>
> **312.82 Conduct disorder, adolescent-onset type:** absence of any criteria characteristic of conduct disorder prior to age 10 years
>
> **312.89 Conduct disorder, unspecified onset:** age at onset is not known

Specify severity:

> **Mild:** few if any conduct problems in excess of those required to make the diagnosis **and** conduct problems cause only minor harm to others
>
> **Moderate:** number of conduct problems and effect on others intermediate between "mild" and "severe"
>
> **Severe:** many conduct problems in excess of those required to make the diagnosis **or** conduct problems cause considerable harm to others

isolated and appeared to lack a conscience or superego. This distinction proved difficult to make in clinical settings. Other classifications differentiate those who behave aggressively from those who engage primarily in covert, nonconfrontational problem behaviors (e.g., stealing and truancy). In addition, whether aggressive behavior is "predatory" (goal oriented, planned) or "affective" (impulsive, reactive) may have implications for etiology and treatment.

DSM-IV-TR specifies two types of CD: childhood onset, in which at least one criterion is met before age 10 years, and adolescent onset. Longitudinal studies (Langbehn et al. 1998) have found that childhood onset is associated with male predominance, more physical aggression, impaired peer relationships, and comorbid ADHD. A typical course for this subtype is ODD in early childhood, which develops into full-blown CD by puberty, followed by risk of persistent CD and development of adult antisocial personality disorder. Those with adolescent onset have few symptoms before puberty and are less likely to be aggressive and more likely to be female than those in the early-onset group. Most of those with adolescent onset have friends but often in the context of a gang or other delinquent peer group. The prognosis for cessation of conduct problems is better if onset is in adolescence; however, course and outcome may be influenced by the nature of the delinquent group and the availability of alternative social supports.

Consequences of truancy and suspensions for violating school rules, as well as coexisting attention problems and specific learning disorders, include loss of interest in school, school failure and drop-out, and eventual unemployment. Youths with CD are at increased medical risk for early pregnancy; sexually transmitted diseases; physical injury from fighting, accidents, rape, or even murder; and the sequelae of smoking, drinking, and drug abuse. Rates of suicidal ideation and behavior are increased, especially when substance use is present.

Despite the diversity of behavioral symptoms and severity, certain psychological characteristics are common (Table 3–6).

Epidemiology

DSM-IV-TR reports prevalence estimates of CD among children and adolescents in the United States ranging from less than 1% to more than 10%. Although the prevalence of CD in girls has increased, boys still outnumber girls by 3–4:1. Less is known about CD in girls than in boys. Boys commit far more violent crimes than girls do (8:1). When self-report data are used, the overall prevalence of misconduct and delinquent behaviors is even greater, and the male predominance for crime declines to about 2:1. Cultural attitudes toward gender, race, and class may affect the relative likelihood of a youth's being identified as having a CD. CD is frequent among youths referred to outpatient psychiatric services.

TABLE 3–6. **Common psychological characteristics of children and adolescents with conduct disorder**

Attention deficits, low frustration tolerance

Impulsivity, recklessness

Learning disorders, especially in reading

Negative mood
  Sullenness
  Irritability
  Volatile anger

Low self-esteem

Impaired cognitions
  Distortions of size and time awareness
  Lack of or distorted connection between prior events and consequences
  Limited ability to generate, evaluate, and implement alternative problem-solving strategies

Use of less adaptive intrapsychic defense mechanisms
  Minimization
  Avoidance
  Externalization
  Denial
  Identification with the aggressor

Emotional deficits
  Minimization of fear and sadness, exaggeration of anger
  Lack of empathy
  Lack of guilt

Impaired interpersonal relations
  Suspiciousness or paranoia, with cognitive distortions
  Attributional bias: misperception of others' actions as hostile
  Preference for nonverbal, action-oriented, aggressive solutions to problems

Comorbidity

Comorbid psychiatric or neurological disorders are common in association with CD and contribute to its severity and chronicity. ADHD occurs in as many as half of children with CD in community surveys. In psychiatric clinical programs, CD without ADHD is rare.

Posttraumatic stress disorder (PTSD) and dissociative disorders are often reported, especially by incarcerated delinquent youth. Hypervigilance, irritability, and flashbacks may contribute to aggression when youths feel threatened. Learning disorders (especially reading disorder and expressive language disorder) are common. Depression or bipolar disorder may be seen. Although it seems contradictory, anxiety disorders are found in many youth with CD, especially girls, at increased rates after puberty. Substance use is often present and may not be recognized. Drug or alcohol use can aggravate impulsivity, risk taking, aggression, suicidality, and school failure.

Etiology

Many etiological factors have been implicated in the development of CD, which is a heterogeneous disorder (Table 3–7). Understanding the contributing factors for the individual patient is important in planning treatment. Current views emphasize an interaction among socioeconomic, cultural, family dynamic, temperamental, genetic, neurobiological, and psychiatric factors to explain the development and persistence of CD and its pattern of transmission from one generation to the next.

Data from a study of male twins suggest that, compared with adult antisocial behavior, juvenile conduct problems are more strongly related to environmental factors and less strongly related to genetic factors (Lyons et al. 1995). The interaction of inadequate and often abusive parenting with characteristics intrinsic to the child results in noncompliant and aggressive behaviors and deficient academic and social skills. Temperamental characteristics such as negative emotions, intense reactions, and inflexibility are associated with higher risk of CD. Multiple studies have found that birth complications combined with early maternal rejection (unwanted pregnancy, attempt to abort fetus, and placement outside the home before age 1 year), poor parenting, or parental mental illness increase the likelihood of violent criminal behavior (Raine 2002). Patterson and colleagues (1989) emphasized the importance of a parent–child negative spiral of ever-increasing aversive and

TABLE 3–7.   **Factors implicated in the etiology of conduct disorders**

Genetic transmission of predisposing psychiatric disorder

Antisocial personality disorder

Oppositional defiant disorder

Attention-deficit/hyperactivity disorder

Substance abuse

Mood disorders

Learning disorders

Neurobiological

Serotonergic dysfunction

Low autonomic activity/arousal (as shown by low resting heart rate)

Intrauterine exposure to alcohol

Maternal smoking (may be correlate or cause)

Birth complications, low birth weight

Psychomotor seizures

Head injuries from accidents or abuse

Temperament

Difficult

Resistant to parental discipline

Poor adaptability to change

Intense activity

High level of novelty-seeking (may relate to dopamine D_4 receptor gene)

Other psychiatric disorders

Attention-deficit/hyperactivity disorder

Mood disorders

Posttraumatic stress disorder

Learning disorders

Communication disorders

Substance abuse

Psychosis, paranoia

TABLE 3–7.	Factors implicated in the etiology of conduct disorders *(continued)*

Parenting characteristics

Failure of parent–child bonding

Large family

Young mother

Absent or alcoholic father

Conflict between parents

Depressed, irritable, substance-using, or psychotic parent

Lack of parental monitoring; inadequate supervision and limit setting

Harsh and inconsistent, unpredictable discipline

Rejection, abandonment, or neglect by parents

Physical or sexual abuse

Modeling of impulsivity, aggression, or antisocial behavior

Lack of enculturation to use of language for problem-solving or to values of larger society

Placement outside of the home as an infant or toddler

Social problems

Poverty and cultural disadvantage

Cultural behavior norms: gang- and drug-infested neighborhoods

Rejection by prosocial peers

Association with antisocial peers

Early puberty (for girls only)

coercive behaviors. In effect, these children train their parents to use harsh but inconsistent discipline, and the parents train the children in noncompliant, defiant, and antisocial behaviors. Although less is known about girls with CD, some data suggest that their families are even more dysfunctional than those of boys with CD. Rejection by peers and school failure encourage affiliation with similarly troubled peers. One study found that approximately one-third of prepubertal children with depressive mood disorders developed a DSM-III diagnosis of CD by age 19 years (Kovacs et al. 1988).

The multiple risk factors appear to have a cumulative effect. Most children with risk factors do not, however, develop CD.

Divorce does not appear to be a major risk factor; family discord rather than separation appears to mediate the risk for CD. Protective factors are not well understood, but an easy or behaviorally inhibited temperament, areas of competence, adequate supervision at home, or a good relationship with one parent or another adult can reduce an at-risk child's chance of developing CD. Associating with nondelinquent peers and attending a school with a positive environment also offer some protection.

Course and Prognosis

The first signs of behavior problems—aggression, impulsivity, and noncompliance—may be seen as early as age 4 years. Several studies have found that the combination of aggression and shyness in first grade predicts adolescent delinquency and substance abuse. Symptoms tend to emerge in a predictable developmental sequence, with milder behaviors followed by more severe ones. Progression may stop at any stage. Early onset; greater frequency, number, and variety of conduct symptoms; and comorbid ADHD are associated with more severe and prolonged CD.

CD remits in many youths, but some lead lives of delinquency or develop antisocial personality disorder. Low IQ score and parental antisocial personality disorder predict persistence of CD (Loeber et al. 1995). A relatively small number of chronic offenders account for most juvenile crime. Recidivists are more likely to have early onset, poor school grades, and low socioeconomic status. In a 7 year follow-up of clinic-referred boys ages 7–12 years with CD, the majority showed fluctuating or increasing CD behaviors. At baseline, the minority with a more positive outcome were more likely to have lower severity of CD, fewer symptoms of ADHD, higher verbal IQ, greater family socioeconomic advantage, and biological parents who were not antisocial. Treatment or incarceration did not account for improvement (Lahey et al. 2002).

Despite the high risk for major psychiatric symptoms, substance abuse, functional impairment, and incarceration, many children with CD achieve a favorable adult adjustment. More adaptive social skills, more positive peer experiences, and adolescent onset predict a better long-term outcome. Head Start and several innovative elementary school–based programs have been able to reduce delinquent outcomes and improve academic achievement in children at risk for CD.

Evaluation

Youths with more severe and complex forms of CD require a comprehensive biopsychosocial evaluation by a multidisciplinary team that might include a child and adolescent psychiatrist, a clinical psychologist, a social worker, a pediatrician or specialist in adolescent medicine, a neurologist, an educational diagnostician and school consultant, a speech and language pathologist, occupational and recreational therapists, a legal advisor, and a case manager or probation officer.

Conventional diagnostic interviews may be difficult, because many youths with CD are uncomfortable or hostile when talking with adults in roles of authority and have a limited ability to express themselves verbally and to think abstractly. Efforts to establish rapport and careful questioning are essential to identify comorbid psychiatric disorders and a history suggestive of neurological impairment. Patients often underreport deviant behaviors as a result of either unconscious denial or lying. Sources of information in addition to the patient are essential. Youths generally report more of their covert behaviors, such as lying, stealing, vandalism, and fire setting, whereas parents are more likely to report their child's overt behaviors, such as fighting, assault, and rape. However, parents who are trying to shield their child from legal consequences may not disclose behaviors.

Evaluation of neurological history is needed because of the frequency of head trauma (both contributing to and resulting from the CD) and seizures. Cognitive and educational assessment are essential because of the high association with specific learning disorders and borderline intellectual functioning or mental retardation. In addition, truancy, comorbid ADHD, and lack of socialization to the value and culture of school may contribute to educational deficits.

Differential Diagnosis

CD is a heterogeneous descriptive diagnosis that is made if the symptoms meet the behavioral criteria. Because virtually any psychiatric disorder can present with disturbance of conduct, the clinician must evaluate the full range of Axis I psychiatric diagnoses, intelligence, neuropsychological performance, language and speech abilities, social competence, and family functioning. During an episode of depression or mania in bipolar disorder, irritability and impaired judgment can lead to behavior problems that can be distinguished from primary CD by their time course and associated mood symptoms. Psychosis in children and adolescents may result in behaviors consistent with CD. Differential diagnosis also includes intermittent explosive disorder and a spectrum of less severe disorders: ODD, adjustment disorder with disturbance of conduct, and child or adolescent antisocial behavior (a DSM-IV-TR V code), as well as normal mischief. Although many cases of CD (especially childhood onset) also meet criteria for ODD, a diagnosis of ODD is preempted if criteria for CD are met.

Treatment

Despite the cost of CD to individuals, families, and society, few treatments with proven efficacy are available. The patient is rarely motivated to change, and the family and social environments may lack the necessary resources. Early-onset CD becomes increasingly resistant to treatment as the child enters adolescence; therefore, early intervention with young children is crucial. Treatment may take a variety of forms: family interventions, social support, behavior modification, psychopharmacology, or legal sanctions. The treatment setting may be the home; a school, clinic, hospital, or residential treatment program; or a specialized delinquency program. Complex cases of CD often require lengthy multimodal therapeutic interventions. The environment in which the patient is living or to which he or she will return must be considered. Comorbid conditions also require attention.

A containment structure and effective limit setting must be established quickly to provide a safe and stable environment for treatment. Limit setting at home may be compromised by parental conflict, parental absence, inconsistent discipline, vague or low expectations for appropriate behavior, or parental depression or other psychiatric illness. Creating or reinforcing limits for the child with CD may require counseling of parents, treatment of parents' psychiatric problems, increased supervision at home, surveillance at school, or use of legal mechanisms. Guardianship, hearings before judges, supervision by parole officers, and brief incarceration may be required for effective limit setting and communicating the significance of behavioral violations. Families may need concrete assistance with income, housing, legal matters, or medical care. Hospitalizing the youth briefly may be useful for containment and intensive evaluation, perhaps including a trial of medication. More stringent criteria for "medical necessity" have decreased the frequency of hospitalization for CD unless it is comorbid with other psychiatric disorders, in part because hospitalization is not effective as definitive treatment.

Psychotherapeutic Interventions

Several treatments based on cognitive, behavioral, and family systems principles have shown efficacy, when youth and families can be motivated to participate in and complete treatment programs. Even with treatment, many remain outside the normal range of problem behavior, however. Intensive cognitive problem-solving skills training (PSST) that teaches children to generate and use alternative solutions to manage interpersonal problems and incorporates behavior modification techniques such as practice, modeling, role playing, corrective feedback, and social and concrete reinforcement can decrease aggressive and delinquent behavior and increase social skills (Kazdin 1997). Parental involvement appears to be key to the use, generalization, and maintenance of the skills learned. The addition of parent management training to PSST leads to greater improvement in the child's behavior and reduction of parental stress and depression.

Parent management training (PMT) and functional family therapy (FFT) can be helpful for relatively motivated and intact families. Principles of behavior modification and family systems theory are used to improve communication and negotiation skills, encourage positive reinforcement, correct dysfunctional parent–child interaction patterns, and promote more effective and less damaging methods of discipline. Long-term positive effects have not been shown, however. Younger children are more likely than adolescents to benefit from parent training interventions. Multisystemic therapy (MST) (see Henggeler et al. 1998 in "Additional Reading"), a comprehensive treatment combining systemic family therapy with behavior modification and direct intervention into the youth's social system, has been shown to be an effective treatment of delinquency in youths, even those from chaotic, multiproblem families; it improves adjustment of patients and family members and reduces future criminal behavior. The therapist empowers parents; enlists social service agencies; and actively reaches out into the home, school, and neighborhood. Individual supportive therapy or pharmacotherapy for the identified patient or a family member is added when necessary.

Group therapy, particularly in residential treatment or group-oriented facilities, uses peer pressure to promote positive change and to improve socialization skills. Caution is needed, because treating antisocial youth together in groups can lead to contagion and worsening of problem behaviors. Insight-oriented individual psychotherapy is not useful.

Pharmacotherapy

Medication treatment of CD can include virtually any psychotropic drug, depending on the individual patient's target symptoms and co-morbid disorders (see Chapter 8). In patients with coexisting

ADHD, stimulants and clonidine, alone or in combination, can decrease impulsive conduct symptoms, verbal and physical aggression, overactivity, and inattention. Bupropion also may be effective.

CD that is secondary to a major depression may remit when the depression is successfully treated. Lithium may be considered in the treatment of severe impulsive aggression, especially when it is accompanied by explosive, irritable, labile affect. In a well-designed controlled study, lithium was shown to be equal or superior to haloperidol in reducing aggression, hostility, and tantrums and to have fewer side effects (Campbell et al. 1995). Lithium may be the first pharmacological choice if the patient with CD has a family history of bipolar disorder. Trazodone is sometimes used to reduce aggression, but the risk of priapism limits its use in adolescent boys.

Patients who have severe impulsive aggression with emotional lability and irritability, an abnormal electroencephalogram, a strong clinical suggestion of epileptic phenomena, or nonresponse to lithium may benefit from a trial of carbamazepine or valproate. Propranolol, a β-adrenergic blocker, may be useful in patients with otherwise uncontrollable rage reactions and impulsive aggression, especially those with evidence of organicity. Antipsychotic medications may decrease aggressive symptoms that result from psychosis. Even in nonpsychotic, severely aggressive children, atypical antipsychotics such as risperidone may reduce aggression, hostility, negativism, and explosiveness, although the side-effect profile (cognitive dulling and risk of tardive dyskinesia) may be problematic.

School and Juvenile Justice Interventions

School interventions include special attention to behavior control; individualized educational programming; vocational training; and remediation of language, speech, and other specific learning disorders. Despite their political popularity, "boot camps" are not effective in reducing future crimes committed by juvenile delinquents (Henggeler and Schoenwald 1994).

■ OPPOSITIONAL DEFIANT DISORDER

Clinical Description

ODD is considered to be the developmentally earlier, less severe form of disruptive behavior disorder. Children with ODD show argumentative, disobedient, and defiant behavior, without serious violation of the rights of other people. These children are stubborn, negativistic, and provocative. Anger-related symptoms are typically directed at parents and teachers. A lesser degree of anger dyscontrol may be seen in peer relationships.

DSM-IV-TR defines ODD as a pattern of negativistic, hostile, disobedient, and defiant behavior lasting at least 6 months, during which at least four of the behavioral criteria are present at a frequency greater than that typical for the child's age and developmental level. Data from a community survey provide guidance in determining when a behavior occurs more frequently than expected for age (Angold and Costello 1996). DSM-IV-TR criteria and suggested cutoff frequencies are listed in Table 3–8. To diagnose ODD, the symptoms must not occur exclusively during the course of a psychotic or mood disorder.

TABLE 3–8. **DSM-IV-TR criteria and suggested cutoff frequencies for oppositional defiant disorder**

DSM-IV-TR criteria	**Suggested cutoff frequency**
1. Often loses temper	Twice a week
2. Often argues with adults	Twice a week
3. Often actively defies or refuses to comply with adults' requests or rules	Twice a week
4. Often deliberately annoys people	Four times a week
5. Often blames others for his or her mistakes or misbehavior	Once in 3 months
6. Is often touchy or easily annoyed by others	Twice a week
7. Is often angry and resentful	Four times a week
8. Is often spiteful or vindictive	Once in 3 months

Source. American Psychiatric Association 2000; Angold and Costello 1996.

A crucial feature of ODD is the self-defeating stand that these children take in arguments. They may be willing to lose something they want (a privilege or toy) rather than lose a battle or lose face. The oppositional struggle takes on a life of its own in the child's mind and becomes more important than the reality of the situation. The child may experience "rational" interventions as continuing arguments. Disobedience can take the form of overt defiance and provocation or dawdling and procrastination, as well as "sneaky" behavior. Parents, and sometimes teachers, become exhausted, frustrated, and angry. As a result, discipline veers between overly punitive and hopelessly lax. By the time of clinical referral, the findings are the result of an interactive, negative spiral between parents and child.

Epidemiology

The changing criteria for ODD have prevented stable prevalence estimates. Perhaps 3%–15% of children have ODD, with equal or slightly higher rates in boys than girls. ODD is common in psychiatric clinics and in classes for children with emotional disturbances and learning disabilities. It often occurs concurrently with ADHD.

Etiology

Several psychosocial mechanisms have been hypothesized to contribute to ODD:

- Parents use inconsistent methods of disciplining, structuring, and limit setting.
- Children identify with a stubborn and impulsive parent who acts as a role model for oppositional and defiant interactions with other people.
- Parents have insufficient time and emotional energy for the child.

Marital problems are common in the parents of children with ODD, but it is difficult to distinguish the cause from the effect of raising such a child. Genetic, neurobiological, and temperamental factors may also contribute. The features of ODD and difficult temperament overlap significantly. One study of adopted high risk youth suggests that symptoms of ODD in adolescent males may be linked to genetic traits leading to adult antisocial personality (Langbehn et al. 1998).

Course and Prognosis

Some children with ODD develop CD, but many do not. In one sample of 7- to 12-year-old clinic-referred boys with ODD, 44% developed CD over a 3-year period (Loeber et al. 1995). Risk factors for progression of ODD to CD include poverty and parental characteristics such as a mother who is young when her first child is born and parents who abuse substances, discipline children inconsistently, and supervise children inadequately. Risk factors in the child are low IQ, physical fighting, and resistance to parental discipline (Lahey et al. 1992).

Evaluation and Differential Diagnosis

Psychiatric evaluation of the child and family is needed to rule out alternative or comorbid disorders and to seek family and psychosocial contributing factors. The ODD symptoms are generally reported by parents and caregivers. The children may not view themselves as defiant or argumentative and often externalize blame onto parents, authority figures, and peers. Symptoms are more prominent when the child is with familiar people.

Although these behaviors can be normal for children in phases during toddlerhood and adolescence, the 6-month duration criterion for ODD ordinarily excludes these developmental phenomena. Some children are simply temperamentally stubborn but lack the pattern of more severe disturbance characteristic of ODD. Children with ODD are often annoying or spiteful but stop short of the pattern of serious behavior problems seen in CD. A diagnosis of CD precludes a diagnosis of ODD.

Severe separation anxiety disorder, panic disorder, or obsessive-compulsive disorder may lead to temper tantrums and dramatic resistance, but in these disorders the problem behavior is restricted to the feared situations, and in most cases these children can verbalize specific triggers of anxiety.

A key to the diagnosis of ODD is its lifelong pattern. Discrete periods of irritability and resistance to adult direction may be secondary to major affective episodes (depression or hypomania), psychosis, or an adjustment disorder. The intentional and provocative noncompliance characteristic of ODD should be differentiated from the noncompliance resulting from impulsivity and inattention in ADHD, although both disorders are often present. If criteria for both ODD and ADHD are met, both are diagnosed.

Oppositional behavior that is restricted to the school setting may be a result of mental retardation, borderline intelligence, or a specific developmental disorder or lack of training in cultural norms and expectations.

Treatment

Multimodal programs such as Fast Track can reduce progression to CD in young children identified as at-risk (Conduct Problems Prevention Research Group 2002). PMT in behavior modification techniques such as positive reinforcement, giving more effective commands, "time-out," and token economies can reduce power struggles and modify oppositionality. Maximal improvement may result from combining the use of a social skills, problem-solving, and conflict management training group for the child with a behavior modification training group for parents (Webster-Stratton and Hammond 1997). Traditional individual or family systems psychotherapy is not helpful for the primary symptoms of ODD.

In children with coexisting ADHD, anxiety, or mood disorder, medication may reduce oppositional behavior and improve compliance.

■ REFERENCES

American Psychiatric Association: Diagnostic and Statistical Manual of Mental Disorders, 3rd Edition. Washington, DC, American Psychiatric Association, 1980

American Psychiatric Association: Diagnostic and Statistical Manual of Mental Disorders, 4th Edition, Text Revision. Washington, DC, American Psychiatric Association, 2000

Angold A, Costello EJ: Toward establishing an empirical basis for the diagnosis of oppositional defiant disorder. J Am Acad Child Adolesc Psychiatry 35:1205–1212, 1996

Barbaresi WJ, Katusic SK, Colligan RC, et al: How common is attention-deficit/hyperactivity disorder? Arch Pediatr Adolesc Med 156:217–224, 2002

Barkley RA: Attention Deficit Hyperactivity Disorder: A Handbook for Diagnosis and Treatment. New York, Guilford, 1990

Barkley RA: Attention-Deficit Hyperactivity Disorder: A Handbook for Diagnosis and Treatment, 2nd Edition. New York, Guilford, 1998

Biederman J, Faraone S, Milberger S, et al: A prospective 4-year follow-up study of attention-deficit hyperactivity and related disorders. Arch Gen Psychiatry 53:437–446, 1996

Biederman J, Wilens T, Mick E: Is ADHD a risk factor for psychoactive substance use disorders? Findings from a four-year prospective follow-up study. J Am Acad Child Adolesc Psychiatry 36:21–29, 1997

Campbell M, Adams PB, Small AM, et al: Lithium in hospitalized aggressive children with conduct disorder: a double-blind and placebo-controlled study. J Am Acad Child Adolesc Psychiatry 34:445–453, 1995

Conduct Problems Prevention Research Group: Evaluation of the first 3 years of the Fast Track prevention trial with children at high risk for adolescent conduct problems. J Abnorm Child Psychol 30:19–35, 2002

Henggeler SW, Schoenwald SK: Boot camps for juvenile offenders: just say no. Journal of Child and Family Studies 3:243–248, 1994

Kazdin AE: Practitioner review: psychosocial treatments for conduct disorder in children. J Child Psychol Psychiatry 38:161–178, 1997

Kovacs M, Paulauskas S, Gatsonis C, et al: Depressive disorders in childhood, III: a longitudinal study of comorbidity with and risk for conduct disorders. J Affect Disord 15:205–217, 1988

Lahey BB, Loeber R, Quay HC, et al: Oppositional defiant and conduct disorders: issues to be resolved for DSM-IV. J Am Acad Child Adolesc Psychiatry 31:539–546, 1992

Lahey BB, Loeber R, Burke J, et al: Adolescent outcomes of childhood conduct disorder among clinic-referred boys: predictors of improvement. J Abnorm Child Psychol 30:333–348, 2002

Langbehn DR, Cadoret RJ, Yates WR, et al: Distinct contributions of conduct and oppositional defiant symptoms to adult antisocial behavior: evidence from an adoption study. Arch Gen Psychiatry 55:821–829, 1998

Loeber R, Green SM, Keenan K, et al: Which boys will fare worse? Early predictors of the onset of conduct disorder in a six-year longitudinal study. J Am Acad Child Adolesc Psychiatry 34:499–509, 1995

Loney J, Milich R: Hyperactivity, inattention, and aggression in clinical practice. Advances in Developmental and Behavioral Pediatrics 3:113–147, 1982

Lyons MJ, True WR, Eisen SA, et al: Differential heritability of adult and juvenile antisocial traits. Arch Gen Psychiatry 52:906–915, 1995

Patterson GR, DeBaryshe BD, Ramsey E: A developmental perspective on antisocial behavior. Am Psychol 44:329–335, 1989

Pelham WE, Milich R, Murphy DA, et al: Normative data on the IOWA Conners Teacher Rating Scale. Journal of Clinical Child Psychology 18:259–262, 1989

Raine A: Biosocial studies of antisocial and violent behavior in children and adults: a review. J Abnorm Child Psychol 30:311–326, 2002

Tallmadge J, Barkley RA: The interactions of hyperactive and normal boys with their fathers and mothers. J Abnorm Child Psychol 11:565–579, 1983

Webster-Stratton C, Hammond M: Treating children with early-onset conduct problems: a comparison of child and parent training interventions. J Consult Clin Psychol 65:93–109, 1997

■ ADDITIONAL READING

American Academy of Child and Adolescent Psychiatry: Practice parameters for the assessment and treatment of children, adolescents, and adults with attention-deficit/hyperactivity disorder. J Am Acad Child Adolesc Psychiatry 36 (10 suppl):85S–121S, 1997

American Academy of Child and Adolescent Psychiatry: Practice parameters for the assessment and treatment of children and adolescents with conduct disorder. J Am Acad Child Adolesc Psychiatry 36 (10 suppl):122S–139S, 1997

Barkley RA: Attention-Deficit Hyperactivity Disorder: A Handbook for Diagnosis and Treatment, 2nd Edition. New York, Guilford, 1998

Burke JD, Loeber R, Birmaher B: Oppositional defiant disorder and conduct disorder: a review of the past 10 years, part II. J Am Acad Child Adolesc Psychiatry 41:1275–1293, 2002

Henggeler SW, Schoenwald SK, Borduin CM, et al: Multisystemic Treatment of Antisocial Behavior in Children and Adolescents. New York, Guilford, 1998

Hill J: Biological, psychological and social processes in the conduct disorders. J Child Psychol Psychiatry 43:133–164, 2002

Loeber R, Burke JD, Lahey BB, et al: Oppositional defiant and conduct disorder: a review of the past 10 years, part I. J Am Acad Child Adolesc Psychiatry 39:1468–1484, 2000

4

OTHER AXIS I DISORDERS USUALLY FIRST DIAGNOSED IN INFANCY, CHILDHOOD, OR ADOLESCENCE

This chapter covers several disorders from the childhood-onset section of DSM-IV-TR (American Psychiatric Association 2000). These disorders always begin prior to adulthood, although they may not be diagnosed until later. Separation anxiety disorder, pica, rumination, encopresis, enuresis, and selective mutism nearly all remit by adulthood. Tourette's and other tic disorders typically become less severe by adulthood but may persist. It is assumed that children with reactive attachment disorder remain impaired in adulthood, but longitudinal studies have not been done to demonstrate what adult psychopathology might develop.

■ SEPARATION ANXIETY DISORDER

Clinical Description

In separation anxiety disorder (SAD), cognitive, affective, somatic, and behavioral symptoms appear in response to genuine or fantasized separation from the individual(s) to whom the child is most attached (Table 4–1). The symptoms of SAD are first observed when the child experiences a sense of separation from the "attachment object," usually a parent or caregiver, but sometimes a favorite toy or familiar place. Typically, even a young child with SAD can specify

TABLE 4–1.	**DSM-IV-TR diagnostic criteria for separation anxiety disorder**

A. Developmentally inappropriate and excessive anxiety concerning separation from home or from those to whom the individual is attached, as evidenced by three (or more) of the following:

    (1) recurrent excessive distress when separation from home or major attachment figures occurs or is anticipated

    (2) persistent and excessive worry about losing, or about possible harm befalling, major attachment figures

    (3) persistent and excessive worry that an untoward event will lead to separation from a major attachment figure (e.g., getting lost or being kidnapped)

    (4) persistent reluctance or refusal to go to school or elsewhere because of fear of separation

    (5) persistently and excessively fearful or reluctant to be alone or without major attachment figures at home or without significant adults in other settings

    (6) persistent reluctance or refusal to go to sleep without being near a major attachment figure or to sleep away from home

    (7) repeated nightmares involving the theme of separation

    (8) repeated complaints of physical symptoms (such as headaches, stomachaches, nausea, or vomiting) when separation from major attachment figures occurs or is anticipated

B. The duration of the disturbance is at least 4 weeks.

C. The onset is before age 18 years.

D. The disturbance causes clinically significant distress or impairment in social, academic (occupational), or other important areas of functioning.

E. The disturbance does not occur exclusively during the course of a pervasive developmental disorder, schizophrenia, or other psychotic disorder and, in adolescents and adults, is not better accounted for by panic disorder with agoraphobia.

Specify if:

    Early onset: if onset occurs before age 6 years

the attachment object that gives a sense of protection or safety. The anxiety can be experienced and expressed as an unrealistic fear of the child or parent being injured, kidnapped, or killed. Resulting symptoms can include inability to sleep alone, attend school, visit friends, go on errands, or stay at camp. In order to avoid leaving home, children with SAD will often complain of somatic symptoms such as stomachaches or headaches (which they may actually be experiencing) or claim that peers or teachers pick on them.

Not all children with school absenteeism have SAD, and not all children with SAD miss excessive amounts of school. However, approximately three-quarters of children with SAD exhibit school avoidance (Last et al. 1987a). The historical term for school avoidance or school refusal secondary to SAD is *school phobia*. School absenteeism has various etiologies (Table 4–2). In a large clinical sample of children and adolescents with school refusal, 25% had both an anxiety and a depressive diagnosis, and half of the total group had either an anxiety or a depressive disorder (Bernstein et al. 1996).

TABLE 4–2.   **Causes of school absenteeism**

Separation anxiety disorder
Other psychiatric disorders
   Mood disorder
   Anxiety disorder
      Generalized anxiety disorder
      Phobic disorder (such as social phobia)
      Panic disorder
      Obsessive-compulsive disorder
   Psychotic disorder
Truancy (often associated with conduct disorder)
Substance abuse
Sociocultural conformity
   Permission granted by family (overt or covert)
   Normative peer behavior
Realistic fear
   Excessive teasing or humiliation
   Physical bullying–intimidation or bodily harm

Epidemiology

SAD has a reported prevalence of 2.4%–4.7% in nonreferred samples (American Academy of Child and Adolescent Psychiatry 1997). The female-to-male ratio is probably equal. As with other anxiety disorders, SAD appears to aggregate in families.

Etiology

A wide variety of theoretical perspectives on the etiology of SAD exist. The high familial concurrence of anxiety disorders makes it difficult to separate the contributions of genetic inheritance, temperament, family dynamics, and other environmental factors. An interactive model is most likely.

Developmental theorists focus on the interplay between the exploring toddler's normal uncertainty about the location of the caregiver and the at-risk child's anxious or insecure attachment. Behaviorally oriented theories emphasize the maintenance of symptoms by conditioned fear, based on stimulus generalization and reinforcement. The psychoanalytic view sees the parent and child bound to each other by fears of separation related to unconscious internal conflicts.

Biological theories focus on temperamental, genetic, and physiological factors. The parents and other relatives of many children with SAD have mood or anxiety disorders. In particular, children of parents with panic disorder are at high risk for anxiety disorders. "Behavioral inhibition to the unfamiliar" is a temperament construct (describing shy, cautious, introverted children) that has been associated with anxiety. Family studies of anxiety disorders support the proposition that behavioral inhibition is correlated with proneness to anxiety. Recent work by Rosenbaum et al. (2000) further supports prior findings that children whose parents suffer from panic disorder and depression may be at increased risk for behavioral inhibition.

Course and Prognosis

SAD typically begins around school age and is usually recognized in early or middle childhood. The disorder is often recurrent, with acute exacerbations at the beginning of the school year, following holiday breaks from school, or when starting a new school. Precipitants include actual separations, deaths, family moves, or crises. Symptoms may worsen during or after medical illnesses or procedures.

As in most childhood psychiatric disorders, comorbidity is common. More than 92% of children with SAD have additional psychiatric disorders, typically mood or other anxiety disorders (Last 1989). Up to one-third of anxious children in one study also had attention-deficit/hyperactivity disorder (ADHD), oppositional defiant disorder (ODD), or both (Last et al. 1987b). As many as one-third of children with an anxiety disorder meet criteria for two or more anxiety disorders.

Most children with SAD in the community never receive psychiatric treatment. A substantial proportion of children with SAD eventually recover, with or without treatment. Another group experiences repeated remissions and relapses. The remainder have a chronic course, with impairment extending into adulthood. Follow-up studies of childhood school absenteeism have reported a high prevalence of adult maladaptation and psychiatric symptoms. Although these children tend to return to school, many have poor overall emotional and social functioning. Based on the heterogeneity of children with excessive school absences, there is a spectrum of symptomatology. These adults frequently manifest somatization and tend to be excessively dependent and home-oriented. School absentees often have academic underachievement and social avoidance and can be at risk for excessive absenteeism from work or chronic unemployment in adulthood. A link between childhood SAD and adult agoraphobia or panic disorder has been suggested, although SAD may be considered a general risk factor for depression and anxiety disorders. A significant proportion of adults with agoraphobia report a childhood history of SAD.

Evaluation and Differential Diagnosis

A parent may need to be present with the child for the entire initial interview, if separation is too difficult. Evaluation should include probing for symptoms of anxiety disorders or mood disorders in both the child and the parents. Physical symptoms such as nausea, vomiting, abdominal pain, or headaches require medical evaluation. In SAD, somatic symptoms are typically worse on evenings and mornings before school and absent on weekends and holidays, except as separations threaten.

Separation anxiety is a normal developmental phenomenon at ages 18–30 months. In children younger than 6 years, separation anxiety typically reappears in stressful situations. In an older child, this may represent an *adjustment disorder with anxiety.* Other anxiety disorders in the differential diagnosis include *generalized anxiety disorder, panic disorder,* and *simple or social phobia.* A *depressive disorder* may cause clinginess and refusal to separate from the parent. Children with *schizophrenia, autistic disorder,* or *pervasive developmental disorder not otherwise specified* may present with separation anxiety features.

When evaluating the patient with chronic school absenteeism, the clinician should investigate causes other than separation anxiety (see Table 4–2). The most common cause of school absenteeism in adolescents is truancy, a feature of *conduct disorder.* Youngsters with truancy typically show delinquent behavior. They may leave home in the morning and spend the day with friends, while their parents are unaware of or not concerned about their activities, in contrast to children with SAD, who remain at home with their parents' knowledge.

Treatment

Psychosocial Treatments

SAD is treated with individual educational/supportive, cognitive-behavioral (Kendall 1994), and/or psychodynamic psychotherapy, combined with parent guidance, behavior modification, family therapy, and school consultation. Cognitive-behavior therapy is becoming more widely used but lacks systematic study in SAD.

School absenteeism requires prompt intervention because, regardless of the cause, the longer the child is out of school, the higher the likelihood of treatment resistance, chronicity, and school failure. The goals are age-appropriate separation of parent and child and a rapid return to school. Referral to a partial hospitalization program (day treatment) may be warranted in more extreme cases to be used as a transition to prompt school reentry. Treatment typically focuses on behavioral or cognitive-behavior therapy, enlisting the cooperation of the family and the school. Techniques include limit setting, eliminating secondary gain for staying home, relaxation training, gradual exposure to increasing lengths of time at school, and rewarding the child for graduated successful attendance. Home schooling is contraindicated. Limit setting in the treatment of SAD must be done sensitively, with understanding of the child's internal psychological world. If the child also has a panic disorder or a major depressive episode, then limit setting prior to addressing these comorbid issues can make symptoms painfully worse. A thoughtful treatment plan for school reentry includes the use of new cognitive-behavioral skills by children and parents, as well as safety features in the environment (such as a school social worker providing support during the school day).

Firm limit setting is necessary in treating truancy. When school absenteeism is based on family permission, socializing with peers, fear of physical danger, or substance abuse, social interventions are appropriate.

SAD-related sleep disturbance or resistance to sleeping alone is generally treated behaviorally. Techniques include systematic monitoring of bedtime behavior, teaching the child relaxation skills, and supporting parents while training them to positively reinforce the child for sleeping in his or her own bed (McMenamy and Katz 1989).

Individual psychodynamic psychotherapy may help children with SAD to resolve conflicts and achieve improved self-esteem and mastery over separation and autonomy. Psychotherapy for children with SAD is organized around the child's experience of actual separations within therapy. The therapist should pay special attention to planned and unplanned absences (e.g., vacations by the patient or therapist, school transitions, pregnancy in the therapist or teacher, unavailability of parents, illness of the therapist, deaths of friends or family members) and to the termination of treatment.

Preparation of the parents and the child with guidance regarding expected separations help reduce these patients' symptoms. Therapy must actively include parents so they can reassure the child as he or she achieves more independence and autonomy. The therapy should also emphasize termination work with the parents, whose own separation issues and psychopathology may lead them to remove the child from treatment abruptly because they have difficulty tolerating their own emotions elicited by the loss of the child's therapist. Once treatment is completed, the therapist should be specific about when and how to return to treatment, particularly for parents with mood and anxiety disorders who may be psychologically vulnerable at times of loss.

Pharmacotherapy

An antidepressant may be added to the treatment of separation anxiety or comorbid mood disorder when psychosocial interventions do not result in reduction in symptoms and prompt return to school. Selective serotonin reuptake inhibitors (SSRIs) have replaced imipramine and other tricyclic antidepressants (TCAs) as a result of their more favorable side-effect profile and improved tolerability. Benzodiazepines (alprazolam and clonazepam) have been used occasionally as adjuncts to psychological interventions, although behavioral disinhibition is a serious potential side effect, along with sedation and dependence/withdrawal. These agents should be used sparingly and only for a short time, if indicated.

Other Interventions

If a parent's anxiety or mood disorder is causing difficulty in separating from the child, then the parent should also receive direct psychiatric treatment (possibly including an antidepressant or anxiolytic) as well as guidance in child management in the context of individual or family therapy.

Severe SAD that results in total avoidance of school and does not respond to environmental, psychotherapeutic, and pharmacological interventions may require psychiatric hospitalization. However, prompt initiation of partial hospitalization treatment can often prevent the need for inpatient hospitalization.

■ FEEDING AND EATING DISORDERS OF INFANCY OR EARLY CHILDHOOD

Pica

Clinical Description

Pica, a pattern of eating nonfood materials, may occur in young children, mentally retarded individuals, chronically anxious persons, and pregnant women. It is culturally normative in certain regions of the world. Pica is minimally documented in the psychiatric literature, despite the presumed biopsychosocial etiology and major potential behavioral, cognitive, neurological, and developmental complications. Pica in children most often comes to clinical attention in association with other behavior and medical problems.

Epidemiology

Up to one-third of young children are believed to exhibit pica at some point in their lives. It may be normative in children younger than 3 years. Low socioeconomic status, environmental deprivation, and parental psychopathology appear to be risk factors. The prevalence of the problem in mentally retarded individuals increases with the severity of the retardation.

Etiology

Etiological possibilities include nutritional deficiencies, insufficient stimulation, parent–child relationship difficulties, or cultural tradition, although there is no definitive support for any of these.

Course and Prognosis

Pica usually starts at age 12–24 months and resolves by school age except in mentally retarded persons who may have pica into adulthood. Common forms of pica include ice, lead, clay, or soil ingestion. Delayed motor and mental development, neurological deficits, and behavioral abnormalities may predate (and perhaps contribute to) or result from pica.

Pica has numerous potentially severe medical complications, including heavy metal poisoning, parasitic infections, or intestinal obstruction. Lead toxicity (from ingestion of peeling paint, dust from home renovation, plaster, or soil) can lead to learning disorders, hyperactivity, fatigue, weight loss, or constipation, and even to toxic encephalopathy.

Evaluation and Differential Diagnosis

Pica should be considered in all cases of developmental delays, learning difficulties, mental retardation, unusual behavioral symptoms, and chronic constipation. In order to diagnose pica, the clinician must do a behavioral and psychiatric evaluation of the child and parents, and determine the child's nutritional status and feeding history. Inadequate supervision of children or parental neglect should be considered. Questions should be asked about peeling paint or renovation in the home that might increase lead exposure.

Unexplained fatigue or weight loss, learning impairments, mental retardation, or gingival "lead lines" can be signs of lead poisoning; however, most children with elevated blood lead levels have no symptoms. Periodic blood tests in children with pica are recommended. Consultation with pediatric colleagues is indicated if blood lead levels are elevated (>10 μg/dL).

Treatment

Behavior therapy has been successful in mentally retarded individuals with pica and may be applicable to other children. Components include education, the rewarding of appropriate eating, and teaching the differentiation of edible foods. Appropriate responses to instances of pica include overcorrection (enforced immediate oral hygiene) and negative reinforcement (time-outs, restriction of privileges), combined with a positive reinforcement contingency behavior plan (reward system). Additional interventions include increased supervision, promotion of appropriate stimulation, improvement of play opportunities, or placement in day care. Concomitant treatment of medical complications may be required.

Rumination Disorder of Infancy

Clinical Description

Rumination disorder of infancy is a rare but potentially fatal eating disorder. Ruminating infants regurgitate and rechew their food in the absence of an associated gastrointestinal illness or dysfunction. Rumination may start with the infant placing fingers or clothes in the mouth to induce vomiting, with rhythmic body or neck motions, or without any apparent initiating action. During rumination, the infant generally lies quietly and looks happy or "spacey"; the body and head may be held in a characteristic arching position while sucking. When not ruminating, the infant may appear apathetic and withdrawn, become irritable and fussy, or seem quite normal. Various self-stimulatory behaviors, such as thumb sucking, cloth sucking, head banging, and body rocking, are commonly seen in association with rumination disorder.

Etiology

The etiology is unknown, although theories include adverse psychosocial factors. Genetic influences are not established. A recent study (Whelan and Cooper 2000) found a strong relationship between maternal eating disorders and childhood feeding problems, although it is unclear whether this is genetically and/or environmentally mediated. Rumination is highly associated with gastroesophageal reflux.

Clinicians generally presume that the infant, lacking external sources of gratification, uses rumination for self-stimulation or social reinforcement. Although an understimulating or overstimulating environment can contribute to the appearance of rumination disorder, some infants with the disorder appear happy and have emotionally supportive and interactive parents. Thus, this disorder is a heterogeneous one. Children with severe and persistent feeding problems tend to have mental retardation, physical disabilities, medical illnesses, or developmental delays.

Course and Prognosis

Rumination typically occurs during the first year of life. It usually resolves by the end of the second year but may persist for another year or two. Spontaneous remissions are common. Indigestion, halitosis, tooth decay, failure to thrive, dehydration, electrolyte imbalance, and malnutrition can be complications.

A major complication is the parental reaction to the symptoms. A parent's typical immediate response to the observance of rumination is acute anxiety and distress, with ongoing reactions that impair parental attachment to the child. The parents' frustration and disgust, particularly at the odor, may lead to further avoidance and understimulation of the child.

Evaluation and Differential Diagnosis

Behavioral and psychiatric evaluation of the child and parents emphasizes developmental history and psychosocial assessment, feeding and eating history, nutritional status, attachment, and observation of parent–child interactions during feeding. Medical conditions must be considered. Usually, children with rumination disorder appear happy and enjoy the regurgitation, whereas children with gastrointestinal disorders vomit with discomfort and experience pain, but this distinction is often not clear in practice. The clinician should carefully evaluate esophageal and gastric function in conjunction with the psychiatric evaluation.

Treatment

Behavioral consultation is highly recommended in treating rumination disorder. Parent training focusing on behavioral techniques including positive attention and interaction (cuddling and playing with the child before, during, and after mealtimes) will reduce social deprivation and behavioral withdrawal. Negative attention, such as shouting or physical discipline, can actually reinforce the behavior, especially if other forms of reinforcement and attention are lacking or ineffective. Negative reinforcement (ignoring) combined with a reward for time not ruminating (parental attention and social interaction, such as playing) can be used in outpatient treatment.

Pediatric hospitalization may be necessary for severe cases of malnutrition. By providing a partial separation of the child from the primary caregiver, an alternative feeding environment for the child (to "decondition" the symptoms), and a period of respite for the parent (to reduce anxiety), hospitalization can be effective. Reassurance, education, and support of the parents help to reduce their anxiety and avoidance, diminish their acute stress at times of the infant's rumination, and reestablish the parents' comfort in the feeding process. Continuing treatment facilitates attachment between infant and parent, monitors the psychosocial environment at home, and provides support in the event of emerging mental retardation or other developmental problems.

■ TOURETTE'S DISORDER AND OTHER TIC DISORDERS

Clinical Description

"A *tic* is a sudden, rapid, recurrent, nonrhythmic, stereotyped motor movement or vocalization" (American Psychiatric Association 2000, p. 100). Although tics are experienced as involuntary, they may be temporarily suppressed by conscious effort. They are often preceded by an "urge" to make a certain tic. DSM-IV-TR subdivides tic disorders into Tourette's disorder, chronic motor or vocal tic disorder, and transient tic disorder. Tourette's disorder is characterized by its chronicity and the presence at some time of both motor and vocal tics. Unlike other DSM-IV-TR disorders, functional impairment is not required (American Psychiatric Association 2000).

Epidemiology

Simple tics are extremely frequent, especially in school-age boys. Tourette's disorder is up to 3 times more prevalent in boys than girls. The prevalence of Tourette's disorder may be higher than traditionally thought, according to a population-based epidemiological study in 13- to 14-year-olds in mainstream schools that found a rate of 0.76%–1.85% (Hornsey et al. 2001). Milder forms of chronic tics are far more common than full Tourette's disorder.

Comorbidity

Comorbid disorders are common and are often more disabling than the tics. About one-half of children with Tourette's disorder referred to psychiatric clinics also have ADHD. Oppositional behavior is also common, and anger dyscontrol can impede functioning. Obsessive-compulsive symptoms are often present, with up to 60% of patients with Tourette's disorder meeting criteria for obsessive-compulsive disorder (OCD) at some time. OCD is typically associated with a more severe Tourette's presentation. Other anxiety disorders may correlate with tic severity in Tourette's disorder (Coffey et al. 2000; State et al. 2000).

Etiology

The neurological basis of Tourette's disorder is not known, although it is considered to be a neuropsychiatric illness with a variety of etiologies. There is increasing evidence suggesting frontal subcortical circuitry involvement. Numerous neurotransmitters have been implicated in this illness.

Twenty years of genetic research support the heritability of this disorder. Siblings of affected individuals have a 10- to 100-fold increased risk of developing Tourette's disorder, compared with the general population. The interactions of genetic and (biological) environmental influences are complex. Genetic linkage studies have not been conclusive, although a recent research suggests linkage for a locus on chromosome 4q and possible 8p. The heterogeneity of the disorder is becoming more apparent.

Pediatric autoimmune neuropsychiatric disorders associated with streptococcal group A β-hemolytic streptococcal infections (PANDAS) are characterized by a relapsing-remitting symptom pattern with significant psychiatric comorbidity including affective, behavioral, anxiety, and cognitive symptoms. Some cases of Tourette's disorder (and of OCD), particularly those with sudden onset or exacerbation, have been linked to antineuronal antibodies resulting from group A β-hemolytic streptococcal infections (Allen et al. 1995). Although there is significant evidence for this association, the immunological mechanism is unclear.

The nature of the association with ADHD has been controversial, but approximately 10% of children with ADHD have tics, regardless of treatment with stimulant medication. Stimulants and some antidepressants may temporarily aggravate tics, but it is unclear whether they can cause tic disorders or hasten the appearance of tics in a vulnerable child or whether the medication use is simply coincidental with the onset of tics.

Course and Prognosis

Symptoms of tic disorders typically wax and wane, and the location of tics changes over time. Transitions or stressors, such as the start of the school year, vacations, and family disruption or geographic move, typically precipitate increased frequency and severity of tics. Anxiety, excitement, boredom, or fatigue can exacerbate tics.

Onset of Tourette's disorder is typically during childhood (ages 2–15 years) and is rarely postpubertal. Symptoms of ADHD often appear before any tics. Seven years is the mean age at onset of motor symptoms, which usually begin as a single motor tic and have a rostrocaudal (head before trunk and limbs) progression over time. Motor tics can include eye blinking, eyebrow raising, facial grimacing, head jerks, abdominal tics, and leg/foot movements. Complex gestures may appear later. Complex motor tics may appear purposeless or may be camouflaged by being blended into purposeful movements. They may mirror someone else's movements (echokinesis). By age 9–10 years, many patients with Tourette's disorder can describe premonitory sensory urges (uncomfortable feelings in a specific part of the body that are relieved with the performance of a tic).

At an average age of 11 years, phonic and vocal tics may appear, along with obsessions and compulsive behaviors. Vocal tics may start as a single syllable or sounds such as throat clearing, grunting, sniffing, snorting, or barking, and progress to longer exclamations. Classic coprolalia (swearing or obscene language) is present in fewer than 10% of patients with Tourette's disorder. Other complex vocal tics include palilalia (repeating one's own sounds) and echolalia (repeating others' words). Copropraxia (complex obscene gestures) may appear later, as coprolalia resolves.

In most cases, the severity of symptoms diminishes after puberty; about one-third recover by late adolescence, and another one-third significantly improve by adulthood. In the remaining one-third, moderately to severely disabling symptoms persist.

Complications of Tourette's disorder include self-consciousness, shame, impaired self-esteem and social adaptation, and avoidance of social situations that result from being teased and rejected by peers and even parents and teachers. Severe symptoms may interfere with forming satisfying friendships and romantic relationships. The unemployment rate in adults with Tourette's disorder is reportedly as high as 50%. Comorbid illnesses, including mood disorders, self-injurious behavior, or anxiety disorders, can also contribute to impairment. There is some evidence that children with Tourette's disorder and explosivity represent a more comorbid presentation (Budman et al. 2000). Cohrs et al. (2001) observed markedly disturbed sleep in patients with Tourette's syndrome, which correlated with symptom severity during the day.

Evaluation and Differential Diagnosis

Patients with Tourette's disorder often attempt to hide symptoms or are unaware of them. They typically suppress tics while in the physician's office. As a result, the physician may underestimate the severity or overlook the diagnosis altogether. There are often many years between the first symptoms and the diagnosis.

Neurological history and examination are needed to rule out other movement disorders. Baseline dyskinesias should be assessed before medication is started. If myoclonic seizures are suspected, an electroencephalogram may be helpful.

Psychiatric evaluation focuses on identifying concomitant anxiety, mood, behavior, and developmental disorders and stressors that may be exacerbating symptoms. School reports of academic performance, standardized test results, tic severity, social skills, and behavioral observations are useful. If school performance is impaired, psychological testing that includes assessment of intellectual functioning and academic achievement can clarify the diagnosis of a comorbid learning disorder or mental retardation. Other possible interference with school success includes direct effects of tics or premonitory urges, efforts to suppress tics or compulsions, intrusive obsessions, ADHD, anxiety symptoms, social stigmatization, cognitive dulling or anxiety secondary to medication, and excessive absenteeism. The clinician evaluates the child's self-consciousness, ability to manage peer teasing, social ostracism, and assertiveness. Family history of tics and associated disorders is important, and evaluation of relatives for tic disorders may be considered.

The differential diagnosis includes a wide variety of *neurological disorders* that present with involuntary movements. Patients with *autistic disorder* or *stereotypic movement disorder* may have stereotyped movements that resemble tics. *Normal* children may have isolated, fleeting tics, but such twitches (blinks, grimaces) and habits are not diagnosed even as a transient tic disorder unless they persist nearly every day for at least 4 weeks. The clinical boundaries between Tourette's disorder, *ADHD,* and *OCD* are blurred in many patients who have symptoms of all three disorders. Complex tics may be difficult to distinguish from compulsions, and some patients have both.

Treatment

Transient tics do not require treatment. The clinician should advise the family to reduce attention to the symptom and avoid criticism.

The clinician may also educate and reassure the patient and family and encourage them to return if symptoms persist. Chronic tic disorder alone rarely requires specific treatment unless the tics are disabling, in which case the same treatments may be used as for Tourette's disorder (see below). There is evidence that tics are highly associated with school problems; therefore, special education programming may be indicated (Kurlan et al. 2001). Behavioral relaxation techniques, brief psychotherapy, or medication may help manage anxiety and decrease tics.

For Tourette's disorder, a period of initial monitoring helps to establish a baseline of symptom severity. Children are often brought to clinical attention at a time of crisis, and the evaluation itself, along with reassurance about the nature of the illness, may result in a decrease in tic severity.

Psychosocial Treatments

Education of the patient and parents, teachers, and peers ameliorates the social consequences of tics. Referral to a local chapter of the Tourette Syndrome Association may be invaluable to provide information and support. Psychosocial interventions often precede pharmacological treatment. In many cases, the control of tics is less urgent than the treatment of the accompanying attentional, behavioral, or obsessive-compulsive symptoms. Psychotherapy may help an individual cope with the stigma of illness, promote self-esteem, improve interpersonal comfort and social skills, and improve anxiety. Family therapy may assist in reducing the child's stress and helping the family manage associated symptoms. Behavior modification at home and school is recommended for comorbid symptoms of ADHD and ODD but is no longer considered appropriate for the treatment of tics, per se. Cognitive-behavioral modification may be used for obsessive-compulsive symptoms. A school Individualized Education Program (IEP) with tutoring, resource room, or special education classroom may be indicated for children with comorbid learning disabilities or behavior problems.

Pharmacotherapy

Medication treatment is complicated by possible side effects and the difficulty in determining efficacy because of the disorder's natural waxing and waning course. The goal is not to eliminate tics but to reduce them to a level that does not interfere with the child's development and functioning. The first step in treatment planning is to identify the most troubling target symptoms and choose a medication that is likely to address those symptoms while producing the fewest side effects.

In a randomized controlled trial in children with comorbid tics and ADHD, guanfacine improved teacher and clinician ratings but not parent ratings of ADHD symptoms, decreased errors on a continuous performance test (subjects on placebo had increased errors), and decreased tic severity (Scahill et al. 2001). Treatment of tics with clonidine has some empirical support along with improvements in comorbid disorders such as ADHD, sleep disorders, and developmental disorders. Guanfacine is associated with less sedation and vital sign changes than is clonidine.

The use of stimulants to treat symptoms of ADHD in the presence of tics has been controversial. Current practice is to balance the possible risk of tic exacerbation with the impairment caused by the ADHD symptoms. Although stimulants are safe and effective for many children with tics, careful monitoring is prudent to evaluate for possible stimulant-induced tic exacerbation. A recent multisite randomized controlled trial found that methylphenidate and clonidine (particularly in combination) were effective for ADHD in children with accompanying tics (Tourette's Syndrome Study Group 2002). Mean tic severity improved in all three active treatment conditions, but most with combination treatment. Clonidine was most helpful for impulsivity and hyperactivity; methylphenidate was most helpful for inattention. The proportion of subjects whose tics worsened was no higher in those treated with methylphenidate (20%) than in those on clonidine alone (26%) or placebo (22%). Clonidine commonly caused sedation, but there was no evidence of cardiac toxicity, whether used alone or combined with methylphenidate. Amphetamine may be more prone to increase tics.

For more severe tics, risperidone is now more commonly used than the older typical neuroleptic medications such as haloperidol or pimozide, due to fewer and less severe side effects with the newer, atypical agents. Olanzapine and ziprasidone have shown promise in open trials (Budman et al. 2001) and a small randomized controlled trial (Sallee et al. 2000). SSRIs are effective for OCD symptoms but not for tic reduction. A randomized controlled trial in children and adolescents with comorbid chronic tics and ADHD (Spencer et al. 2002) found that desipramine significantly improved both tics and ADHD symptoms. However, given the side-effect profile of TCAs, desipramine is not commonly used. There is recent interest in transdermal nicotine, although conclusive data are not available.

■ ELIMINATION DISORDERS

Functional Encopresis

Clinical Description

Functional encopresis is defined as fecal soiling of clothes or excretion in inappropriate places, occurring at least once a month for at least 3 months. The child's chronological age must be at least 4 years, when full bowel control is developmentally expected. Medical evaluation is necessary before labeling the disorder as "functional."

Encopresis typically occurs during the day. Many children deny the problem even when the odor is obvious or stool is discovered in their underwear. In half of these patients, bowel control is not yet learned, so the encopresis is termed *primary*. In *secondary* encopresis, the child learned bowel control, was continent for at least 1 year, and then regressed. Between 50% and 60% of encopretic children have secondary encopresis. Boys with primary encopresis are more likely than those with the secondary form to also have developmental delay and enuresis. Children with secondary encopresis experience higher levels of psychosocial distress and are more frequently diagnosed with conduct disorder.

Children may have constipation with continuous leaking overflow incontinence, a problem that resolves with treatment of the constipation. This problem is classified as "retentive encopresis." Children with incontinence without constipation, or "nonretentive encopresis," tend to produce formed stools that they may leave for discovery.

Epidemiology

Prevalence of encopresis gradually decreases with age and is reported in approximately 3% of 4-year-olds, 2% of 6-year-olds, and 1.6% of 10- to 11-year-olds. The problem is rare in adolescents. Among school-age children, males predominate in ratios from 2.5:1 to 6:1. Higher rates are observed among individuals with moderate or severe mental retardation and those in lower socioeconomic classes.

Etiology

Retentive encopresis may initially be triggered by painful defecation, inadequate or punitive toilet training, fear of using the school bathroom, or toilet-related fears. Once retention and constipation are initiated by emotional or medical factors, bowel physiology may maintain them independently. Parents may not recognize that the soiling is related to chronic constipation rather than reluctance to use the toilet. Pathophysiological mechanisms include altered colon motility and contraction patterns, obstruction, stretched and thinned colon walls (megacolon), and decreased sensation or perception secondary to a neurological disorder. Liquid stool leaks around the impaction, and the child is unaware and unable to exert control. Studies that examine the physiological causes of encopresis do not clearly differentiate between problems caused by primary organic pathology and those due to emotionally initiated chronic constipation.

Encopresis may result from stress-induced diarrhea, a problem related to irritable bowel syndrome in adulthood. Nonretentive encopresis may be a deliberate attempt by the child to effect change, as a means of avoiding stressors or communicating anger. These cases are typically more complicated and difficult to treat.

Course and Prognosis

Secondary encopresis usually starts by age 8 years. Among patients who have constipation and encopresis before age 4 years, 63% recover with treatment. Of children older than 5 years who were placed on a laxative protocol in an encopresis clinic, 50% were able to discontinue the laxatives with no symptom recurrence after 1 year; another 20% discontinued the laxatives after 2 years (Loening-Baucke 1989). Psychiatric or medical comorbidity may be the primary determinant of prognosis.

Behavior problems such as conduct disorder are more common in the psychiatrically referred population than in those seen by pediatricians. In the psychiatric population, 25% of children with functional encopresis also have functional enuresis. In the pediatric population, patients will occasionally suffer from a symptom complex that includes urinary tract infection, encopresis, and constipation. Treatment of the constipation and urinary tract infection may resolve all of the symptoms, without a need for further urologic examination. Some children withhold both urine and feces and may have megabladder and megacolon.

Evaluation and Differential Diagnosis

A detailed history of bowel function, nature and pattern of soiling, attempts to train or treat, and bathroom habits and environment is needed. Physical examination should include an abdominal examination for evidence of a fecal mass, an anal examination for evidence of fecal material, a rectal digital examination for stool consistency, and a neurological examination with perianal sensation testing. The need for additional laboratory tests is based on the history and physical examination. A barium enema is not necessary in uncomplicated cases of encopresis but may be helpful in diagnosing *Hirschsprung's disease* (congenital megacolon). Urinalysis will detect a secondary urinary tract infection, which is common in girls with encopresis. *Medical causes of fecal incontinence* (preempting the diagnosis of functional encopresis) include thyroid disease, hypercalcemia, lactase deficiency, pseudo-obstruction, myelomeningocele (spina bifida), cerebral palsy with hypotonia, rectal stenosis, anal fissure, Hirschsprung's disease (which is usually associated, however, with large feces rather than incontinence), and anorectal trauma.

Psychiatric evaluation includes assessment for associated psychiatric disorders. Oppositional children may soil willfully. Children with ADHD do not plan ahead, so they may be caught by an urge to defecate when a bathroom is not available. They also may be prone to constipation (because of spending insufficient time toileting) or fecal soiling of underwear (due to careless hygiene). Timid or phobic children may be intimidated by perceived or real dangers or humiliations in school bathrooms and avoid defecation, only to have an "accident" on the way home.

Treatment

Most cases of functional encopresis can be treated by a pediatrician, but more complex cases need psychiatric intervention. The pediatrician must educate the child and parents about bowel function. For encopresis without constipation, a behavior shaping program gives rewards first for just sitting on the toilet and later for moving the bowels appropriately. A negative consequence for soiling may be used. Patients with chronic diarrhea may benefit from stress reduction techniques, including systematic desensitization, hypnosis, and relaxation training. Manipulative soiling requires parent management training and a reduction of reinforcers for maladaptive behavior. For children with severe stool retention, impaction, and loss of bowel tone, initial bowel cleaning (e.g., with enemas or suppositories) followed by "retraining" the bowel (e.g., with mineral oil, a high-roughage diet, development of a toileting routine, and use of a mild suppository if necessary) may be used in conjunction with the behavioral program (see "Additional Reading"). Repeated administration of enemas by parents is harmful to the parent–child relationship. Children have benefited from the use of hypnosis and biofeedback to improve sphincter control, although no systematic studies have examined either of these techniques. They are primarily considered to be adjunct treatments to more conventional modalities. Individual and family psychiatric interventions are indicated in resistant cases, in which the focus of treatment shifts to the associated psychiatric disorders. The role of psychopharmacology in the treatment of these children is relatively insignificant. Recent studies of cisapride (Propulsid) for the treatment of encopresis with constipation are encouraging, but the medication is not yet available in the United States.

Functional Enuresis

Clinical Description

Urinary incontinence in young children, and occasionally in older children after toilet training has been completed, may be a normal developmental phenomenon. The mechanisms involved in learning bladder control are not well understood. Functional enuresis is diagnosed when wetting occurs after the chronological or developmental age of 5 years either at least twice a week for 3 months or sufficiently often to cause distress or impairment. The addition of subjective criteria allows the clinician to make the diagnosis in children who do not meet either the frequency or the duration criterion, but wetting is accompanied by emotional upset or social consequences.

Bed wetting is more common than daytime incontinence. Nocturnal enuresis typically occurs 30 minutes to 3 hours after sleep onset but may occur at any time during the night. The child may sleep through the episode or be awakened by the moisture. Daytime bladder control usually precedes nocturnal control by 1–2 years. Most children with daytime enuresis also have nocturnal enuresis. Some clinicians do not diagnose nocturnal enuresis until the child is age 6 or 7 years. If bladder control has not yet been achieved, the enuresis is *primary*. In *secondary* enuresis, wetting reappears after a period of established urinary continence.

Epidemiology

Enuresis is seen in 5%–10% of 5-year-olds and around 3%–5% of 10-year-olds (American Psychiatric Association 2000). The male predominance of primary enuresis decreases with age. After age 5 years, the prevalence of enuresis in both boys and girls spontaneously decreases by 5%–10% per year. Between 3% and 9% of school-age girls experience daytime wetting (Mattsson and Gladh 2003). The general prevalence in older adolescents and adults is 1%. Few of the children with nocturnal enuresis also have diurnal enuresis or encopresis. In contrast, 50%–60% of patients with diurnal enuresis are likely to experience nocturnal problems. Enuresis is of the primary type in more than 85% of cases, a percentage that gradually decreases with age. Secondary enuresis is equally prevalent in boys and girls.

Etiology

Approximately 70% of children with enuresis (particularly boys) have a first-degree relative with functional enuresis. Studies of monozygotic and dizygotic twins show a strong genetic factor, although the mode of transmission is unclear. A "maturational" etiology is suggested in patients with primary enuresis who have small-volume voidings, short stature, low mean bone age, and delayed sexual maturation. Some patients have a relative inability to concentrate urine. In these cases the spontaneous remission rate is 15% per year (Forsythe and Redmond 1974). Research has not established, however, that children suffering from enuresis have a smaller than average bladder capacity. Excessive fluid intake may contribute to the problem. Anatomical abnormalities of the urinary tract are not typical causes of enuresis and rarely warrant surgical interventions. Common physiological causes of diurnal enuresis in girls are vaginal reflux of urine, "giggle incontinence," and urgency incontinence. Possible links between sleep architecture and bladder physiology in the development of enuresis are currently under investigation. Enuresis may be a side effect of certain medications.

Children experiencing enuresis are often emotionally upset, but the relationship between psychiatric disorder and enuresis is not clear. No study has yet associated a particular psychological disturbance with enuresis. Response to imipramine is not dependent on comorbid psychiatric symptoms. Although a recent study found higher rates of behavior problems in children suffering from primary enuresis when compared with a nonclinical control sample, the level of disturbance was lower than in a psychiatrically referred comparison group. In addition, mean standardized behavior rating scores for the enuretic population were below the clinically significant cutoff (Friman et al. 1998). Anxious children may experience urinary frequency, resulting in daytime incontinence if toilet facilities are not readily available or if the child is fearful of certain bathrooms. In ODD, refusal to use the toilet may be part of the child's battle for control. Children with either primary or secondary enuresis are more likely to meet diagnostic criteria for ADHD, although the connection is probably situational rather than physiological or genetic. For example, many children with ADHD wait until the last minute to urinate and then lose control on the way to the bathroom. Enuresis may be associated with psychiatric disturbance (e.g., ODD, conduct disorder, psychosis) but causality may be difficult to discern in individual patients. Secondary enuresis may be related to stress, trauma, or psychosocial crisis. Enuresis that continues into adolescence is associated with increased rates of psychopathology.

Course and Prognosis

Primary enuresis has a high rate of spontaneous remission. Only about 1% of boys (and fewer girls) still have this condition at age 18 years. Secondary enuresis usually begins between ages 5 and 8 years. Onset in adolescence, however, may signify more psychiatric problems and less favorable outcome.

Complications include embarrassment, anger from and punishment by caregivers, teasing by peers, avoidance of overnight visits and camp, social withdrawal, and angry outbursts. The development of psychiatric disorders is higher in enuretic children than in the general population.

Evaluation and Differential Diagnosis

Initial medical evaluation is required to rule out medical causes (Table 4–3), especially in secondary and diurnal enuresis. This includes a medical history (including questions about polyuria, dribbling, and urgency), a physical examination, observation of the size and velocity of the urine stream, and a urine culture and urinalysis. The osmolality result can help rule out diabetes mellitus or diabetes insipidus. In the absence of suggestive findings on the history and physical examination, additional evaluation of the urinary tract is not indicated. Enuresis during both day and night and difficulty with voiding are indications of urinary tract abnormalities that may warrant ultrasonography. Family history should investigate the presence of diabetes or renal disease; positive findings may suggest additional testing. A family history of enuresis is generally reassuring and implies that it will eventually be outgrown.

TABLE 4–3.   **Medical causes of enuresis**

Urinary tract infection
Urethritis—bubble bath, sexual abuse
Diabetes mellitus
Diabetes insipidus
Sickle cell trait
Seizure disorders
Neurogenic bladder—myelodysplasia, trauma, other neurological disorder
Physiological genitourinary abnormality
Congenital malformation of the genitourinary tract
Urinary obstruction—stone, pelvic mass

Psychiatric evaluation of the child and family includes assessment of associated psychiatric symptoms, recent psychosocial stressors, and family concern about and management of the symptoms. Psychological and developmental evaluation can identify the child who is not mature enough to achieve continence. When a psychiatric disorder is suspected, management of the enuresis should await effective treatment of the primary disorder.

Treatment

Successful treatment of enuresis improves self-esteem. Many cases of functional enuresis can be managed successfully by the pediatrician. For younger children who wet only at night, the most useful strategy is to minimize symptoms by discouraging the parents from punishing or ridiculing the child, while awaiting maturation. Children can be taught to change their own beds to reduce negative parental reactions. Rewards for successful dry nights may help. Restricting fluids before bedtime and waking the child after 2–3 hours of sleep to urinate are only occasionally useful.

For older children who are motivated to stop bed wetting, a monitoring and reward procedure (a chart with stars to be exchanged for rewards) may be effective. Daytime urinary continence may be achieved rapidly with a behavioral program. A program of "bladder training" exercises may be helpful. Practice in delaying bladder emptying may increase bladder capacity. Interruption of the stream while urinating may strengthen sphincter muscles and improve awareness of bladder sensations. Instruction on adapted voiding posture and hygiene may be effective for urethrovaginal reflux (Mattsson and Gladh 2003).

If simple interventions are unsuccessful, a urine alarm is recommended. This device, an improvement on the "bell and pad," has a high success rate of 75% at 6 months and 56% at 12 months. This compares favorably to rates of 6% at 6 months and 16% at 12 months using observation alone. If the alarm is set up to awaken the parents so they awaken the child, then the relapse rate is low. A combination of the urine alarm, cleanliness training, retention control, and overlearning can stop bed wetting in two-thirds of children with primary enuresis (Houts et al. 1983). (The PALCO Wet-Stop enuresis alarm may be ordered from PALCO Laboratories; 1-800-346-4488 or see Web site at http://www.wet-stop.com.)

Although behavioral treatments consistently demonstrate higher success rates than medication, DDAVP (desmopressin) or low doses of a TCA at bedtime can be helpful in the short term in patients who are resistant to behavioral interventions, who need a rapid result (e.g., for camp), or who have daytime as well as nighttime enuresis. The mechanism of action of TCAs is not known. The majority of patients relapse when either type of medication is withdrawn (unless maturation has intervened). DDAVP is available in nasal spray and a newer oral form. It is preferred to imipramine because of the risk of overdose of a TCA.

Psychotherapy is rarely useful in the treatment of enuresis. However, it may be indicated for the treatment of psychosocial sequelae of enuresis. Children who experience enuresis as a consequence of trauma or stress may also benefit from psychotherapeutic interventions. Hypnotherapy may be an effective adjunct to treatment. Associated disorders may require psychiatric treatment.

Surgical procedures are not indicated in the absence of demonstrated structural abnormalities of clear etiological significance.

■ SELECTIVE MUTISM

Clinical Description

Children with selective mutism do not speak in one or several important settings despite having the ability to comprehend spoken language and to speak in other situations. Symptoms persist for at least 1 month and are severe enough to affect educational and interpersonal functioning. These children have an adequate knowledge of the language yet may experience specific developmental communication disorders. Typically, speech is normal at home when the child is alone with parents and siblings, but partial or total muteness appears in the presence of teachers, peers, and strangers or selectively in unfamiliar places or particular social situations. When these children are separated from a familiar or comfortable setting, they might use gestures, nods, monosyllabic responses, written notes, or whispers but avoid full vocalization. Many of these children are shy, anxious, submissive, and excessively dependent. They cling to their parents, sulk with strangers, throw temper tantrums, and are prone to immature behaviors when under stress.

Epidemiology

Selective mutism is estimated to occur in fewer than 1% of school-age children and typically begins between 3 and 8 years of age. Prevalence ranges from 0.06% to 0.7%, depending on the age of the population studied and the length of their exposure to school. Recent studies note a female to male ratio of 2:1. Increased prevalence in immigrant families is reported.

Etiology

Explanations for the development of selective mutism vary widely. Emotional and physical trauma, such as witnessing or being victimized by physical or sexual abuse, are rarely a primary precipitant. Biological factors including temperament and anxiety disorders are more important contributors to etiology. Early hospitalization and family instability characterized by divorce, death, and frequent moves could also contribute to the development of these symptoms.

There may be a link between selective mutism in children and social phobia in adults. These adults recall feeling intensely anxious as children when they were asked to speak, with accompanying symptoms that approximate panic. Selective mutism may have been an early observable form of developing social phobia. Parents of selectively mute children tend to have a variety of anxiety disorders including panic, separation anxiety, and social/performance anxiety.

Selectively mute children typically also experience developmental delays in speech and language. Approximately 25% of children with selective mutism also have delayed onset of speech, and 50% have a speech disorder or speech immaturities. The prevalence of mental retardation and neurological disorders is increased. These associations suggest a neurodevelopmental etiology or that developmental disorders may worsen communication impairments. Global mutism can result from cerebellar lesions and is known to accompany cerebellar hemorrhages, subarachnoid hemorrhages, vertebral artery injuries, basilar artery occlusion, and head trauma.

Course and Prognosis

The disorder is usually discovered when the child attends kindergarten or first grade and demands for speech increase. Excessive shyness may be identified retrospectively. The diagnosis is typically made between 3 and 8 years of age. Symptoms may last for weeks, months, or years and usually resolve by age 10. When selective mutism persists beyond age 12, patients are less likely to completely recover. Complications of selective mutism include academic underachievement, impaired peer relationships, and reliance on the secondary gains of illness (excessive protection and attention). The child's persistent silence may lead to inappropriate special class and school placements. Many of these children have comorbid psychiatric problems, including social phobia, avoidant disorder, OCD, and school avoidance.

Evaluation and Differential Diagnosis

Standard psychiatric evaluation (including familial patterns of communication, silence, and anger), neurological assessment for possible brain damage, physical examination for oral–facial abnormalities, psychometric assessment for mental retardation, and speech and language evaluation are warranted. The clinician should review the child's medical history for evidence of neurological injury or delay or hearing deficit, with neurological evaluation or audiological testing if indicated. Family history is evaluated for selective mutism or anxiety disorders. Although the child may not speak directly to the clinician, observation of the quality of interaction and ability to communicate nonverbally can yield valuable information. The clinician should evaluate the possible presence of physical or sexual abuse, depression, and shyness in the child and the family.

The differential diagnosis of failure to speak includes *hearing impairment, mental retardation, communication disorder, aphasia, pervasive developmental disorders, schizophrenia,* and *conversion disorder.* Global impairment of speech is characteristic of all but the latter three disorders.

Treatment

Treatment, particularly in cases involving anxiety, behavioral difficulties, or developmental delay, should involve a team of professionals. The comprehensive plan may include behavioral, family systems, psychodynamic, pharmacological, and speech and language therapy approaches. Therapy is based on the assumption that the child will speak again. Any form of communication is encouraged through behavioral plans that shape behavior by reinforcing attempts to speak. Short-term therapy may be effective, although more resistant cases may require longer-term treatment. Behavior therapy and parent counseling generally are more effective than individual psychotherapy for treatment of selective mutism. Family therapy may help to identify and then change dysfunctional patterns that maintain symptoms. Although teachers and parents often make accommodations to the child's muteness, it is better to maintain a clear expectation that the child talk and communicate, at least for a structured period of each session. The parents, especially the protective parent, should be explicit with the child about these expectations: to talk at school and in therapy.

Pharmacological interventions have paralleled those used to treat social phobia, particularly SSRIs such as fluoxetine or fluvoxamine.

■ REACTIVE ATTACHMENT DISORDER OF INFANCY OR EARLY CHILDHOOD

Clinical Description

Reactive attachment disorder of infancy or early childhood (RAD) is characterized by an inability to form normal interpersonal relationships and a persistent disturbance in the child's responsiveness in all social situations. The disorder appears before age 5 years and is preceded by a history of maltreatment, deprivation, or repeated changes in primary caregiver. The *inhibited type* includes children with inhibited, hypervigilant, or contradictory behaviors. Their responses to caregivers include a mixture of approach, avoidance, and resistance to comforting, or frozen watchfulness. The *disinhibited type* is characterized by excessive and inappropriate sociability with relative strangers and lack of selectivity in choice of attachment figures. These children may lack empathy and show limited eye contact, poor impulse control, lack of conscience, and abnormal speech patterns.

The clinical presentation changes with age. In early infancy, diagnosis is based on the failure to achieve social developmental expectations: lack of eye tracking or responsive smiling by age 2 months, failure to play simple games or to reach out to be picked up by age 5 months, or failure to show overt behavioral signs of attachment and bonding to a parent by age 8 months. Infants appear lethargic, have a weak cry, show little body movement or activity, have excessive or disrupted sleep, gain weight slowly, and resist being held. There may be associated feeding disorders.

In childhood, odd social responses, weak interpersonal attachment, inappropriate excitability, and mood abnormalities are seen. The children may appear withdrawn, passive, and disinterested in people (inhibited type) or, in the disinhibited type, may display overly rapid familiarity, inappropriate touching and clinging, and immediate emotional involvement that seems odd or unusual.

Epidemiology

RAD is considered to be extremely rare, although there are no good studies of prevalence. There are suggestions of increasing prevalence, but this may reflect changes in reporting of neglect and abuse or increased awareness of the diagnosis.

Etiology

By (DSM-IV-TR) definition, RAD requires evidence of pathogenic care. This can take the form of abuse, neglect, or impaired parenting. Frequent changes in the primary caregiver with a resulting inability of the child to form stable attachments are presumed to contribute to the disorder. Parents or caregivers may have major depression, psychosis, substance abuse, or mental retardation. They may be poor, uneducated, or isolated from social and emotional supports. They may be hostile or indifferent to the child or simply have insufficient skills, supports, and frustration tolerance to deal with a "difficult" child. RAD is not inevitable in the presence of abuse, neglect, and inadequate parenting. Other disorders may result, or resilient children who are placed in nurturing environments can eventually develop normal attachments and social relationships.

Course and Prognosis

The prognosis of RAD varies from spontaneous remission to malnutrition, infection, and death. Nutritional or psychosocial deprivation may result in long-term behavior changes, short stature, and lowered intelligence quotient (IQ). If emotional deprivation continues but food intake is adequate, children may have improved body growth but show emotional problems and developmental delays (Whitten et al. 1969).

Evaluation

RAD is diagnosed by observation of parent–child interactions and a decrease in the child's symptoms in response to adequate emotional and physical care. The clinical observer assesses physical and emotional nurturance, including the adult's capacity for empathy, appropriateness of level and timing of stimulation, attentiveness to the child's behavior, matching of expectations with the child's developmental level, and emotional reactions (e.g., anxiety, anger, indifference) to the child. A home visit may be indicated to evaluate the adequacy of housing, safety, and nutrition. Psychiatric evaluation of the parents is essential. Physical or sexual abuse or neglect may not be quickly or easily identifiable.

A medical examination is required to rule out chronic physical illness or disability that may be causing organic failure to thrive and to diagnose associated medical conditions that require treatment.

Pediatric hospitalization of infants or very young children helps to make the diagnosis. Removal from the home environment may permit normal feeding and sleeping patterns to be reestablished and parental caregiving capacity to be evaluated and remediated. Clinical improvement in response to hospitalization or treatment confirms the diagnosis. Lack of improvement implies that a different disorder is present or that medical complications with physical damage occurred before treatment.

Differential Diagnosis

Reactive attachment disorder can be differentiated from *pervasive developmental disorders* (including *autistic disorder*) by the remission of cognitive and social deficits in a caring environment and the absence of characteristic abnormalities in speech, language, and social communication. *Depression* is an alternative psychiatric disorder to consider for the inhibited type. Some of the behaviors in the disinhibited type may resemble *ADHD*.

Treatment

Basic medical care, provision of adequate nurturance, and education and psychiatric treatment of parents are needed. Legal intervention may be indicated. If parents are unavailable or unable to improve the quality of care, placement in therapeutic foster care may be indicated. Hospitalization is often justified by the complexity of medical and psychiatric interventions. Outpatient therapy is recommended when the parent understands the nature and consequences of the disorder and actively and reliably participates in the treatment program. Parents may require a great deal of practical assistance in establishing a nurturing environment. These children are resistant to typical psychotherapeutic interventions because of an inability to form reciprocal relationships and lack of previous exposure to helpful adults.

■ REFERENCES

Allen AJ, Leonard HL, Swedo SE: Case study: a new infection-triggered, autoimmune subtype of pediatric OCD and Tourette's syndrome. J Am Acad Child Adolesc Psychiatry 34:307–311, 1995

American Academy of Child and Adolescent Psychiatry: Practice parameters for the assessment and treatment of children and adolescents with anxiety disorders. J Am Acad Child Adolesc Psychiatry 36 (suppl):69S–84S, 1997

American Psychiatric Association: Diagnostic and Statistical Manual of Mental Disorders, 4th Edition, Text Revision. Washington, DC, American Psychiatric Association, 2000

Bernstein GA, Rapoport JL, Leonard HL: Separation anxiety and generalized anxiety disorders, in Textbook of Child and Adolescent Psychiatry, 2nd Edition. Edited by Wiener JM. Washington, DC, American Psychiatric Press, 1996, pp 471–485

Budman CL, Bruun RD, Park KS, et al: Explosive outbursts in children with Tourette's disorder. J Am Acad Child Adolesc Psychiatry 39:1270–1276, 2000

Budman CL, Gayer A, Lesser M, et al: An open-label study of the treatment efficacy of olanzapine for Tourette's disorder. J Clin Psychiatry 62:290–294, 2001

Coffey BJ, Biederman J, Smoller JW, et al: Anxiety disorders and tic severity in juveniles with Tourette's disorder. J Am Acad Child Adolesc Psychiatry 39:562–568, 2000

Cohrs S, Rasch T, Altmeyer S, et al: Decreased sleep quality and increased sleep related movements in patients with Tourette's syndrome. J Neurol Neurosurg Psychiatry 70:192–197, 2001

Forsythe WI, Redmond A: Enuresis and spontaneous cure rate: study of 1129 enuretics. Arch Dis Child 49:259–263, 1974

Friman PC, Handwerk ML, Swearer SM, et al: Do children with primary nocturnal enuresis have clinically significant behavior problems? Arch Pediatr Adolesc Med 152:537–539, 1998

Hornsey H, Banerjee S, Zeitlin H, et al: The prevalence of Tourette syndrome in 13–14-year-olds in mainstream school. J Child Psychol Psychiatry 42:1035–1039, 2001

Houts AC, Liebert RM, Padawer W: A delivery system for the treatment of primary enuresis. J Abnorm Child Psychol 11:513–520, 1983

Kendall PC: Treating anxiety disorders in children: results of a randomized clinical trial. J Consult Clin Psychol 62:100–110, 1994

Kurlan R, McDermott MP, Deeley C, et al: Prevalence of tics in school children and association with placement in special education. Neurology 57:1383–1388, 2001

Last CG: Anxiety disorders of childhood or adolescence, in Handbook of Child Psychiatric Diagnosis. Edited by Last CG, Hersen M. New York, Wiley, 1989, pp 156–169

Last CG, Francis G, Hersen M, et al: Separation anxiety for school phobia: a comparison using DSM-III criteria. Am J Psychiatry 144:653–657, 1987a

Last CG, Hersen M, Kazdin AE, et al: Comparison of DSM-III separation anxiety and overanxious disorders: demographic characteristics and patterns of comorbidity. J Am Acad Child Adolesc Psychiatry 26:527–531, 1987b

Loening-Baucke V: Factors determining outcome in children with chronic constipation and faecal soiling. Gut 30:999–1006, 1989

Mattsson S, Gladh G: Urethrovaginal reflux: a common cause of daytime incontinence in girls. Pediatrics 111:136–139, 2003

McMenamy C, Katz RC: Brief parent-assisted treatment for children's nighttime fears. J Dev Behav Pediatr 10:145–148, 1989

Rosenbaum JF, Biederman J, Hirshfeld-Becker DR, et al: A controlled study of behavioral inhibition in children of parents with panic disorder and depression. Am J Psychiatry 157:2002–2010, 2000

Sallee FR, Kurlan R, Goetz CG, et al: Ziprasidone treatment of children and adolescents with Tourette's syndrome: a pilot study. J Am Acad Child Adolesc Psychiatry 39:292–299, 2000

Scahill L, Chappell P, Kim YS, et al: A placebo-controlled study of guanfacine in the treatment of children with tic disorders and attention deficit hyperactivity disorder. Am J Psychiatry 158:1067–1074, 2001

Spencer T, Biederman J, Coffey B, et al: A double-blind comparison of desipramine and placebo in children and adolescents with chronic tic disorder and comorbid attention-deficit/hyperactivity disorder. Arch Gen Psychiatry 59:649–56, 2002

State MW, Lombroso PJ, Pauls DL, et al: The genetics of childhood psychiatric disorders: a decade of progress. J Am Acad Child Adolesc Psychiatry 39:946–962, 2000

Tourette's Syndrome Study Group: Treatment of ADHD in children with tics: a randomized controlled trial. Neurology 58:527–536, 2002

Whelan E, Cooper PJ: The association between childhood feeding problems and maternal eating disorder: a community study. Psychological Medicine 30:69–77, 2000

Whitten CF, Pettit MG, Fischhoff J: Evidence that growth failure from maternal deprivation is secondary to under eating. JAMA 209:1675–1682, 1969

■ ADDITIONAL READING

Separation Anxiety Disorder

American Academy of Child and Adolescent Psychiatry: Practice parameters for the assessment and treatment of children and adolescents with anxiety disorders. J Am Acad Child Adolesc Psychiatry 36 (suppl):69S–84S, 1997

Tourette's Disorder and Other Tic Disorders

Leckman JF, Cohen DJ: Tourette's Syndrome—Tics, Obsessions, Compulsions: Developmental Psychopathology and Clinical Care. New York, Wiley, 2001

Elimination Disorders

Butler RJ: Annotation: night wetting in children: psychological aspects. J Child Psychol Psychiatry 39:453–463, 1998.

Levine MD: Encopresis, in Developmental-Behavioral Pediatrics, 2nd Edition. Edited by Levine MD, Carey WB, Crocker AC. Philadelphia, PA, WB Saunders, 1992, pp 389–397

Maizels M, Gandi K, Keating B, et al: Diagnosis and treatment for children who cannot control urination. Curr Probl Pediatr 23:402–450, 1993

Mikkelsen EJ: Enuresis and encopresis: ten years of progress. J Am Acad Child Adolesc Psychiatry 40:1146–1158, 2001

Selective Mutism

Dow SP, Sonies BC, Scheib D, et al: Practical guidelines for the assessment and treatment of selective mutism. J Am Acad Child Adolesc Psychiatry 34:836–846, 1995

5

"ADULT" DISORDERS THAT MAY BEGIN IN CHILDHOOD OR ADOLESCENCE

The disorders covered in this chapter are described in the general sections of DSM-IV-TR (American Psychiatric Association 2000), Axis I. Eating disorders may begin in adolescence (and, very rarely, prior to puberty), but bulimia typically begins in young adulthood. Substance-related disorders and schizophrenia have a similar pattern of peak incidence in early adulthood, becoming increasingly rare with decreasing age. The early onset of mood disorders is more apparent than in the past, but the most common time of onset is in adulthood. The anxiety disorders in this section and the adjustment disorders can begin at any age. Gender identity disorder is presumed to appear early in development, but may not become clinically apparent until much later. The sleep disorders are a heterogeneous group in time course and etiology.

■ EATING DISORDERS

Anorexia Nervosa

Clinical Description

Anorexia nervosa is characterized by a refusal to maintain normal weight or a failure to reach expected weight gain as a result of purposeful strict dieting or other extreme measures. Patients have either a distorted perception of their body shape and size or a denial of the seriousness of the weight loss. The preoccupation with food and body shape is obsessive. In severe cases, these patients may appear delusional. The appetite is not lost, but there is an intense fear of gaining weight. Postmenarchal females cease menstruating. The *restricting type* of anorexia is characterized by strict dieting, fasting, or excessive exercise. In the *binge-eating/purging type,* huge quantities of food are eaten and then purged.

The physiological process of starvation leads to the development of additional psychological symptoms. Patients may become socially withdrawn, irritable, and anhedonic, with a decreased interest in sex, low self-esteem, and recurrent feelings of helplessness and inadequacy; this picture is consistent with major depression. Depression impairs the individual's ability to function in the classroom, in social situations, and within the family. The patient's increasing sense of incompetence further impairs self-esteem. In addition, patients tend to be controlling, not only of their own habits but also of those around them. Patients are often preoccupied with personal academic overachievement and exercise. An accompanying diagnosis of obsessive-compulsive disorder (OCD) should be made if criteria are met.

Epidemiology

More than 90% of patients with anorexia nervosa are female, and they constitute about 1%–2% of adolescent females and young adult women in the United States. The exact prevalence of anorexia nervosa in prepubertal children is unknown, but it is much less. The incidence is greatest in the 15- to 24-year age group. Milder forms of eating disorders are even more common. Anorexia nervosa is found predominantly in Western industrialized nations, and the prevalence of anorexia is probably significantly affected by social and societal factors.

Etiology

Anorexia nervosa has a multifactorial etiology. Patients experience a variety of psychological, physical, academic, and social problems, leading to a diminished sense of self-esteem and self-control. These patients tend to be dissatisfied with their bodies at puberty. Dieting is chosen as a socially acceptable method to improve the patient's sense of well-being and control.

Genetic and neurophysiological mechanisms contribute to the development of anorexia and bulimia nervosa. First-degree relatives of anorexic and bulimic patients are 6–10 times more likely to have an eating disorder than are control populations. However, it remains difficult to separate environmental from heritable causative factors. Studies examining hormonal and neurohormonal relationships in adult and late adolescent eating disordered patients are promising. It is not clear whether these studies are identifying risk factors or simply measuring the effects of the disorder. In many cases, hormone levels return to normal with refeeding and weight gain.

Although a history of sexual abuse may be present in patients with eating disorders, it is not clear that this risk is different from that in other psychiatric disorders, except perhaps for adolescents with bulimia. Family dynamics, including parental overinvolvement, lack of appropriate boundaries within the family, and insufficient autonomy, have received much attention in the literature, particularly from theorists such as Minuchin and Schwartz (Minuchin et al. 1978; R.C. Schwartz et al. 1985). However, few studies have tested these theories, and these characteristics are also present in families in which eating disorders do not develop. The effect on a family of having a child starving herself to death must not be confused with family characteristics that might have contributed to the disorder.

Course and Prognosis

Anorexia nervosa usually presents during adolescence, between ages 14 and 18 years, a time of rapid growth with accompanying weight gain and changes in body shape. Onset before puberty is less common, in part because symptoms of amenorrhea and pubertal changes in body image do not apply to children. Nevertheless, prepubertal children may have anorexia nervosa or problem eating behaviors, including food avoidance, body image disturbance, inappropriate dieting, overeating, ritualistic behavior during meals, and selective eating. The first evidence of dissatisfaction with body shape may be found in a preoccupation with dieting. In one survey, between one-half and two-thirds of all girls considered themselves to be overweight, although only 15% were actually overweight (Mellin et al. 1992).

Physiological changes are common. Medical complications may require hospitalization (Palla and Litt 1988; Table 5–1). The course of anorexia nervosa is typically prolonged. One review estimated prognosis to be 50% with a good outcome, 21% with intermediate outcome, and 26% with poor outcome (Theander 1985). The disorder does not remit without treatment. Continuing symptoms include low weight for height and age, peak bone mass reduction, excessive concern with weight or appearance, pubertal delay or interruption, amenorrhea, and troubled social and sexual relationships. Poor outcome is associated with longer duration of illness, older age at onset, extreme weight loss, and poor interpersonal relationships.

Mortality in part depends on chronicity. Risk of death from medical complications of anorexia nervosa is estimated at between 5% and 6%, with some of these deaths due to suicide. Additional psychiatric diagnoses contribute to a poor prognosis, and partial remission rather than recovery is common, especially in those patients with psychiatric comorbidity. Recovered patients have rates of other psychiatric disorders comparable to those in nonclinical control groups.

Evaluation and Differential Diagnosis

A complete history, physical examination, and routine laboratory studies are necessary to rule out a medical cause for loss of weight or appetite. In addition, starvation can produce physiological disturbances that should be identified through laboratory studies (see Table 5–1). Hypoglycemia is a particularly poor prognostic sign. Dehydration can lead to elevations in blood urea nitrogen, liver function tests, and serum cholesterol levels. Signs of infection may be masked by leukopenia and hypothermia. Abnormal thyroid

TABLE 5–1. **Physical signs and symptoms and complications associated with anorexia nervosa and bulimia nervosa**

Cardiovascular	Hypotension (especially postural)
	Bradycardia (rates between 40 and 50 beats per minute)
	Arrhythmias (prolonged QT interval may be a marker for risk of sudden death)
	Mitral valve prolapse
	Cardiac arrest
	Edema and congestive heart failure during refeeding
	Cardiac failure secondary to cardiomyopathy from ipecac (emetine) poisoning
Neuroendocrine	Amenorrhea or irregular menses (low levels of FSH and LH despite low estrogen levels)
	Low basal metabolism rate
	Abnormal glucose tolerance test with insulin resistance
	Hypothermia
	Elevated levels of growth hormone and cortisol
	Sleep disturbances
Bone	Osteopenia
Fluid disturbance	Dehydration
	Electrolyte imbalance
	Abnormal urinalysis
Gastrointestinal	Constipation
	Diarrhea

TABLE 5–1. Physical signs and symptoms and complications associated with anorexia nervosa and bulimia nervosa *(continued)*

Hematological	Leukopenia
	Anemia
	Thrombocytopenia
	Low sedimentation rate
Dermatological	Dry skin
	Lanugo (baby-fine body hair)
Oral, esophageal, and gastric damage from vomiting and/or binge eating	Loss of dental enamel
	Enlarged salivary glands
	Gastritis
	Esophagitis
	Increased rates of pancreatitis

Note. FSH=follicle-stimulating hormone; LH=luteinizing hormone.
Source. Adapted from Palla and Litt 1988.

function studies are classified as euthyroid sick syndrome, with normal to low levels of thyroxine (T4) and free T4 and variable levels of thyroid-stimulating hormone.

The psychiatric interview of a patient with suspected anorexia nervosa includes details about the onset and course of the eating disorder, the highest and lowest weight, and the weight identified by the patient as most comfortable. The clinician should also explore daily eating patterns, including not only amounts of food but also times for meals. Questions about the use of laxatives, emetics, or diuretics can be incorporated into this eating history. Although anorexic patients learn to disguise their continuing wish to lose weight, hide excessive exercise and purging, and claim to eat more than they do, they may inadvertently reveal important diagnostic information during an eating history.

In addition to individual assessments, a family evaluation is essential when treating young patients. The therapist may ask family members about their impressions of the illness and its origins. A review of at-home treatment attempts uncovers family alliances and individual perceptions about the problem's origins and possible solutions. A family eating or weight history may show patterns of behavior imitated by the child or adolescent. Family history of psychiatric illness may suggest similar diagnoses in the patient.

The differential diagnosis of anorexia nervosa is shown in Table 5–2.

Treatment

The treatment of anorexia nervosa should be comprehensive and emphasize a return to normal eating patterns. In most cases, the initial focus of treatment is on acceptance of the disorder and subsequent weight gain. This initial phase may take place on an inpatient unit. No controlled studies define indications for inpatient hospitalization, but typical indications include weight more than 25%–30% below ideal body weight, rapid and severe weight loss refractory to outpatient treatment, symptomatic hypotension or syncope, heart rate below 40 beats per minute, or evidence of arrhythmia or a pro-

TABLE 5–2.　Differential diagnosis of anorexia nervosa

Normal thinness

Physical disorders causing weight loss

Hyperthyroidism

Other endocrine disorders

Gastrointestinal disorders resulting in vomiting, loss of appetite, and/or malabsorption

Malignancy

Chronic infection

Psychiatric disorders causing loss of appetite and weight loss

Depression

Peculiar eating behavior secondary to obsessive-compulsive disorder or to delusions in schizophrenia or psychotic depression

Avoidance of eating caused by phobia of choking, with or without psychosis

Vomiting secondary to conversion disorder

Hypothyroidism producing hypothermia and amenorrhea

longed QTc interval. The denial and fears of loss of control and of becoming fat generate severe resistance to treatment, even when the patient and family acknowledge the diagnosis. A firm focus on a target weight within 90% of the ideal body weight is helpful. The patient should reach this goal through gradual weight gain of 1 pound per week as an outpatient or 2–3 pounds per week while hospitalized (Mehler 2001). Anorexic patients usually require a large amount of calories early in treatment to accomplish this goal. Appetite stimulants are not recommended and may be contraindicated. Involvement of a pediatric dietitian with experience in eating disorders is essential, whether treatment is inpatient or outpatient. Psychotherapeutic approaches can act as an adjunct to the refeeding regimen. Forced weight gain alone is futile, and too-rapid weight gain exacerbates fears of loss of control and may be medically hazardous. Tube or intravenous feeding should be reserved for medical emergencies, because these methods are viewed by patients as punitive. The patient's sabotage of these methods can be dangerous (e.g., bleeding from the site of a pulled intravenous line, aspiration of tube feedings). Regardless of the success of refeeding, a comprehensive treatment plan that includes an exploration of underlying psychological factors is essential.

Family therapy is particularly effective when symptoms appeared prior to age 18. Issues range from struggles for autonomy by the patient to deterioration of the parents' marriage. Families are affected secondarily by the presence of the eating disorder, and the clinician should not assume that every family has premorbid problems. Psychoeducational programs for family members greatly facilitate treatment and may be done in an individual or group setting. Family involvement in treatment, whatever the primary modality, clearly benefits young patients.

Behavior modification facilitates an initial gain to a minimal healthy weight, which decreases the medical risk and the negative emotional and behavioral effects of starvation. Privileges and activities are made contingent on weight gain. The benefits of this intervention appear to be short lived, however. Cognitive-behavioral modification initially emphasizes changing incorrect beliefs and dysfunctional cognitions about food and eating. The focus of treatment eventually extends to include issues of body weight, appearance, peer relationships, and individual control. Cognitive-behavioral interventions (e.g., the use of food diaries) have been effective, particularly in preventing relapse in patients whose weight had returned to normal.

Individual psychodynamic psychotherapy is not recommended as the sole treatment of anorexia, especially early in the refeeding or weight gain period. However, once the patient's eating patterns have normalized, interpersonal psychotherapies may provide insight for the patient that will facilitate long-term recovery. Older patients tend to do well with individual therapies, while younger patients respond best to family interventions.

Medication may contribute to the effective treatment of anorexia nervosa. Anorexic patients occasionally become anxious when required to eat, and the addition of a benzodiazepine or major tranquilizer may facilitate their recovery. Unfortunately, patients may become dependent on anxiolytics. Patients plagued by obsessional thinking may benefit from low-dose neuroleptics. However, these medications can contribute to the initiation of bingeing behavior, and no controlled studies exist on their effectiveness. Although not yet systematically studied, selective serotonin reuptake inhibitors (SSRIs) may stabilize patients and prevent symptom relapse. The anxiety and agitation that accompany treatment of anorexia may be so extreme that medications are not effective. Patients may also have postprandial bloating and discomfort that may compromise treatment. Prokinetic agents such as cisapride and domperidone may provide relief and improve compliance. Concomitant psychiatric disorders, including depression and OCD, can be effectively treated with medication.

Bulimia Nervosa

Clinical Description

Bulimia nervosa is characterized by repeated episodes of uncontrollable binge eating of huge amounts of food in a short time (2-hour period) accompanied by excessive attempts to compensate for this caloric intake. Bingeing and compensatory behaviors occur at least twice a week for at least 3 months. Binge eating is typically done secretly and may initially be pleasurable. The patient may engage in the behavior during a dysphoric episode or in response to a recent stressor. The binge usually brings the patient relief, but self-deprecatory thoughts return. Patients feel that their eating is out of control.

Vomiting has been considered a hallmark of bulimia nervosa; 80%–90% of clinically referred patients induce vomiting. Some patients become particularly adept at purging at will; however, only one-third of all persons with bulimia induce vomiting. Exercise and strict fasting are the most common compensatory behaviors. The use of laxatives, diuretics, or thyroid medication is less common, particularly in the pediatric population.

Adolescent patients gradually increase the frequency of binges as the disorder develops. Patients with bulimia nervosa are generally of normal weight but may be slightly over or under their ideal weight. Bulimic patients may be prone to obesity before the onset of the disorder. The patient's self-image is unduly influenced by body shape and weight.

Epidemiology

Studies on the prevalence of bulimia nervosa are affected by changing diagnostic criteria, the short history of the diagnosis, and the secrecy of the behavior. Bulimia nervosa is more common than anorexia nervosa, and almost 50% of cases appear before age 18 years. Binge eating is common among adolescents, but relatively few meet diagnostic criteria for bulimia. Approximately 1%–3% of adolescent females and young adult women and 0.2% of adolescent males and young adult men in the United States have bulimia. Males account for 10%–15% of all clinically referred bulimic patients. Rates are highest in the 15- to 40-year age group in both males and females, with an older mean age at onset for boys. Patients generally become ill in the latter half of adolescence. The disorder is more common in elite athletes whose activity emphasizes thinness. Bulimic patients have increased rates of drug and alcohol use, tend to be of higher socioeconomic status, and are typically white or Hispanic. Japan is the only non-Western country with rates of eating disorders comparable to those in the United States. Recent studies have noted an increasing prevalence of bulimia and purging with laxatives in the African American population. The prevalence of mild eating disorders is much higher among adolescents, with many meeting criteria for a diagnosis of eating disorder not otherwise specified. Studies of adolescent females note that between 40% and 60% are "dieting" to lose weight. This is particularly true among white adolescent girls from high-income families. The definition of dieting varies, however, and in more than 10% may include induced vomiting or the use of diet pills and diuretics. Dieting behavior clearly increases the risk for eating disorders.

Etiology

Anorexia nervosa and bulimia frequently present on a continuum, and many patients demonstrate symptoms of each. Approximately 50% of anorexia patients will develop bulimic symptoms, and bulimic patients commonly become anorectic. Identical twins of patients with bulimia have higher rates of the disorder. Monozygotic twins have higher concordance rates than do dizygotic twins. Data on the vulnerability of first-degree female relatives to the disorder are inconsistent. A family history of obesity, depression, or alcoholism is common. Serotonin has become a focus in studies of the neurophysiological etiology of bulimia, principally because of the treatment success with SSRIs. Sexual and physical abuse predispose children to various psychiatric disorders but not preferentially to the development of eating disorders.

Course and Prognosis

Dieting usually precedes the development of bulimia. The patient first begins to binge-eat as a direct result of food restriction; the behavior then becomes a compulsion or an addiction. The patient regards bingeing as abhorrent behavior, which contributes to feelings of depression and self-criticism. The patient once again begins dieting, often augmented with vigorous exercise or purging, in an attempt to undo the damage of the bingeing episode. Although these behaviors give the patient temporary relief from the emotional pain, they become part of a vicious cycle that maintains bulimia and symptoms of depression. A constant state of semistarvation results, which places the patient at additional risk for affective disorders.

Few studies have examined either the short- or the long-term prognosis for treated bulimic patients. Relapse rates are 30%–50% when patients are followed for 6 months to 6 years. Some speculate that improvement continues for 10–15 years. In one study that followed bulimic patients for 6 years after treatment, the outcomes of 60% were considered good, 29% intermediate, and 10% poor, with 1% deceased (Fichter and Quadflieg 1997). Risk factors for relapse include induced vomiting and the use of alcohol or drugs. Patients with milder symptoms at the onset of therapy appear to have a better prognosis. Among bulimic adolescents, comorbid anxiety or affective disorders predict continued eating-disordered behaviors. No factors have been identified as predictive of treatment success. Studies on bulimia nervosa note a mortality rate of approximately 5%.

Social complications can be severe, with time and finances depleted by obtaining food, binge eating, and purging. School functioning and peer relationships typically deteriorate. Associated disorders include depression, substance abuse, and borderline personality disorder. The presence of a comorbid medical diagnosis (i.e., diabetes, cystic fibrosis) may cause otherwise benign levels of symptoms to become dangerous. The risk of suicide or death from medical complications is significant. Risk factors for death from bulimia include a greater than 2-year duration; daily vomiting or bingeing; and use of laxatives, diuretics, ipecac, and stimulants (diet pills).

Evaluation and Differential Diagnosis

The clinician should evaluate the patient by 1) obtaining a detailed history of weight changes, noting periods of greatest fluctuation in the patient's life; 2) inquiring about current eating patterns in a typical day, including the number of calories consumed and any use of diet pills; 3) determining the onset and current status of bingeing and purging behaviors; and 4) asking about possible use of thyroid hormone, excessive exercise, laxatives, and diuretics. The medical history may suggest a neurological, endocrinological, or genetic (e.g., Prader-Willi syndrome) etiology of binge eating. Patients may have medical complications (see Table 5–1). The abuse of laxatives can lead to abdominal cramping, diarrhea, or rectal bleeding. Vomiting or abuse of diuretics or laxatives can produce metabolic alkalosis, elevations in serum amylase, hypomagnesemia and hypophosphatemia, and hypokalemia. A review of psychiatric history focuses on comorbidity and on previous treatment attempts. The individual's social and personal history may reveal contributing factors. Family assessment considers dynamics; attempts to help the patient; eating habits; and a review of significant social, medical, and psychiatric family history.

Treatment

Goals of treatment include eliminating the binge–purge cycle, establishing healthy eating habits, and promoting new strategies and skills to deal with emotions and problematic situations. The treatment plan progresses in a stepwise fashion, beginning with nutritional rehabilitation. Nutritional consultation can facilitate eating regular, well-balanced meals to avoid the hunger that triggers the urge to binge. Bulimic patients who maintain a normal weight generally do not require hospitalization. Hospitalization is indicated when the patient is suicidal, has out-of-control eating and vomiting, has metabolic instability, or does not respond to outpatient treatment. In the hospital, a behavior contract can be implemented, with activities and privileges contingent on eating regular meals and not vomiting. Patients must be watched closely for hiding or stealing food and for secretive vomiting.

Cognitive-behavioral modification, conducted in an individual or group setting, can help patients overcome feelings of helplessness and the habit of using food to deal with all of their uncomfortable feelings. The patient learns skills and strategies for problem solving, coping with stress, identifying feelings, and avoiding relapse. Patients are more successful when they are from less-controlling families, have lower weights, and do not abuse laxatives or diuretics. Family therapy appears to be particularly effective in the adolescent population. The reduction of negative comments and physical forms of punishment in the home are important positive outcome variables.

Pharmacological treatment of bulimia nervosa addresses either the relation between bulimia and mood disorders or the neuroregulation of appetite behaviors in the hypothalamus through norepinephrine or serotonin. No clinical trials exist on clinical or biological predictors of drug response in bulimic patients. Pharmacological treatment of bulimia nervosa in adolescents is not as effective as cognitive-behavioral approaches. Tricyclic antidepressants (TCAs) exert an antibulimic effect, but side effects may be problematic. Monoamine oxidase inhibitors (MAOIs) are effective, but their use is limited by the need to adhere to a dietary regimen. Other antidepressants, such as trazodone and bupropion, have moderate antibulimic effects; however, bupropion is associated with the occurrence of grand mal seizures and should not be used in these patients. The SSRIs (e.g., fluoxetine) may be effective. Anticonvulsants, benzodiazepines, and lithium produce inconsistent results. Experience is based on short-term treatment of binge eating. Longer-term studies do not exist.

■ SUBSTANCE-RELATED DISORDERS

Clinical Description

The DSM-IV-TR criteria for the substance-related disorders do not change with age. The continuum of adolescent substance use ranges from nonusers, through experimental and casual users, to abuse and dependence. The line between use and abuse is crossed more easily by young persons than by adults, and some recommend that any use of alcohol or illicit drugs among people under the legal drinking age be called abuse. Although any use of substances by an adolescent constitutes risk-taking behavior, DSM-IV-TR requires evidence of harmful consequences for a diagnosis of abuse. Physical dependence is rare in adolescents.

Epidemiology

There are two national surveys conducted by agencies of the federal government that provide regularly updated data on substance use in youth. The National Institute on Drug Abuse (NIDA)–sponsored Monitoring the Future survey is an ongoing study of the behaviors, attitudes, and values of American secondary school students, college students, and young adults. Each year, approximately 50,000 8th-, 10th-, and 12th-grade students are surveyed (report available at http://monitoringthefuture.org). The rates are likely underestimates, because many of the heaviest drug users drop out of school or are likely to be absent when surveys are taken. The National Household Survey on Drug Abuse, conducted by the Substance Abuse and Mental Health Services Administration (SAMHSA), uses an interactive, computer-based questionnaire to provide annual reports on the prevalence, patterns, and consequences of drug and alcohol use and abuse in the general U.S. civilian noninstitutionalized population ages 12 years and older (report available at http://www.drugabusestatistics.samhsa.gov).

In the past several years, overall rates of substance abuse by youth have remained stable. More than half of American young people have tried an illicit drug (not including nicotine or alcohol) by the time they finish high school. The use of alcohol and nicotine is even more common. Nearly two-thirds of high school seniors have tried cigarettes, and almost one-third are current smokers. Cigarette smoking and inhalant use have continued to decline since the late 1990s. Use of alcohol and marijuana remain relatively constant. The prevalence of use of MDMA (3,4-methylenedioxy-*N*-methamphetamine; also known as Ecstasy) continues to rise, although at a slower rate than in recent years. The use of heroin has begun to decline after years of increase, due largely to the increase in use by smoking or snorting rather than injection. The use of LSD (lysergic acid diethylamide) has gradually declined for the past 5 years. The use of crack and powdered cocaine peaked in the mid-1980s and continues to slowly decrease. The 2002 Monitoring the Future survey found that the percentage of teenagers smoking, drinking, and using illegal drugs all declined from the previous survey (http://www.monitoringthefuture.org/new.html).

Comorbidity

Virtually all adolescents referred for treatment of substance use have additional disorders, including various combinations of attention-deficit/hyperactivity disorder (ADHD), oppositional defiant disorder (ODD), conduct disorder (CD), depression, anxiety disorders, posttraumatic stress disorder (PTSD) (often as a consequence of physical or sexual abuse), and specific developmental disorders (learning disabilities). Virtually any psychiatric disorder may occur in association with substance use as a cause, an effect, or a correlate. Psychiatric disorders may predate substance abuse or be secondary to pharmacological or situational effects of drug use. In a longitudinal school-based study of adolescents, major depression and heavy smoking each increased the prospective risk for the other. This association does not appear to be due to shared risk factors (Windle and Windle 2001). The presence of ADHD, especially when accompanied by ODD or CD, is associated with early onset of substance abuse.

Etiology

Children of substance abusers appear to be particularly vulnerable to adolescent drug use, likely resulting from a combination of genetic and family dynamic factors with learned attitudes toward substance use (Table 5–3). Genetic contributions to alcoholism are strongest in males. Peer influence mediates avoidance of drugs, as well as both initiation and maintenance of substance use. Sub-

TABLE 5–3.	Risk factors associated with serious substance abuse in adolescence

Rebelliousness
Aggression
Impulsivity
Low self-esteem
Elementary school underachievement
Failure to value education
Absence of strong religious convictions
Experimentation with drugs before age 15 years
Relationships with peers who have behavior problems and use drugs
Alienation from parents
History of physical or sexual abuse
Family lacking in clear discipline, praise, and positive relationships
Family history of substance abuse

stances may be used to produce positive feelings and avoid unpleasant ones, relieve tension and stress, reduce disturbing emotions, alleviate depression or anxiety, and gain peer acceptance. Among youth, determinants of use are often specific to each drug, related to some extent to the perceived risks and benefits of the substance.

Course and Prognosis

Adolescence is the critical period for initiation of drug abuse. Onset is rare in adulthood, except for the abuse of prescription drugs. Substance abuse typically progresses in predictable stages (Kandel 1975). Each stage serves as a "gateway" to the next—from abstinence to cigarettes, then beer or wine, to hard liquor, to marijuana, and then to other illicit drugs. At each stage, many youths do not progress further, but when progression occurs, stages are rarely skipped. In general, drugs from each stage are continued into the next, leading to a pattern of multiple drug abuse. Abuse of inhalants is an exception. Children may begin to use these easily available volatile substances (e.g., glue, freon, propane, aerosols, paint thinner, lighter fluid, gasoline, nitrous oxide, butane, amyl and butyl nitrite) but then desist as they gain access to other drugs. Although many young people experiment with alcohol and drugs, a smaller number proceed to regular use, and only a fraction of those become chemically dependent. Unfortunately, it is difficult to predict which young people will only experiment with substances, or continue social use of alcohol, in contrast to those who will progress to chemical dependency. Early onset and rapid progression appear to increase the risk for subsequent serious problems.

In children and adolescents, substance use interferes with developing cognitive, social, and physical abilities. Chronic use of marijuana may result in apathy and resulting arrest of academic and social development. Critical developmental experiences that are missed may be difficult or impossible to replace, leading to high risk for impairment of future functioning in every sphere. Potential morbidity and mortality from substance use are substantial. Rates of suicidal ideation and behavior are increased. The risk of death from intentional or accidental overdose, dangerous behavior while intoxicated (especially automobile accidents), or homicide related to drug dealing is significant. Injection drug use is the current major vehicle for the spread of human immunodeficiency virus (HIV) among adolescents. Indiscriminate sexual activity (related to direct drug effect on impulse control and judgment or induced by prostitution to buy drugs) places the adolescent at high risk for exposure to HIV and other sexually transmitted diseases. Adolescent female drug users may become pregnant and place the developing fetus at risk for drug-induced damage or HIV infection. Inhalant abuse may result in brain damage, cardiac arrest, liver and kidney damage, or lead poisoning.

Evaluation and Differential Diagnosis

A high index of suspicion for substance use is essential in all clinical settings. Virtually any change in emotional state, behavior, social activities, or academic performance can signal a problem with substance use. The clinician should question all patients older than 9 years about substance use, in a nonjudgmental manner. If there is evidence of substance use, the patient should be asked about every category of substance, including details of amount, frequency, impairment, and social and emotional context. Verification by parents, teachers, other professionals, or peers may be crucial. Specific areas of inquiry should include intoxication at school, missing classes because of substance use, evidence of tolerance, and discriminating preferences that indicate experience. Sequelae of substance use, such as decline in school attendance or grades, increase in family conflict, cessation of previously important activities, association with a marginal peer group, and involvement in risky behavior (especially driving while intoxicated and reckless sexual behavior), should be specifically queried.

Self-report questionnaires are available for use with adolescents, including the Drug Use Screening Inventory (DUSI) (Tarter 1990), the Drug and Alcohol Problem (DAP) Quick Screen (R.H. Schwartz and Wirtz 1990), the CAGE (Dias 2002), and the Adolescent Drinking Inventory (Harrell and Wirtz 1989).

Because most young substance users have "dual diagnoses" (psychiatric disorders in addition to substance use disorders), it is helpful to attempt to establish the chronology of substance use and the emotional and behavioral symptoms. A detailed family history of psychiatric disorders and substance use is essential. The risk of substance abuse in parents and siblings is high.

Physical or neurological examination may disclose effects of substance use. Physical signs and symptoms of inhalant abuse may include spots or sores around the mouth, red or runny eyes or nose, dazed or dizzy appearance, and nausea or loss of appetite. Laboratory screening for drug use can provide valuable information, although false-positive and false-negative results occur, and verification and integration with the rest of the assessment are essential.

Treatment

Medical detoxification is rarely necessary in adolescents. Common features of treatment programs for substance abuse include developmentally appropriate approaches to abstinence, group therapy with other substance abusers, participation in self-help "12-Step" programs such as Alcoholics Anonymous (AA) and Narcotics Anonymous (NA), and the concept of "recovery" rather than cure (see Jaffe 2000 in "Additional Reading"). The effects of denial, lack of motivation, and the peer drug culture make conventional individual psychotherapy unlikely to succeed. Better response to treatment may be associated with motivation and cooperation in the patient and family, the patient's willingness to undergo urine testing, earlier stages of drug use, and remaining in treatment longer. Suggested therapeutic strategies include teaching problem-solving and coping strategies, social skills, and relapse prevention and encouraging structured and supervised recreational activities with drug-free peers. Comorbid psychiatric disorders and specific learning disorders must be addressed and treated, although they cannot be validly assessed without a period of abstinence. Academic deficits need to be remedied, and vocational testing and training may be useful for older adolescents for whom return to school is unlikely.

Family therapy approaches have been shown to be effective, particularly those that use structural and behavioral techniques to address parent–youth relationships and interaction patterns, as well as behavior management skills training for parents. Other effective models add interventions with peers, teachers, and other parts of the youth's social environment, as well as job and school skills training for youth (Henggeler et al. 2002).

Short-term hospitalization (7–30 days) is now used primarily when outpatient treatment has failed or comorbidity with other psychiatric conditions increases the acute risk of harm to self or others. Both the patient and the family should be actively involved in group treatment and education regarding drugs. Psychotropic medications may alleviate concomitant disorders, reduce withdrawal symptoms, or facilitate abstinence. Residential treatment for 3 to 12 months is used only for the most severe, complex, or recalcitrant cases or when a parent is an active drug user.

Long-term continuation of treatment is important, whether as an outpatient or conducted in a day treatment program or halfway house. Intensive participation in AA or NA is often required. Adolescents probably do best in groups with other adolescents rather than mixed with adults. Family therapy is an integral part of treatment. Goals include educating parents about substance abuse and its consequences, thus decreasing denial and facilitating their support of treatment and of abstinence; improving parental skills of firm and consistent, but supportive, limit setting and supervision; and enhancing communication between family members. Parents may require referral for treatment of their own substance use or other psychiatric disorders. Effective treatment results in less substance abuse as well as improved school performance and fewer behavioral and psychological symptoms.

Relapses are common and should be viewed as predictable complications rather than as catastrophes or reasons for terminating treatment. Relapse prevention (i.e., specific attention to situations in which drug use is likely, with training in coping strategies) may reduce the number and severity of relapses. Periodic urine testing can facilitate abstinence.

■ SCHIZOPHRENIA

Clinical Description

DSM-IV-TR criteria for schizophrenia do not change with age, except that in children, failure to reach expected levels of interpersonal or academic functioning may be seen instead of deterioration. Schizophrenia in children is characterized by markedly uneven development and gradual onset. Language and social behavior not only are delayed but also are qualitatively different from those seen in nonschizophrenic children at any developmental stage. Peers rapidly identify schizophrenic children as different. Visual hallucinations are more common in children with schizophrenia than in adults. Delusions and hallucinations may be less complex than those in adults.

Epidemiology

Childhood-onset schizophrenia is quite rare, even less common than autistic disorder. Prevalence prior to adolescence is less than

0.1%. It is somewhat more common in boys than in girls. After puberty, the prevalence increases and approaches adult levels (1%) in late adolescence.

Etiology

Schizophrenia is considered to be a neurodevelopmental disorder. A substantial genetic contribution is evident, and various prenatal neurological insults have been implicated. There is no evidence that psychological or social factors cause schizophrenia.

Course and Prognosis

Very-early-onset schizophrenia (before age 13 years) is more common in males and typically has an insidious onset and chronic course. In very-early-onset schizophrenia, common premorbid symptoms are language and motor delays; academic problems; short attention span, hyperactivity, and disruptive behavior; social withdrawal and isolation; and symptoms usually associated with pervasive developmental disorder, such as echolalia, rituals, and stereotypies. The course appears to be similar to that in chronic poor-outcome adult schizophrenia. In schizophrenia with adolescent onset, premorbid social, motor, and language impairments are often present. Some adolescents have episodes and remissions like those seen in some adults. The range of outcomes for adolescent-onset schizophrenia appears to be similar to that for adult-onset schizophrenia, and most patients remain impaired in social relationships and educational or job skills that would permit independent living. Adolescents with schizophrenia are at increased risk for death from suicide or accidents.

Evaluation and Differential Diagnosis

A careful history is necessary to clarify premorbid functioning and current positive (e.g., delusions, hallucinations) and negative (e.g., apathy, affective flattening, poverty of speech) symptoms. A history of sexual or physical abuse may identify the precipitant of acute symptoms or suggest an alternative diagnosis (e.g., PTSD). In adolescents, a detailed drug and alcohol use history and a urine drug test are needed. The clinician should ascertain the presence and nature of command hallucinations and suicidal ideation. Comorbid disorders should be identified.

Pediatric and neurological evaluations are required to rule out organic psychoses, both acute (delirium or intoxication) and chronic. Causes include brain tumor, congenital malformation, head trauma, seizure disorder; neurodegenerative disorder; metabolic disorder; toxic encephalopathy due to substance abuse, prescribed medication (e.g., stimulants, corticosteroids, anticholinergic agents), or other toxins such as heavy metals; and infections (encephalitis or HIV-related syndromes). The extent of the medical and neurological workup and any neuroimaging or electroencephalography should be guided by the clinical history and neurological examination.

When a psychotic child or adolescent first presents clinically, the clinician often has difficulty making a definitive diagnosis. One of the most difficult distinctions is between schizophrenia and *bipolar disorder with psychosis*. Longitudinal follow-up and periodic reassessment are essential, and a family history may be helpful. Thought disorder is difficult to diagnose prior to age 7 years. In young children who are nonverbal, it is not possible to diagnose schizophrenia. Some of these children appear to have *autistic disorder* or other *pervasive developmental disorder*. As the child develops language, evidence of delusions, hallucinations, and thought disorder emerges, enabling the correct diagnosis to be made. True autistic disorder does not "change into" classic schizophrenia, although very rarely both may be present. Among children referred for presumed very-early-onset schizophrenia, a substantial proportion do not actually meet DSM criteria, but instead have been characterized as *multidimensionally impaired* (McKenna et al. 1994). Their condition does not fit into any of the existing diagnostic categories, but they have a variety of impairing psychiatric symptoms, including poor reality testing, perceptual disturbances, neuropsychological deficits, affective instability, and inability to relate to peers despite attempts to do so.

Most children who have hallucinations are not schizophrenic. Acute hallucinations occur in nonschizophrenic children as a result of *acute phobic reactions, physical illness with fever or metabolic aberration, migraine headaches,* or *medications.* Recurring hallucinations may appear in *dissociative disorder, PTSD, mania,* and *major depressive disorder.* In young children, it may be difficult to differentiate delusions and hallucinations from fantasy play or magical thinking at the extreme end of the normal range, or from play with normal imaginary companions. Children may have difficulty distinguishing between psychotic hallucinations and dreams, illusions, and hallucinations occurring while falling asleep (hypnagogic) or awakening (hypnopompic). Apparent delusions or hallucinations may also be reflections of shared religious or cultural beliefs.

Children who are *mentally retarded* have multiple delays in development, but they are consistent and do not have the peculiarities of thought and behavior characteristic of schizophrenia. Apparent thought disorder may actually be *deafness* or *language disorder.* Children with *schizotypal* or *borderline personality disorder* have severe symptoms that may resemble schizophrenia, but they do not have hallucinations or delusions. Inattention and distractibility may be present, but DSM-IV-TR specifies that *ADHD* is not diagnosed in the presence of schizophrenia. Other differential diagnostic possibilities include *schizophreniform disorder, brief psychotic disorder, schizoaffective disorder, organic syndromes, intoxication or withdrawal due to substance abuse, OCD,* and *depression with psychotic features.*

Treatment

The treatment plan should be comprehensive and reevaluated at regular intervals. The cornerstone of treatment is an intensive program that includes a structured environment, programming in school or day treatment tailored to the child's needs, and social skills training. Treatment must address developmental arrests and regression, as well as specific symptoms of schizophrenia and any comorbid conditions. Hospitalization or long-term residential treatment may be needed, but less so than in the past, largely due to the availability of new medications. Community support services include crisis intervention, respite care, and in-home interventions for the child and family. In the milieu setting, token economies may be useful in shaping adaptive behavior and reducing inappropriate behaviors, once acute psychotic symptoms have abated. Family, individual, or group psychoeducational treatment is important and can reduce the rate and severity of relapse. Advocacy groups such as the National Alliance for the Mentally Ill Child and Adolescent Network (NAMI-CAN) can provide support to families and concrete assistance with accessing resources.

Supportive individual psychotherapy may be useful as a part of a comprehensive treatment plan. The therapist must be prepared to provide structure, to limit regression and fantasy, and to focus on reality testing and development of stronger defense mechanisms and healthier coping skills. The relationship with the therapist may be especially crucial for these youngsters.

Medication (see Chapter 8) is indicated as part of the treatment program if positive psychotic symptoms cause significant impairment or interfere with other interventions. Target symptoms that may respond include overactivity, aggression, agitation, stereotyped movements, delusions, and hallucinations. Disabling negative symptoms (e.g., apathy and social withdrawal) also may be indications for drug treatment, given the potential therapeutic effects of the novel or atypical antipsychotic drugs, such as clozapine, risperidone, olanzapine, and quetiapine. Full efficacy may not appear for many months. In general, adolescents with schizophrenia are less responsive to pharmacotherapy than are adults and continue to have substantial impairment, even if the more florid symptoms abate. Prepubertal children are less likely to respond to antipsychotics, and these children are more likely to have troublesome sedation. The risk of tardive dyskinesia mandates caution in the prescription of neuroleptic drugs. Based on the limited research to date, risperidone, olanzapine, or quetiapine are recommended for the initial medication choice.

■ MOOD DISORDERS

Clinical Description

DSM-IV-TR criteria for mood disorders are the same for children and adults, with a few exceptions (Table 5–4). At all ages, depressed mood inferred from observation of the patient (appears sad or tearful) can be substituted for the patient's report. The anhedonia criterion of diminished interest or pleasure in activities can be met by observed apathy. Children and adolescents often report this as pervasive boredom. Mood-related symptoms may be manifested in different ways at different developmental levels. Key indicators of depression in young people are declining school performance, withdrawal from social activities, somatic symptoms (especially headaches and abdominal pain), sleep difficulties, and conduct problems. Consistent neurovegetative symptoms are rare in childhood depression or dysthymic disorder. Of the criteria for the diagnosis of mania, children have far less opportunity than adults for buying sprees or foolish investments. The classic pattern of alternating episodes of depressed and elated mood with corresponding vegetative (sleep, activity, appetite) symptoms does not typically emerge until late adolescence or adulthood.

Epidemiology

The prevalence of major depression has been estimated at 1%–3% in prepubertal children and 3%–9% in adolescents, although rates vary with the population, the diagnostic criteria, and the methods of assessment. In the Oregon Adolescent Depression Project, Lewinsohn and colleagues (1994) found the lifetime prevalence of at least one episode of major depression by late adolescence to be 20%–25% and of dysthymic disorder to be 3%. Many more youth have depressive symptoms than have full major depression or dysthymia. Before puberty, depression is equally common in boys and girls, with a change in adolescence to the female predominance found in adults.

Mania is rare before middle adolescence but by late adolescence is nearly as common as in adults. A community survey of

TABLE 5–4.	Developmental differences in DSM-IV-TR criteria for mood disorders	
Disorder	**Adults**	**Children**
Major depression	Depressed mood	Can be irritable mood
	Change in weight or appetite	Can be failure to make expected weight gains
Dysthymia	Depressed mood	Can be irritable mood
	2-year duration	1-year duration
Cyclothymia	2-year duration	1-year duration

high school students found a lifetime prevalence of 1% for all bipolar disorders. An additional 5.7% of the sample had persistent subthreshold hypomanic and associated symptoms (Lewinsohn et al. 1995). Approximately 20% of all bipolar patients have their first episode during adolescence.

Etiology

Etiological factors for mood disorders in children are similar to those in adults. Depression in a parent may be a powerful contributing factor to depression in young people, via genetic transmission, plus the parent's modeling, emotional unavailability, and decreased capacity for parenting. Abuse and neglect may be significant precipitants, especially in very young children.

Course and Prognosis

Mood disorders in childhood are serious and potentially fatal problems. In a 15-year follow-up of children with major depression, 4% had died by suicide (Wolk and Weissman 1996). A 10- to 15-year follow-up of a clinical sample of subjects with adolescent onset of major depression found that nearly 8% had committed suicide (Weissman et al. 1999). Over the full age range, earlier age at onset implies a lengthier and more severe course and greater genetic loading. Over the past 25 years, the age at onset of major depression appears to have consistently decreased. In a prospective study of clinically referred prepubertal children, the median length of the major depressive episode was 9 months. The median length of time for recovery from dysthymia was 4 years. Dysthymia often progressed to a major depressive episode before resolving. Risk for subsequent episodes of major depression or dysthymia is high (Kovacs 1996). In a sample of high school students, episodes of major depression lasted as long as 10 years (mean=26 weeks; median=8 weeks). Of those who recovered, one-third had another episode within 4 years. Suicidal ideation was associated with earlier onset, longer episodes, and earlier relapse of depression (Lewinsohn et al. 1994). Follow-up studies of depressed youth consistently find increased risk of repeated mood disorders and other psychiatric disorders and impairment in subsequent educational and vocational achievement and peer and family relationships.

Childhood-onset depression is more likely than adult-onset depression to evolve into bipolar disorder. Among adolescents with major depression, subsequent bipolar mood disorder was predicted by precipitous onset of symptoms, psychomotor retardation, psychotic features, psychopharmacologically precipitated hypomania, and family history of bipolar disorder (Strober and Carlson 1982).

Evaluation and Differential Diagnosis

The clinician should ask children direct questions about depression. Young children have more difficulty recognizing and verbalizing their feelings and may use idiosyncratic words to describe dysphoria or anhedonia. Both parent and child reports are essential. Some children report their mood states more accurately than their parents can, although young children may have limited insight into other symptoms. A trained clinician should observe children for depressed affect. The Children's Depression Inventory (CDI) (Kovacs 1985) may be a useful self-report screening instrument.

Assessment of the degree of potentially dangerous behavior is crucial. The clinician can question children directly regarding suicidal ideation, plans, and attempts. No evidence indicates that inquiries about wishes to die increase the risk of self-destructive behavior. Substance abuse increases the risk of suicide. (See Chapter 7 for discussion of suicidal behavior.) The clinician should ask specifically about emotional or physical abuse or neglect of the child.

Mania and hypomania occurring before adulthood are often misdiagnosed or not recognized. Children and adolescents with bipolar disorder are prone to a chronic mixed state or rapid cycling, with dysphoric, agitated affect and explosive anger. Severe, often aggressive temper outbursts lasting more than 30 minutes, heedless risk taking, highly energized affect, and developmentally inappropriate sexual preoccupation and behavior are useful markers for mania. Precocious sexuality in a bipolar child should not be presumed to be evidence of sexual abuse. Grandiosity is expressed in different terms than in adults, but the experienced clinician can distinguish these beliefs from normal bragging or childhood fantasy (Geller et al. 2002a). Manic or hypomanic decreased need for sleep must be differentiated from insomnia. Family history and longitudinal course may provide important clues.

Anxiety disorders, ADHD, or disruptive behavior disorders frequently coexist with depression, dysthymia, or bipolar disorder, even in nonclinical community epidemiological samples. Their onset may precede or follow the onset of the mood disorder. Alcohol or drug abuse may cause a secondary depression or may represent an attempt to "self-medicate" dysphoria. Diagnosis of a mood disorder may be impossible without observing the patient in a drug-free state. *Separation anxiety disorder* may resemble major depression or dysthymic disorder or may coexist with it. Children younger than 4 years may develop a clinical picture similar to major depression when separated from their parents. Children with *reactive attachment disorder* secondary to parental abuse or neglect who present with lethargy, apathy, and withdrawal may appear depressed.

Both mania and agitated depression may be confused with *ADHD,* but mood disorders are episodic, whereas ADHD is a chronic condition with onset in early childhood. Symptoms that best discriminate juvenile bipolar disorder from ADHD are elation, grandiosity, flight of ideas/racing thoughts, decreased need for sleep, and hypersexuality (Geller et al. 2002b). Mania in childhood and adolescence is frequently misdiagnosed as *schizophrenia.* Manic or depressed youth may have some symptoms of *ODD* or *CD* that are secondary to their mood symptoms. Of course, *disruptive behavior disorder* may precede mood disorder or develop in parallel. *Secondary mania* may result from prescribed medication (e.g., steroids, carbamazepine, antidepressants, stimulants), illegal drugs (e.g., cocaine, amphetamines), metabolic abnormalities (especially hyperthyroidism), or central nervous system disturbances (e.g., tumor, trauma, multiple sclerosis, epilepsy, infections).

The strong family clustering of mood disorders suggests that parents and siblings should be evaluated routinely for mood and anxiety disorders, and treatment should be provided or arranged as necessary.

Treatment

If risk-taking behavior or suicidal ideation is present, close parental and psychiatric supervision is needed. Psychiatric hospitalization may be required for youngsters who are psychotic or seriously suicidal or who do not respond to outpatient treatment.

Early-onset mood disorders often have devastating effects on development. Even after spontaneous remission or successful treatment with medication, reduced coping skills, cognitive patterns associated with depression, and impaired interpersonal relationships with peers and family members may require individual, group, or family therapy to address developmental deficits or sequelae of the depression. Whatever the treatment, involvement of the family is even more crucial than for adult patients. Both patients and families benefit from psychoeducational therapy (provision of information about the disorder and its treatment) and from instruction in relapse prevention (complying with medication, recognizing early symptoms of relapse, avoiding precipitants of relapse such as sleep deprivation and drug abuse).

Fluoxetine is the only medication currently approved by the U.S. Food and Drug Administration (FDA) for the treatment of pediatric major depressive disorder. For nonpsychotic depression, psychotherapy is typically the first treatment. Medication is added if symptoms do not improve in 4–6 weeks. In uncomplicated adolescent depression seen in primary care settings, an SSRI is often the first treatment, with psychiatric consultation and specific therapy added if necessary. Cognitive-behavior therapy (CBT) and interpersonal therapy (IPT) techniques developed for the treatment of depression in adults have been adapted for use in children and adolescents (Mufson et al. 1999) (see "Additional Reading"). Current research (Treatment for Adolescents with Depression Study [TADS]; TADS Team 2003) is comparing the relative efficacy of fluoxetine, CBT, and the combination in depressed adolescents. Data from studies of adults suggest that for severe or chronic depression, both medication and CBT or IPT are needed. Social withdrawal and limited peer relationships may respond to behavior modification and social skills training. Remedial education or tutoring may be needed when the illness has interfered with learning in school.

The use of antidepressants and mood stabilizers is discussed in Chapter 8. Research supports the efficacy in pediatric depression of the SSRIs citalopram, fluoxetine, paroxetine, and sertraline, although a substantial number of subjects do not respond and even many of the responders continued to have symptoms and functional impairment. TCAs are rarely used for depressed youth, due to their side-effect profile and the paucity of research evidence of efficacy. An algorithm for the treatment of pediatric major depressive disorder (Hughes et al. 1999) begins with one of the SSRIs, with change to another SSRI if there is no or only partial response. If that is unsuccessful, an antidepressant from a different class is substituted, such as bupropion, mirtazapine, nefazodone, a TCA, or venlafaxine. If necessary, combinations of antidepressants are used, with an MAOI as the last pharmacological step. Suicidal and impulsive outpatients should be excluded from MAOI treatment because of the risk of interactions with food and drugs. Close supervision and repeated careful dietary instruction are necessary even for responsible youngsters. In severe cases of depression, electroconvulsive therapy

(ECT) may be appropriate if adequate pharmacotherapy trials are ineffective or contraindicated (e.g., in pregnancy).

It is extremely difficult to implement controlled trials in bipolar youth. Based on the limited existing research data and clinical experience, lithium and anticonvulsants (divalproex sodium, carbamazepine) are used for children and adolescents with bipolar affective disorder (mixed or manic) to treat acute episodes and as maintenance prophylaxis or as an adjunct to antidepressants for treatment-resistant depression. Only lithium has an FDA-approved indication for bipolar disorder in youth (adolescents only). Some patients require a combination of mood stabilizers. Several newer antiepileptic agents are being tried as mood stabilizers in treatment-resistant patients, but there are very few data to support their use in youth. Benzodiazepines such as lorazepam may be added briefly for symptomatic treatment of agitation and insomnia in acute mania. Atypical antipsychotic medications are used as an adjunctive treatment for psychotic symptoms and agitation, but the increased risk of tardive dyskinesia in patients with mood disorders must be kept in mind. For depression in bipolar youth, mood stabilizers may not be sufficient, but antidepressants increase the risk of a manic relapse. As a result, antidepressants are not typically used for bipolar depression until treatment with a mood stabilizer is established.

Children and adolescents who have seasonal affective disorder may respond to treatment with bright white light (Sonis et al. 1987).

■ ANXIETY DISORDERS

Phobias, PTSD, OCD, and panic disorder can begin in childhood or adolescence, but they are placed in the "adult" anxiety disorders section of DSM-IV-TR. The childhood DSM-III-R (American Psychiatric Association 1987) diagnosis of overanxious disorder (OAD) was replaced by generalized anxiety disorder (GAD) in DSM-IV [American Psychiatric Association 1994] and DSM-IV-TR. (Separation anxiety disorder is covered in Chapter 4.)

Although fears and anxiety occur normally during development (Table 5–5), anxiety disorders in children can lead to lack of

TABLE 5–5.　**Common normal fears**

Developmental stage	Feared object or situation
Birth to 6 months	Loss of physical support
	Loud noises
	Large rapidly approaching objects
7–12 months	Strangers
1–5 years	Loud noises
	Storms
	Animals
	The dark
	Separation from parents
3–5 years	Monsters
	Ghosts
6–12 years	Bodily injury
	Burglars
	Being sent to the principal
	Punishment
	Failure
12–18 years	Tests in school
	Social embarrassment

social competence, rejection or neglect by peers, academic under-achievement, and eventual inability to succeed in school, work, and relationships. In contrast to the disruptive behavior disorders, anxiety disorders often cause more distress in the child than in the parents and are thus considered "internalizing" disorders.

Specific Phobia and Social Phobia (Social Anxiety Disorder)

Clinical Description

The DSM-IV-TR criteria for these disorders are largely the same in young people and adults, although cognitive immaturity may limit recognition that fear is excessive or unreasonable, and under age 18 years a duration of 6 months is required for specific phobia. Transient developmentally appropriate fears (see Table 5–5) do not usually require treatment. Phobias are distinguished by their severity, irrationality, persistence, and functional impairment, usually secondary to avoidance of the feared object. The DSM-III-R diagnosis of avoidant disorder of childhood is classified by DSM-IV-TR as social phobia. Social phobia is a pervasive fear of social encounters and public performances where there is the possibility of negative evaluation by others.

Epidemiology

Many children with phobias are never seen in a clinical setting. Unfortunately, parents and teachers rarely refer children with excessive shyness for psychiatric treatment. The rate of social phobia in children and adolescents is estimated to be 1%–2%. However, lifetime rates in the general population may be as high as 13%. In community samples of youth, the prevalence of specific phobia averages 5%. While nonreferred youth with simple phobia have less comorbidity than do those with other anxiety disorders, children presenting for treatment of anxiety symptoms tend to be more symptomatic with regard to both anxiety and comorbidity.

Etiology

The etiology of phobias is likely multifactorial, including temperament, genetic predisposition, and family dynamics and modeling. Some phobias have a clear precipitant, but many others appear to arise spontaneously. The aggregation of fears and phobias within families suggests a genetic contribution, particularly for social phobias, although there may well be a learned or imitative component. There is increasing research support for an association between social phobia and behavioral inhibition (see below) (Biederman et al. 2001).

Course and Prognosis

Specific phobias may begin at any time during development. Phobic symptoms may follow association of a stimulus with an unexpected panic attack or a traumatic event. Most simple phobias remit spontaneously, but a proportion persist. Social phobia tends to start in early to middle adolescence and can interfere with social and academic/occupational functioning through school avoidance, substance abuse, and difficulty with dating and intimacy. The disorder seems to persist into adulthood and is associated with professional underachievment, depression, generalized anxiety symptoms, constrained social functioning, and significant disability.

Evaluation and Differential Diagnosis

Parents are often unaware of phobic symptoms or social anxiety in their children, so the clinical interview with the child is especially important. Children may express their phobic anxiety as crying, tantrums, freezing, or clinging, rather than verbalizing it or explicitly avoiding the feared object or situation. The history includes a description of the feared stimulus, circumstances surrounding the development of the phobia, behavior in response to the phobic object or situation, anticipatory or avoidant behaviors, and any secondary gain. Observations of behavior may be useful. A self-report questionnaire such as the Fear Survey Schedule for Children (originally developed in the 1960s by Scherer and Nakamura and revised twice) (Ollendick 1983) can be helpful to measure symptom severity, especially when symptoms are difficult to elicit by interview.

Differential diagnosis includes *panic disorder, agoraphobia, separation anxiety disorder, schizophrenia with delusions, pervasive developmental disorder, PTSD, OCD,* and *eating disorders* (fear of eating or of gaining weight).

Treatment

Clinicians often integrate several approaches to treat phobic disorders. Behavioral and cognitive-behavioral treatments are the best studied, the most efficient, and generally the treatment of choice for children with one or two phobias. For effective behavioral treatment, the therapist must ensure that the child has the skills and the opportunities to deal with the problem situation in other ways and must work with the family and school to eliminate secondary gain.

Systematic desensitization and exposure and response prevention techniques can be used in children as in adults, with techniques adapted for children with various developmental levels. In vivo desensitization appears to be more effective than imaginal techniques, especially in young children who have difficulty learning the relaxation techniques and imagining the stimuli. Emotive imagery—using stories the therapist creates, pairing the child with a powerful hero who helps the child confront the hierarchy of feared stimuli—is appropriate for younger children although lacking empirical support.

A second group of behavioral techniques is based on modeling or observation learning. The patient observes a model—optimally a child of similar age and same sex—who demonstrates an appropriate response to the feared situation, while verbalizing anxiety and explaining strategies for dealing with it. After the demonstration, the patient is helped to imitate the model, with feedback and positive reinforcement for correct performance, thus adding operant techniques and a shaping procedure. This type of treatment has the advantage of teaching coping skills while reducing anxiety.

In operant conditioning approaches, phobic avoidance is eliminated by changing the positive and negative contingencies that maintain the phobia. These contingency management techniques include shaping, positive reinforcement, and extinction.

CBT techniques aim to change feelings and behavior by specifically addressing maladaptive, distorted, self-defeating thoughts or statements. By changing cognitions associated with anxiety, more adaptive behaviors emerge. Children who are fearful of tests and of social situations have been helped by specific training in cognitive restructuring, which may involve producing thoughts that describe the child as competent and able to cope with the situation. Training in social skills, assertiveness, problem-solving skills, and relaxation techniques, as well as gradual exposure to social situations, are important components of treatment for social phobia. Innovative school-based CBT interventions are being developed.

There has been little study of the use of medication to treat phobias in children and adolescents. Open trials of SSRIs (fluoxetine, sertraline) have had positive results in social anxiety. Fluvoxamine was shown to be effective for youth with social phobia, separation anxiety disorder, or GAD in a randomized, double-blind trial by the Research Units on Pediatric Psychopharmacology Anxiety Study Group (Walkup et al. 2001). Imipramine and alprazolam have been studied but are not typically used because of their potential side effects.

Generalized Anxiety Disorder

Clinical Description

Children with GAD have pervasive worries for at least 6 months about a variety of areas (Table 5–6). The DSM-IV-TR criteria require children to have only one accompanying symptom, whereas adults must have three. It is not clear how previous research on children with the DSM-III-R diagnosis of OAD applies to children with a diagnosis of GAD, although the key symptom of both disorders is unrealistic worry about future events.

Children with GAD are shy, self-doubting, self-deprecating, and pessimistic. They may be pseudomature, overly serious, perfectionistic, and excessively compliant with authority, characteristics that may be encouraged by parents and teachers. Habit disturbances, such as nail biting, hair pulling, or thumb sucking, are common. Somatic symptoms such as headache, upset stomach, or fatigue may result in requests for excessive medical evaluations.

Epidemiology

Isolated subclinical anxiety symptoms are common in normal children. The prevalence of GAD is estimated to be 2%–4%, although the rate in adolescents may be higher. GAD is diagnosed more frequently in females than in males, and comorbidity among the anxiety and depressive disorders is common. Many children with GAD never receive treatment.

TABLE 5–6.	**DSM-IV-TR diagnostic criteria for generalized anxiety disorder (includes overanxious disorder of childhood)**

A. Excessive anxiety and worry (apprehensive expectation), occurring more days than not for at least 6 months, about a number of events or activities (such as work or school performance).

B. The person finds it difficult to control the worry.

C. The anxiety and worry are associated with three (or more) of the following six symptoms (with at least some symptoms present for more days than not for the past 6 months). **Note:** Only one item is required in children.

    (1) restlessness or feeling keyed up or on edge

    (2) being easily fatigued

    (3) difficulty concentrating or mind going blank

    (4) irritability

    (5) muscle tension

    (6) sleep disturbance (difficulty falling or staying asleep, or restless unsatisfying sleep)

D. The focus of the anxiety and worry is not confined to features of an Axis I disorder, e.g., the anxiety or worry is not about having a panic attack (as in panic disorder), being embarrassed in public (as in social phobia), being contaminated (as in obsessive-compulsive disorder), being away from home or close relatives (as in separation anxiety disorder), gaining weight (as in anorexia nervosa), having multiple physical complaints (as in somatization disorder), or having a serious illness (as in hypochondriasis), and the anxiety and worry do not occur exclusively during posttraumatic stress disorder.

E. The anxiety, worry, or physical symptoms cause clinically significant distress or impairment in social, occupational, or other important areas of functioning.

F. The disturbance is not due to the direct physiological effects of a substance (e.g., a drug of abuse, a medication) or a general medical condition (e.g., hyperthyroidism) and does not occur exclusively during a mood disorder, a psychotic disorder, or a pervasive developmental disorder.

Etiology

Historically, anxiety was viewed as resulting mainly from psychodynamic factors, especially parental pressure placed on children or identification with parental anxiety. More recent data have suggested neurodevelopmental and genetic contributions. Boys whose temperament at age 3 years is characterized by quick adjustment to new situations, self-confidence, and self-reliance are less likely to have problems with anxiety in late childhood and adolescence (Caspi et al. 1995). Girls who were rated shy, fearful, quiet, and passive as preschoolers are at risk for problems with anxiety in childhood, increasing in adolescence (Caspi et al. 1995). "Behavioral inhibition to the unfamiliar" has been shown to have physiological correlates of high sympathetic arousal (higher resting heart rate and increased acceleration of heart rate with cognitive effort, elevated salivary cortisol) (Kagan et al. 1988). This construct predicts the development of anxiety disorders (Biederman et al. 1993). Both genetics and modeling or "contagion" are likely to contribute to the familial clustering of anxiety disorders.

Course and Prognosis

Many anxious children improve, with or without treatment, but others have a chronic course and may be at risk for anxiety disorders, mood disorders, or somatization disorder in adulthood. GAD appears to have a worse prognosis and a lower remission rate than separation anxiety disorder. Potential complications are impairments of self-esteem, learning, and peer relationships.

Evaluation and Differential Diagnosis

In general, children report their anxiety symptoms more accurately than parents do. Parents may not be aware of the child's symptoms, or parents may report an exaggerated degree of child anxiety, influenced by the parent's own heightened anxiety. Parents and children may actually be reporting different symptoms as "anxiety." Newer self-report instruments such as the Screen for Child Anxiety

Related Emotional Disorders (SCARED) (Birmaher et al. 1997), with both child and parent scales, and the Multidimensional Anxiety Scale for Children (MASC) (March et al. 1997) can aid in assessment of anxiety symptoms and appear to be an improvement over older scales. The Pediatric Anxiety Rating Scale (PARS) (Research Units on Pediatric Psychopharmacology Anxiety Study Group 2002) was developed to assess separation anxiety, social phobia, and generalized anxiety symptoms, particularly in treatment research.

Other anxiety disorders, such as *separation anxiety disorder, panic disorder, phobia,* and *adjustment disorder with anxiety,* and the *depressive disorders* should be considered in the differential diagnosis of GAD. Unlike children with *ADHD,* who are also restless and fidgety, children with GAD worry obsessively or are preoccupied. Children with ADHD tend to become more disruptive as familiarity with a situation or person increases, whereas children with GAD become more comfortable with time. Because children with GAD often have somatic symptoms, a wide variety of physical illnesses are in the differential diagnosis. Determining the extent of an appropriate medical workup for symptoms such as recurrent headache or abdominal pain can be difficult because children with documented physical etiologies also report anxiety and depression. *Medical disorders* that can mimic an anxiety disorder include substance withdrawal or intoxication, hyperthyroidism, and asthma.

Treatment

Behavioral treatment methods include relaxation, desensitization by progressive exposure or by imagining anxiety-provoking situations, modeling, and contingent reinforcement of approach to feared objects or situations. Individual or group CBT is directed at changing self-defeating, pessimistic, and distorted beliefs and developing and practicing strategies to reduce anxiety and promote mastery, which is then self-reinforcing. Supportive or dynamic psychotherapy is often oriented toward promoting psychological individuation and autonomy in both the child and the family. Assertiveness training may be helpful, especially in a group setting. Despite increasing use of SSRIs for anxiety disorder in the last few years, there are few randomized controlled trials of an SSRI in children with GAD as the primary diagnosis. A recent study suggested both safety and efficacy of 50 mg of sertraline daily in the treatment of GAD in children and adolescents (Rynn et al. 2001). There are no randomized controlled trials of buspirone in children and adolescents.

Treatment of the parents is often important, particularly if a parent also has an anxiety or mood disorder. The therapist should work with the parents to anticipate future developmental events that may lead to parental overprotectiveness or unrealistically high expectations for the child's performance.

Posttraumatic Stress Disorder

Clinical Description

PTSD involves specific, persistent emotional and behavioral symptoms following direct or observed exposure to a traumatic event that makes the individual feel intensely fearful, helpless, or horrified. Symptoms are from three board categories: reexperiencing the traumatic event, avoidance of reminders of the event and/or generalized emotional numbing, and increased arousal.

Although the DSM-IV-TR criteria for PTSD are essentially the same at all ages, symptoms in children differ in some ways (Terr 1987). Immediate effects can include fear of separation from parent(s), of death, and of further fear. Additional fears may develop regarding repetition of the experience, situations that involve separation or danger, or other reminders of the event. Children often withdraw from new experiences or develop various new fears. Perceptual distortions occur, most commonly in time sense and in vision, but auditory, touch, and olfactory misperceptions are also described. Although children accurately remember many details of the experience, sequencing or duration of events is often distorted and they may become more distractible.

Children often reexperience the event in the form of nightmares, daydreams, or repetitive and potentially dangerous reenactment in symbolic play or in actual behavior (rather than in flashbacks). Despite obvious similarities between the reenactments and the original event, most children are unaware of the connection. Even children younger than 3 years demonstrate, through play or dreams, memories of traumatic events that they cannot describe verbally. The denial, repression, and psychic numbing that occur in many adults are not typically seen in children who experience a single traumatic event; however, their behavior may become disorganized.

Children manifest increased arousal by sleep disturbances, which may add to functional impairment (Pynoos et al. 1987). They may have somatic symptoms, particularly headaches and stomachaches. Regression (behavior characteristic of a previous developmental stage) is common as is agitation or irritability. Children often feel guilty because they survived but others did not, or because they failed to save others. This guilt may be exacerbated by shame or children's normal cognitive egocentricity and magical thinking, which may contribute to a belief that they caused the event by thought or action. Constricted affect and diminished interest in activities may be elicited from interviews with parents, teachers, or caregivers.

Epidemiology

The general prevalence of PTSD among children and adolescents following either a single event or chronic repeated trauma is not known, and there has been controversy about the diagnostic criteria in children. Rates vary greatly depending on which criteria are used. Standardized diagnostic interviews for PTSD in children are relatively new. In the general population, the prevalence of PTSD varies from 1% to 14%. A study of 337 school-age children found that one-quarter of the children who were exposed to trauma met criteria for PTSD (McCloskey and Walker 2000). In this study, death or illness of a loved one was the top risk factor for PTSD, and these children had a variety of other psychiatric comorbidity. Rates of trauma exposure and PTSD are higher in girls than boys.

Etiology

Knowledge of predisposing or protective factors in the development of PTSD in children is limited. Children who have experienced multiple stressors, prior loss, disturbances in family functioning, or psychiatric comorbidity are vulnerable to more severe and prolonged symptoms, but a sufficiently severe stressor can produce the disorder in a person without any predisposition. The rate of PTSD increases with the degree of proximity to the traumatic event.

PTSD likely involves a complicated interaction of neuroendocrine dysregulation with psychological and social factors. Proposed mechanisms for the development of PTSD symptoms include destruction of "basic trust," cognitive information overload, and a classical conditioning model to explain extension of anxiety to otherwise harmless stimuli present at the time of the traumatic event. Neurodevelopmental factors have also been considered in the induction or maintenance of PTSD. Abuse or neglect of children may cause cognitive and developmental delays as well as increased arousal or withdrawal secondary to changes in brain physiology. Given the high degree of comorbidity with both internalizing and externalizing disorders, it is possible that trauma affects functioning in a more generalized manner.

Course and Prognosis

In addition to the initial trauma, disasters often result in loss of home, isolation from usual social supports, and loss of parents or other family members, which exacerbate PTSD. Symptoms may be partially ameliorated by a stable, cohesive, and supportive family and safe environment.

Anxiety (especially separation anxiety disorder) or depression may be prominent symptoms. Impulsivity, difficulty concentrating, and decreased motivation may interfere with school performance. Many traumatized children develop a chronic sense of pessimism and hopelessness about the future. These children may create a screen or cover memory, which loses the emotional intensity of the original memories. Even years after the event, children with chronic prolonged symptoms remain fearful, many with continuing disturbances of sleep and play, and deeply ashamed of their helplessness in the face of danger. A history of sexual or physical abuse during childhood is associated with increased risk of lifetime psychopathology, particularly for women (MacMillan et al. 2001).

Evaluation and Differential Diagnosis

At the time of clinical presentation, a traumatic event may or may not be obvious. PTSD should be suspected in any child or adolescent who has had a significant change in behavior or emotional state. The clinician should question both the parents and the child, because the child may have difficulty describing the symptoms and the parents may not be fully aware of the trauma or of the child's emotional reaction. Developmental history may show sources of increased vulnerability. Teacher observations regarding changes in school behavior or achievement can contribute to the evaluation. Consideration should be given to the child's developmental level and cognitive and expressive language skills when evaluating for symptoms. In addition, cultural factors, gender, and family issues can influence the manifestation of symptoms.

Given the increased interest in PTSD in youth, rating scales and structured interviews have been developed for both clinical and research assessment. A multidimensional approach to assessment of PTSD includes evaluation of cognitive, emotional, and behavioral symptoms; social and cognitive development; family and community factors; and overall functioning.

Projective measures can be useful in exploring fears, coping styles, and traumatic themes but should be administered only by qualified professionals who are well trained in this approach.

A mood disorder or an additional anxiety disorder is also diagnosed if criteria are met. PTSD is distinguished from *adjustment disorder* by the severity of the stressor and the distinctive symptoms, such as repetitive reexperiencing of the traumatic event. Some of the symptoms of PTSD may be mistaken for *ADHD, ODD, psychosis,* or *seizures.*

Treatment

There is limited empirical evidence for specific treatments for children with PTSD, with the exception of CBT. The use of a trauma-focused approach is important. Treatment models include focused psychotherapy for the PTSD symptoms, strengthening coping skills in anticipation of further grief or trauma, and the treatment of any other psychiatric disorders. Treatment strategies include direct exploration (in a safe and supportive setting) of the traumatic event and its impact on the child. The therapist carefully and sensitively encourages the child to review the trauma, after using relaxation and desensitization techniques as needed. Stress management techniques such as muscle relaxation, positive imagery, deep breathing, and thought stopping can enable the child to develop control over overwhelming thoughts and affective responses. Understanding cues that trigger symptoms and repairing emotional consequences encourage mastery of the situation and facilitate diminished hyperarousal is beneficial. Individual insight-oriented play and verbal psychotherapy are commonly used. Interpretation of the child's compulsively repetitive reenactment play may be facilitated by the use of toys that the child has incorporated into the stereotyped play. Trauma-focused discussion with the child about techniques to cope with the danger and feeling of helplessness may help in reducing the child's guilt regarding the event. Exploration and correction of inaccurate attributions is important. Systematic desensitization of specific trauma-related fears may be useful in conjunction with other interventions. There is strong consensus that directly involving parents and other supportive individuals in treatment is important. This can include group or community crisis intervention programs.

There are no randomized controlled trials to support pharmacological treatment of childhood PTSD. However, SSRIs are generally used as first-line drugs when medication is required, based on extrapolation from adult studies and safety and efficacy in other mood and anxiety disorders in youth. Medication should be considered when symptoms are severe, functioning is very impaired with comorbid mood/anxiety symptoms, or when symptoms persist despite active psychotherapy. Other agents used to treat children and adolescents with PTSD, such as clonidine or β-blockers, are suggested only by case reports or open trials.

Outreach may be required to reach those in need of psychiatric services, because parents and children are unlikely to seek help spontaneously. A quick response by agencies and schools may moderate the severity of the response to traumatic events. Group therapy with victims who have been exposed to the same event may be helpful in decreasing distortions and reducing the spread of post-traumatic fears and symptoms, but groups that include victims of different traumatic events may actually lead to contagion of fears.

Supportive therapy for parents and siblings can provide information about the child's symptoms, address vicarious trauma experienced by family members, and reduce contagion. Parents may also have PTSD symptoms that require therapeutic attention. The therapist should help the parents to respond supportively to their child's symptoms, including reenactments. Otherwise, psychological denial of the severity of the impact of the event by parents may cause them to avoid talking with the child about the event and the child's reactions, and interfere with the family's ability to assist in the resolution of the child's symptoms.

Obsessive-Compulsive Disorder

Clinical Description

The DSM-IV-TR criteria for OCD include recurrent and persistent thoughts (or impulses or images) and behaviors (or mental acts) that are acknowledged as unreasonable and are accompanied by distress. The child may have either obsessions or compulsions, although most patients have both. Because children may not recognize the senseless or excessive quality of OCD (specified as "with poor insight" in DSM-IV-TR), the requirement that the patient have insight into the nature of the disorder has been waived for youth.

Epidemiology

OCD is more common than clinical populations would suggest. The disorder is underdiagosed principally because symptoms are poorly understood by and embarrassing to children and therefore are hidden from parents and caregivers. In community samples, the prevalence of OCD in children and adolescents has been reported to range from 1% to 4%. However, mild or transient rituals, obsessions, or compulsions are common in the general population. At various stages of development, children commonly exhibit ritualistic behaviors and recurrent worries. The mean age at onset of OCD is 10 years. Boys may tend to have earlier onset than girls; however, by adolescence gender distribution is likely equal (Swedo et al. 1989). Earlier onset OCD is associated with more severe OCD symptoms, higher rates of comorbid tic disorders, and possibly more resistance to medication treatment (Rosario-Campos et al. 2001).

Etiology

OCD is a model neuropsychiatric disorder. The "serotonin hypothesis" for the etiology of the disorder developed following the success of SSRIs in the treatment of OCD. Family studies indicate a genetic link, and neuroimaging suggests abnormalities in connections between the basal ganglia and the cortex. A frontal-striatal-thalamic circuitry mechanism has been proposed. It may eventually be established that the pathophysiology of OCD varies depending on age at onset (Busatto et al. 2001). Changes in neurotransmitter and neuroendocrine function have been implicated in the etiology of OCD, which may follow neurological disorders affecting the basal ganglia, such as Sydenham's chorea, due to group A β-hemolytic streptococcal infection (March et al. 1995). In PANDAS (pediatric autoimmune neuropsychiatric disorders associated with streptococcal infections), streptococcal infection may precipitate the onset or exacerbation of OCD and/or tics, even in the absence of neurological symptoms (Swedo et al. 1998).

Course and Prognosis

OCD in children (as in adults) appears to be a chronic condition with a waxing and waning course. The onset of symptoms is generally gradual but may be more acute. Children typically hide rituals from adults initially, until progressive severity makes this impossible. Partial control of symptoms is common, with suppression of rituals outside of the home but inability to do so with the family. Over time, rituals increase in number and severity, change in content and context, and increasingly interfere with daily activities. OCD tends to be chronic and extend into adulthood, often with functional impairment.

No demographic or clinical outcome predictors have been identified for pediatric OCD. Patients who acknowledge the senselessness and emotional cost of the behavior are considered better candidates for CBT. Complications of OCD include interference with school achievement and peer relationships and physical sequelae such as dermatitis secondary to washing rituals.

OCD in children is often accompanied by other psychiatric disorders. These can include anxiety disorders, depression, eating disorders, trichotillomania, tics or Tourette's disorder, specific developmental disorders, ADHD, or ODD. Children with pervasive developmental disorder or nonverbal learning disorder often have symptoms of OCD. The relationship of body dysmorphic disorder and OCD is unclear.

Evaluation and Differential Diagnosis

Children and adolescents are often secretive about obsessions and compulsions. Temper outbursts, academic struggles, or changing eating patterns may be the presenting concerns until obsessions and compulsions are carefully elicited with specific questions to the child, parents, and teachers. Fears of contamination or danger and compulsive repetitive checking, arranging, counting, or touching are common symptoms. Pathological rituals need to be distinguished from normal developmental childhood routines. Impairment should be assessed periodically. The Children's Yale Brown

Obsessive-Compulsive Scale (C-YBOCS) (Scahill et al. 1997) can aid in diagnosis and in symptom monitoring during treatment.

Alternative diagnoses include *phobic disorder, Tourette's disorder, anorexia and bulimia nervosa,* and *schizophrenia. Neurological conditions* can precipitate OCD symptoms. If PANDAS is suspected, a throat culture and streptococcal antibody (e.g., DNAse B) titers may be indicated for diagnosis and to guide treatment. *Complex tics* may be hard to distinguish from compulsions. Patients with *pervasive developmental disorder* can exhibit obsessive-compulsive symptoms. *Stimulant medication* can induce overfocused or perseverative behaviors, especially at higher doses.

Treatment

CBT and SSRIs are efficacious treatments for OCD and are often used in combination. CBT is often the initial treatment for milder cases; however, depending on the comorbidity or other factors, pharmacological intervention may be indicated.

Due to the problematic side-effect profile of clomipramine, the SSRIs (fluoxetine, fluvoxamine, paroxetine, sertraline, citalopram) are now the first-line treatment agents, with support from randomized controlled trials of safety and efficacy in youth with OCD for all but citalopram.

CBT, which can include hierarchy-based exposure and response prevention, modeling, relaxation techniques, and habit reversal/thought-stopping skills can be effective in motivated patients. Therapy is usually implemented gradually and targets specific behaviors, with strategies to generalize across symptoms. Family participation in treatment is crucial. Advocacy groups such as the Obsessive Compulsive Foundation or Tourette's Syndrome Association can provide additional support.

Panic Disorder

Clinical Description

Panic disorder and agoraphobia are rare in children and more common in adolescents, with the same DSM-IV-TR diagnostic criteria and physical symptom profile as in adults. Family studies and retrospective reports note a continuity between pediatric and adult presentations. Panic symptoms include both physiological and psychological features that occur spontaneously. In youth, cognitive immaturity may preclude some characteristic cognitions during an attack (fear of dying, going crazy, doing something uncontrolled). Studies of pediatric populations emphasize psychosomatic symptoms, including shortness of breath, palpitations, chest pain, paresthesias, trembling, dizziness, tachycardia, sweating, and hyperventilation. Panic disorder can occur with or without agoraphobia.

Epidemiology

Rates of panic disorder vary depending on the nature of the assessment and source of information. Interview-based diagnosis appears to be reliable. Although 11.6% of ninth graders have had at least one four-symptom panic attack (Hayward et al. 1989), the full syndrome of panic disorder is less common than other anxiety disorders in youth. Panic disorder is more common in women than men.

Etiology

Twin studies suggest genetic contributions. Modeling may also contribute. Offspring of parents with panic disorder are at high risk for anxiety disorders.

Course and Prognosis

The evolution of panic symptoms and natural history of the disorder in children are not clear but emerging evidence supports chronicity (Biederman et al. 1997). Children with panic disorder and agoraphobia seem to have high rates of other anxiety and mood disorders as well as ADHD (Biederman et al. 1997). Prepubertal onset may signal greater severity (Vitiello et al. 1990). Youth with the somatic symptoms of panic disorder are likely to first seek the help of a pediatrician or an emergency room. Panic attacks often begin at the onset of or during an episode of major depression or separation anxiety disorder.

Evaluation and Differential Diagnosis

Children can report current panic attacks, but parent report is helpful to verify duration and history. Self-monitoring techniques may be useful in children, as in adults. Panic disorder in children is likely underdiagnosed, with the symptoms attributed to separation anxiety disorder, hyperventilation syndrome, or situational or "normal" anxiety. Panic can be distinguished from *separation anxiety disorder* by the lack of association between initial symptom presentation and separation from a major attachment figure.

Treatment

Education is essential for patients, families, and even school staff if symptoms interfere with school functioning. If the cause of physical symptoms is unclear, consultation with the primary care physician is indicated. There are no controlled trials of any treatment for panic disorder in youth. Psychotherapy may include CBT, or individual, group, or family therapy, depending on the patient's presentation. SSRIs should be considered for panic symptoms that are persistent and/or disturbing despite therapeutic interventions.

■ GENDER IDENTITY DISORDER

In normal development, the child establishes a *core gender identity* (the usually unshakable conviction of being a boy or a girl) by age 3–4 years. *Gender role behavior* (cultural norms of mannerisms, gait, clothing, toys, play activities, and sex of playmates) is established as early as age 1 year and is set by age 6 years. In general, girls are permitted a great deal more latitude in gender role behavior. In nonclinical populations of boys, cross-gender behavior is rare after age 6 years.

Clinical Description

Boys with gender identity disorder (GID) (Table 5–7) display effeminate mannerisms, dress in female clothes (improvising if necessary), and avoid rough-and-tumble play. Girls refuse to wear skirts or dresses or to engage in culturally expected female play, such as dolls, dress up, or house (except as the father). The onset is typically before age 5 years. Parents often tolerate or even encourage cross-gender behavior early on but later become more concerned. Parents frequently disagree on the seriousness of their child's problem.

Epidemiology

There are no epidemiological data on the prevalence of true GID in children. More boys than girls come to clinical attention, perhaps because of greater cultural permissiveness regarding gender roles and behavior for females than for males. Cross-gender behavior of clinical significance, but not meeting full criteria for GID, is common in 5- to 12-year-old boys referred to a psychiatric clinic for various other emotional and behavioral symptoms (Pleak et al. 1989). These patients might fall into the category of GID not otherwise specified, comorbid with their primary diagnosis.

Etiology

Various biological, psychodynamic, and psychosocial causative factors for GID have been proposed. No genetic or hormonal factor has yet been identified, although some evidence suggests that gender identity is determined by prenatal hormones acting on the developing brain. Family characteristics, such as lack of appropriate gender role modeling; parental wish for opposite-sex child; parent who treats child as opposite sex; same-sex parent who is absent, distant, or depressed; disturbance in mother–child relationship; mother who is dissatisfied with her own gender or gender role; and violence in the family, are suggested as etiological factors in individual patients. However, many patients with GID do not have these factors, and many children

TABLE 5–7.   **DSM-IV-TR diagnostic criteria for gender identity disorder**

A. A strong and persistent cross-gender identification (not merely a desire for any perceived cultural advantages of being the other sex).

In children, the disturbance is manifested by four (or more) of the following:

(1) repeatedly stated desire to be, or insistence that he or she is, the other sex

(2) in boys, preference for cross-dressing or simulating female attire; in girls, insistence on wearing only stereotypical masculine clothing

(3) strong and persistent preferences for cross-sex roles in make-believe play or persistent fantasies of being the other sex

(4) intense desire to participate in the stereotypical games and pastimes of the other sex

(5) strong preference for playmates of the other sex

In adolescents and adults, the disturbance is manifested by symptoms such as a stated desire to be the other sex, frequent passing as the other sex, desire to live or be treated as the other sex, or the conviction that he or she has the typical feelings and reactions of the other sex.

B. Persistent discomfort with his or her sex or sense of inappropriateness in the gender role of that sex.

In children, the disturbance is manifested by any of the following: in boys, assertion that his penis or testes are disgusting or will disappear or assertion that it would be better not to have a penis, or aversion toward rough-and-tumble play and rejection of male stereotypical toys, games, and activities; in girls, rejection of urinating in a sitting position, assertion that she has or will grow a penis, or assertion that she does not want to grow breasts or menstruate, or marked aversion toward normative feminine clothing.

In adolescents and adults, the disturbance is manifested by symptoms such as preoccupation with getting rid of primary and secondary sex characteristics (e.g., request for hormones, surgery, or other procedures to physically alter sexual characteristics to simulate the other sex) or belief that he or she was born the wrong sex.

TABLE 5–7.	DSM-IV-TR diagnostic criteria for gender identity disorder *(continued)*

C. The disturbance is not concurrent with a physical intersex condition.
D. The disturbance causes clinically significant distress or impairment in social, occupational, or other important areas of functioning.

Code based on current age:

   302.6   **Gender identity disorder in children**
   302.85 **Gender identity disorder in adolescents or adults**

exposed to these dynamics do not develop GID. Contrary to popular belief, children raised in transsexual or lesbian households show no evidence of confusion about gender identity or role behavior.

Course and Prognosis

Peer relationships are usually significantly impaired. Children generally have rigid gender role expectations and do not tolerate a child who does not conform to these, although tomboys have somewhat more latitude than effeminate boys, who are teased and ostracized. Adolescents can be particularly cruel to peers who do not conform to conventional notions of gender role. The pervasive discomfort of the young patient with GID leads to low self-esteem and interferes with school performance.

As a group, patients with GID have levels of comorbid psychiatric disorders equal to those of other clinically referred patients, although some youngsters with GID have few symptoms of other disorders. Separation anxiety is common in boys with GID.

Follow-up studies of clinical populations show that some effeminate boys become transsexual adults and generally have serious difficulty in social adaptation. A larger number of boys with gender-atypical characteristics develop a homosexual orientation in adulthood, which does not warrant a psychiatric diagnosis. Clinically referred girls with GID show a variety of gender and sexual orientations as adults, although nonreferred tomboys almost always develop more typically feminine interests at puberty. Treatment of GID appears to be more effective in childhood than in adolescence. For children who subsequently develop transsexualism as adolescents or adults, treatment is medically and psychiatrically difficult.

Evaluation and Differential Diagnosis

Sensitive clinical evaluation is required. Older children or adolescents with GID learn from repeated negative feedback not to verbalize their wishes or beliefs about their gender and their anatomy. Children with GID must be differentiated from those who simply do not meet the gender role expectations of their families or their culture. Children with GID can be distinguished from tomboys or boys who have more studious or musical interests (rather than rough-and-tumble play and sports) by the rigidity of their avoidance of the expected gender role, their profound unhappiness with their physical gender, and their discomfort with or dislike of their sexual anatomy. Pediatric evaluation is indicated to rule out a *physical or hormonal abnormality* such as hermaphroditism, congenital adrenal hyperplasia, or androgen insensitivity syndrome.

Treatment

The best documented treatment of childhood GID is behavior modification. Changes in role behavior can lead to changes in gender identity, as well as improved self-esteem and decreased depression. Techniques include social reinforcement of gender-concordant behaviors, ignoring of cross-gender behaviors, reinforcement of play with appropriate toys, response cost (loss of points or privileges) for gender-inappropriate speech or play, and modeling and shaping of skills the child does not have. Generalization is not automatic, and results are best if the program is conducted at home, in school, and at the clinic and several behaviors are addressed. Years of intensive treatment may be required. Cognitive-behavioral self-monitoring of mannerisms also may be useful.

Dynamic individual psychotherapy has been successful in

some patients. Family therapy is often indicated, as is treatment of coexisting mood or conduct disorders. Parent counseling is always needed.

■ SLEEP DISORDERS

Evaluation of Sleep-Related Complaints

Nearly 25% of all children experience a sleep disorder. The most common problems are sleep talking, nightmares, nighttime waking, difficulty falling asleep, enuresis, bruxism, sleep rocking, restless legs syndrome, and night terrors. Assessment of sleep disorders includes pediatric history and physical examination, particularly seeking evidence of obesity, enlarged tonsils, middle ear problems, a seizure disorder, allergies, asthma, and medication use. The evaluation of the airway includes tonsillar size, nasal airflow, and facial abnormalities. Abnormal physical findings in a child with a sleep continuity disorder are relatively infrequent, however. A sleep history includes details of the patient's physical environment for sleeping and inquiries about whether the patient uses a pacifier, sucks his or her fingers while asleep, has nighttime feedings, awakens screaming and confused, walks or talks while asleep, has frequent nightmares, has enuresis, grinds his or her teeth, has nighttime fears, snores, experiences restless legs or nocturnal leg jerks, and rocks or bangs his or her head at night. Sleep habits are reviewed and include co-sleeping, sleep schedules, and intake of caffeinated beverages. Children may resist bedtime or develop diurnal patterns that include difficulty awakening, daytime sleepiness, fatigue, naps, and feelings of anxiety or depression. Developmental and psychiatric histories are necessary to assess possible psychiatric etiology or comorbidity. In addition, details of recent stressors, parental reactions to sleep-related problems, substance abuse (in older children or adolescents), and the effects of prior behavioral and pharmacological interventions are needed. When there is persistent nighttime waking or persistent sleep loss, or sleep apnea or nocturnal epilepsy are suspected, a sleep laboratory evaluation (polysomnography) may be indicated, including sleep electroencephalogram (EEG), eye movements, electromyogram, airflow, respiratory effort, electrocardiogram, and video monitoring. A sleep-deprived EEG is useful in the evaluation of possible seizures. A drug screen may be needed in adolescents. Sleep deprivation is particularly prevalent during adolescence, when late-night activities and early-morning academic schedules limit the available hours for sleep.

Dyssomnias

Dyssomnias, including insomnia, narcolepsy, and breathing-related sleep disorder, are characterized by disturbance in the initiation or maintenance of sleep, or by an excessive amount of daytime sleepiness.

Insomnia

Clinical description.   Patients with insomnia have persistent difficulty initiating or maintaining sleep (compared with norms for age) that results in impaired functioning.

Epidemiology.   Most infants sleep through the night (or at least do not fuss when they awaken) by age 6–9 months. Up to one-half of all infants, however, have irregular sleep patterns and occasional or persistent night wakening throughout the first year. A study of children without sleep disorders found that 21% of 18- to 23-month-olds awakened during the night. Of the 24- to 29-month-olds, 31% took more than 30 minutes to fall asleep on more than 3 nights per week. Children ages 30–36 months are most likely to have difficulty settling for the night (16%) and express fears of the dark (24%) (Crowell et al. 1987). At age 5 years, more than 20% of children surveyed continued to wake during the night and call out to their parents. Parental reinforcement may have contributed to this behavior, however. By school age, children are asleep for 95%–97% of the time they are in bed (Carskadon and Dement 1987).

Etiology.   Sleep patterns in infants and toddlers may be affected by perinatal complications, colic, separation anxiety, the absence of a favorite transitional object, and parent–child interactions. The schedule of daytime naps for preschoolers can contribute to problems sleeping at night. Young children with sleep continuity disorders have a higher rate of family stressors, including parental absence because of employment, family illness, and maternal depression.

Chronic insomnia is much more frequent in children with psychiatric disorders. It is often related to behavior or habit problems in settling for the night (especially in the child with ADHD, ODD, or separation anxiety disorder) or may be a symptom of mood disorder, pervasive developmental disorder, or schizophrenia.

Insomnia may be secondary to the use of caffeine or prescribed or over-the-counter medication such as phenobarbital, theophylline, decongestants, and stimulants, or substance abuse. Patients suffering from physical discomfort may have difficulty staying asleep.

Treatment.   After any psychiatric or medical cause is addressed, in young children the first steps are to remove any factors that interfere with sleep and to enhance structure that encourages sleep (e.g., a bedtime routine, the use of a transitional object, or a night light for the child who is afraid of the dark). Behavior modification removes the secondary gain of parental attention at night and provides positive reinforcement for the child who stays quietly in his or her own room. Older children and adolescents may benefit from hypnosis or relaxation techniques. Consistency among all family members is critical to success. Caregivers should choose a single approach to the sleep disorder and avoid rapidly changing interventions.

In adolescents with insomnia, behavior therapy can disrupt the conditioned association between bedtime habits and anxiety regarding inability to sleep. Sleep hygiene is improved by using the bed only for sleeping, establishing a regular sleep schedule, and avoiding naps.

Chloral hydrate or an antihistamine (e.g., diphenhydramine hydrochloride) may be indicated for short-term use in a crisis. Hypnotic medications are not recommended for chronic use. Many children respond to sedatives with paradoxical agitation. If the child has extreme fear or anxiety, a short-acting benzodiazepine (e.g., triazolam) may be used briefly.

Narcolepsy

Clinical description.   Narcolepsy is characterized by sudden, uncontrollable attacks of rapid eye movement (REM) sleep during wakefulness. Sleep is usually resisted, but the patient eventually succumbs. Features in children are similar to those seen in adults, including excessive daytime sleepiness, cataplexy, hypnagogic visual hallucinations, and sleep paralysis. Children and adolescents have variable presentations, with few experiencing all four symptoms simultaneously. The diagnosis is made by polysomnography.

Epidemiology.   The prevalence of narcolepsy is 1 per 10,000 individuals.

Etiology.   Narcolepsy may have an autosomal dominant genetic transmission but with very low penetrance. Although a family history of narcolepsy can support the diagnosis, many cases have no evidence of family predisposition.

Course and prognosis.   Onset of narcolepsy is typically in late adolescence or early adulthood, although one-fifth of narcoleptic adults have an onset before puberty. Sleep attacks and cataplexy may interfere significantly with schoolwork and peer relationships. Behavioral and emotional changes can develop early in the clinical presentation.

Differential diagnosis.   The most likely alternative diagnosis to narcolepsy is the *normal* increase in daytime sleep and reports of sleepiness in adolescence. Truly excessive daytime sleep may be an *avoidance* mechanism, even in the classroom, or secondary to *insomnia, environmental interference with sleep,* or *sleep apnea.* Sleep-onset or waking hallucinations may be misidentified as symptoms of *psychosis,* and cataplexy or sleep attacks may be confused with a *sei-*

zure disorder or *conversion disorder. Substance use* or *withdrawal* should also be suspected when sleep continuity is disrupted.

Treatment.   Treatment of narcolepsy begins with educating the patient and family members about the nature and course of the disorder. A regular sleep schedule should be maintained to improve sleep hygiene. Short-acting stimulant drugs (methylphenidate, amphetamine) are used to reduce sleep attacks, particularly while the child is at school. Modafinil (Provigil) is a nonstimulant wakefulness-promoting agent that has recently been approved for use in narcolepsy. Very low doses of REM suppressant medications, such as protriptyline or clomipramine, are useful treatments for cataplexy or hypnagogic hallucinations.

Breathing-Related Sleep Disorder (Sleep-Disordered Breathing)

Clinical description.   Breathing-related sleep disorder is characterized by episodes of partial or complete upper airway obstruction and is part of a spectrum of disorders that includes primary snoring and upper airway resistance syndrome (usually due to adenotonsillar hypertrophy). Children may show behavior problems that typically present as inattention or excessive daytime sleepiness or activity. They are, however, less likely to have daytime somnolence than are adults. Actual apnea is rare in children. The preferred term is sleep-disordered breathing (SDB).

Epidemiology.   The prevalence of sleep apnea is thought to be approximately 2% for children between ages 2 and 6 years. SDB is likely more common, and often is unrecognized. There is an increased risk during midadolescence, with symptoms that mirror the adult presentation. Prior to puberty, SDB is equally likely in males and females.

Etiology.   SDB is caused by the loss of patency of the upper airway. This may be caused by structural or neurological factors. With obstruction, respiratory efforts increase and the central nervous system is activated, leading to greater muscle activity and relief of the obstruction. Additional medical causes of SDB include obesity, nocturnal asthma, lax upper airway structures, maxillofacial abnormalities, neuromuscular disease, Down syndrome, hypothyroidism, and dysfunction of central control of breathing.

Course and prognosis. SDB is rarely diagnosed before age 6–12 months. The degree of adenotonsillar hypertrophy does not correlate with the symptomatology. Overnight polysomnography is required to make the diagnosis. Children with sleep apnea may have medical complications, including pulmonary hypertension, systemic hypertension, right heart failure, cor pulmonale, failure to thrive, short stature, and enuresis. Greater awareness of the disorder has dramatically decreased the incidence of medical complications. Psychiatric and academic difficulties may include developmental delay, irritability, aggressiveness, distractibility, inattention, hyperactivity, and enuresis.

Treatment. The treatment of SDB is generally surgical. A tonsillectomy and adenoidectomy successfully treats nearly 70% of pediatric cases. Continuous positive airway pressure (CPAP) is well accepted by young patients. If the cause is central, a home apnea monitor may be required. Tracheostomy is a treatment of last resort.

Parasomnias

These disorders disrupt sleep with abnormalities of arousal, partial arousal, or sleep-stage transitions. The patient does not complain of insomnia or sleepiness. Parasomnias include nightmare disorder, sleep terror disorder, and sleepwalking disorder.

Nightmare Disorder

Clinical description. Occasional nightmares are normal in children and adolescents. Nightmares occur during REM sleep, more commonly in the second half of the night. If the youngster awakens, he or she rapidly becomes oriented and alert, can recount the dream, and rapidly falls back to sleep. Frequency of nightmares waxes and wanes as the child develops. DSM-IV-TR criteria for nightmare disorder require "repeated" awakenings caused by nightmares with "significant distress" and "detailed recall." The child frequently cannot return to sleep and will ask to sleep with the parents. The boundary between normally occurring frightening dreams and nightmare disorder is not clear.

Epidemiology. Among children ages 3–5 years, 10%–50% have recurrent nightmares that disturb their parents. Symptoms typically begin during preschool years and decrease in frequency with age. Occasionally, the disorder persists into adulthood.

Etiology. No psychiatric conditions are associated consistently with nightmare disorder in children. Nightmares tend to increase with stress, sleep deprivation, fatigue, and change in sleep environment. Medications, especially β-blockers, TCAs, alcohol, barbiturates, and benzodiazepines, may also produce nightmares.

Differential diagnosis. The main alternative diagnoses to nightmare disorder are *sleep terror disorder, breathing-related sleep disorder, narcolepsy, panic disorder,* and *drug-induced nightmares* (e.g., as a result of antidepressant or caffeine use).

Treatment. Reassurance is generally the best approach. The child should not be pressured to describe the nightmare but should be given an opportunity to talk about his or her fears. Sleep schedules should be normalized and sleep time increased for patients suffering from sleep deprivation. Children and adolescents with more persistent problems may require anxiety reduction techniques, such as relaxation, imagery combined with systematic desensitization, and dream reorganization.

Sleep Terror Disorder (Pavor Nocturnus)

Clinical description. Episodes of sleep terror disorder typically occur during the first third of the night, in Stage 3 and 4 delta (non-REM) sleep, and last 1–10 minutes. The child looks terrified, screams, and appears to be staring, with dilated pupils, sweating, rapid pulse, and hyperventilation. The child is agitated and confused and cannot be comforted. Subsequently, when alert, the child typically has no memory of the episode but may have brief recall of a feeling of terror or of dream fragments. The child rapidly returns to sleep when the episode is over and in the morning has no memory of the event. The parents are far more distressed than the child.

Epidemiology.   Sleep terror disorder is often seen in children ages 3–6 years, but isolated episodes are common throughout childhood. The estimated prevalence of the full disorder in children is 1%–6%, and it is more common in boys than in girls. A study of sleep habits in middle-class 1- to 3-year-olds found the 1-week prevalence of at least one episode to be 7% (Crowell et al. 1987).

Etiology.   Sleep terror disorder is considered to be developmental and is not caused by anxiety or distress during the day. Sleep terrors can be increased by sleep deprivation or anything that fragments sleep, including fever, illness, a full bladder, SDB, and several medications, including lithium, prolixin, and desipramine. Patients may experience symptoms due to cumulative sleep loss, if night terrors are frequent. Family history of sleep terror is common.

Course and prognosis.   The age at onset is typically between 4 and 12 years, with spontaneous resolution by adolescence. The number and frequency of episodes are highly variable. Consecutive episodes may be separated by days or weeks, but in rare instances they may occur on consecutive nights. No psychiatric conditions are typically associated with nightmare disorder in children.

Differential diagnosis.   Simple *nightmares* or *nightmare disorder* usually occur in the latter half of the night. Those children remember the dream and show less physiological arousal and confusion than do those with sleep terror disorder. Other alternatives are *hypnagogic or hypnopompic hallucinations* or *epileptic seizures* during sleep with postictal confusion. Occasionally, patients with *breathing-related sleep disorder* will awaken in a state of panic that resembles sleep terror disorder.

Treatment.   Parents should be educated about the disorder and reassured that the episodes do not indicate a serious psychiatric or neurological problem. The child's sleep schedule is monitored to provide a sufficient amount of time spent in bed. The patient's safety should be assured by erecting gates across stairs and locking doors and windows to prevent leaving the house. Waking the child before the usual time of the night terror may abort attacks. However, waking the child during the event should be avoided because it may exacerbate or prolong the episode. Medication is used only if the episodes are frequent, put the child in physical danger, severely disrupt the family, or interfere with daytime functioning. A low dose of imipramine or diazepam decreases delta sleep and may temporarily treat sleep terror disorder. However, when the medication is discontinued, delta sleep rebounds and the disorder may recur (Crowell et al. 1987). If SDB is diagnosed, surgery can relieve both SDB and night terrors.

Sleepwalking Disorder (Somnambulism)

Clinical description.   Sleepwalking disorder is characterized by repeated episodes of arising from bed and engaging in motor activities while still asleep. Episodes, which last a few minutes to a half hour, typically occur 1–3 hours after the child falls asleep, during Stage 3 and 4 delta (non-REM) sleep. The child or adolescent arises quietly and engages in perseverative, stereotyped movements (such as picking at blankets), which may progress to walking and other complex behaviors. He or she is difficult to awaken, and coordination is poor. Although the child may be able to see, the risk of injury is high. Speech, when present, is usually incomprehensible. The youngster may awaken and be confused, may return to bed, or may lie down somewhere else and continue sleeping. Morning amnesia is typical. Occasionally, the patient engages in inappropriate behavior, such as urinating in the closet. Young children tend to walk toward a light or sound. Older children may wake in an agitated state with garbled speech and a tendency to recoil when touched.

Epidemiology. A longitudinal study of children and adolescents between ages 6 and 16 years found a 40% incidence of sleepwalking and a yearly prevalence of 6%–17%. Only 2%–3% had more than one episode per month. Sleepwalking continued for 5 years in 33% and for 10 years in 12% of the group.

Etiology. Likelihood of sleepwalking is increased when the child is overtired or under stress. Internal stimuli (e.g., urinary urgency, SDB, or restless legs syndrome) or external stimuli (e.g., noise) may precipitate an episode. Sleepwalking tends be familial. Of patients who sleepwalk, 10%–20% have first-degree relatives with the disorder.

Course and prognosis. The onset of sleepwalking is usually between ages 4 and 8 years, with the peak prevalence at age 12 years. Most cases remit spontaneously by age 15 years.

Differential diagnosis. Diagnostic alternatives to sleepwalking disorder include nocturnal *seizures* and *waking and wandering.* During a *sleep terror,* children occasionally walk in an attempt to escape frightening stimuli. *Breathing-related sleep disorder* may also cause sudden confusion and agitation that will lead the patient to wander.

Treatment. Parents should be guided to remove hazards in the environment. They may need to lock the child's door. Children should maintain regular sleep schedules. If sleepwalking is frequent or dangerous, a low dose of imipramine at bedtime may be used. Pharmacological treatments are limited because symptoms tend to return after the medication is discontinued.

■ ADJUSTMENT DISORDERS

Clinical Description

Adjustment disorder is characterized by the development of a dysfunctional reaction that occurs within 3 months of the onset of a stressor and that adversely affects functioning. An adjustment disorder may be diagnosed in a person with another mental disorder only if an identifiable stressor leads to the development of symptoms that are not characteristic of the original disorder. Adjustment disorders have six subtypes, classified by symptoms of depression, anxiety, and behavior (conduct).

Common stressors in childhood and adolescence include parental divorce, change in schools, physical illness, the birth of a sibling, parental unemployment, and abuse or neglect. Adolescents may be particularly vulnerable to disruptions in a relationship with a boyfriend or girlfriend.

Epidemiology

The prevalence of adjustment disorders in community samples of youth is between 2% and 8%. Populations with particularly severe stressors (i.e., surgical patients) have high rates of adjustment disorder. Children and adolescents usually have mixed presentations with symptoms that are not predominantly affective or behavioral.

Etiology

The adjustment disorder is presumed to be precipitated by the identified stressor. The child's reaction to the stressor rather than the characteristics of the stressor determine whether the diagnosis is present. Even in cases where the patient's emotional response to the stressor may be expected, if the symptom presentation is causing significant impairment, a diagnosis of adjustment disorder is made.

Course and Prognosis

Symptoms of adjustment disorder will typically remit when the stressor is removed or when a new level of adaptation is reached. By definition, if the disorder lasts for more than 6 months after the stressor or its consequences have stopped, then a different diagnosis is warranted. The prognosis depends on the severity and duration of the stressor and its meaning to the child; the vulnerability of the individual; and the response of the family, school, and peers to both the stressor and the young person's reaction. In general, the prognosis is assumed to be benign, although patients can present with active and passive suicidal behavior, substance abuse, and recurrent somatic complaints. Patients with adjustment disorder are more frequently admitted to medical emergency rooms and inpatient units than are control groups without psychiatric symptoms.

Follow-up of adolescents 5 years after receiving a (DSM-II [American Psychiatric Association 1968]) clinical diagnosis of adjustment disorder found that 57% were well, although 23% of these patients had qualified for another psychiatric diagnosis during the intervening period. Research diagnoses at follow-up included schizophrenia, affective disorders, antisocial personality disorder, and substance abuse disorders. One patient committed suicide (Andreasen and Hoenk 1982).

Evaluation and Differential Diagnosis

The clinician should examine the patient thoroughly and obtain reports from the child, parent, and teacher to identify stressors, rather than assuming that the first reported or obvious stressor is the crucial one. Other psychiatric diagnoses should be sought. Adjustment disorder is a residual category and should be used only if the patient's symptoms do not meet criteria for another DSM-IV-TR disorder. In the past, overuse of the diagnosis of adjustment disorder (in an effort to avoid "labeling" children) has often obscured another psychiatric diagnosis. Expectable reactions to the death of a loved one should be classified as *uncomplicated bereavement.* If functional impairment is not evident, or if the degree of emotional or behavioral reaction is considered "normal and expectable," then a V code, such as *relationship problem* or *phase of life problem,* should be used. If the primary reaction to a stressor is exacerbation of a pediatric disorder (e.g., asthma or diabetes), the appropriate diagnosis is *psychological factor affecting medical condition.* If the stressor is sudden and catastrophic or potentially so, *PTSD* or *acute stress disorder* should be diagnosed if the other criteria are met.

Treatment

Crisis intervention and time-limited psychotherapy techniques may be useful for treatment of adjustment disorder. Cognitive therapy to improve coping skills and problem-solving abilities and to reduce dysfunctional thoughts and beliefs in reaction to the stressor may be beneficial. Environmental intervention may be indicated to remove or ameliorate the stressor and to mobilize family and community support systems. Explanations to parents and teachers of the child's or adolescent's reactions may reduce impairment and shorten the course of the disorder. Active treatment of these disorders may reduce subsequent morbidity. For example, if adjustment disorder with depressed mood is debilitating, the same treatments as for major depression may be indicated.

■ REFERENCES

American Psychiatric Association: Diagnostic and Statistical Manual of Mental Disorders, 2nd Edition. Washington, DC, American Psychiatric Association, 1968

American Psychiatric Association: Diagnostic and Statistical Manual of Mental Disorders, 3rd Edition, Revised. Washington, DC, American Psychiatric Association, 1987

American Psychiatric Association: Diagnostic and Statistical Manual of Mental Disorders, 4th Edition. Washington, DC, American Psychiatric Association, 1994

American Psychiatric Association: Diagnostic and Statistical Manual of Mental Disorders, 4th Edition, Text Revision. Washington, DC, American Psychiatric Association, 2000

Andreasen NC, Hoenk PR: The predictive value of adjustment disorders: a follow-up study. Am J Psychiatry 139:584–590, 1982

Biederman J, Rosenbaum JF, Bolduc-Murphy EA, et al: A 3-year follow-up of children with and without behavioral inhibition. J Am Acad Child Adolesc Psychiatry 32:814–821, 1993

Biederman J, Faraone SV, Marrs A, et al: Panic disorder and agoraphobia in consecutively referred children and adolescents. J Am Acad Child Adolesc Psychiatry 36:214–223, 1997

Biederman J, Hirschfeld-Becker DR, Rosenbaum JF, et al: Further evidence of association between behavioral inhibition and social anxiety in children. Am J. Psychiatry 158:1673–1679, 2001

Birmaher B, Khetarpal S, Brent D, et al: The Screen for Child Anxiety Related Emotional Disorders (SCARED): scale construction and psychometric characteristics. J Am Acad Child Adolesc Psychiatry 36:545–553, 1997

Busatto GF, Bushpiguel CA, Zamignani DR, et al: Regional cerebral blood flow abnormalities in early onset obsessive-compulsive disorder: an exploratory SPECT study. J Am Acad Child Adolesc Psychiatry 40:347–354, 2001

Carskadon MA, Dement WC: Daytime sleepiness: quantification of a behavioral state. Neurosci Biobehav Rev 11:307–317, 1987

Caspi A, Henry B, McGee RO, et al: Temperamental origins of child and adolescent behavior problems: from age three to age fifteen. Child Dev 66:55–68, 1995

Crowell J, Keener M, Ginsburg N, et al: Sleep habits in toddlers 18 to 36 months old. J Am Acad Child Adolesc Psychiatry 26:510–515, 1987

Dias PJ: Adolescent substance abuse assessment in the office. Pediatr Clin N Am 49:269–300, 2002

Fichter MM, Quadflieg N: Six-year course of bulimia nervosa. Int J Eat Disord 22:361–384, 1997

Geller B, Zimerman B, William M, et al: Phenomenology of prepubertal and early adolescent bipolar disorders: examples of elated mood, grandiose behaviors, decreased need for sleep, racing thoughts and hypersexuality. J Child Adolesc Psychopharmacol 12:3–9, 2002a

Geller B, Zimerman B, Williams M, et al: DSM-IV mania symptoms in a prepubertal and early adolescent bipolar disorder phenotype compared to attention-deficit hyperactive and normal controls. J Child Adolesc Psychopharmacol 12:11–25, 2002b

Harrell AV, Wirtz PW: Screening for adolescent problem drinking: validation of a multi-dimensional instrument for case identification. Psychol Assess 1:61–63, 1989

Hayward C, Killen JD, Taylor CB: Panic attacks in young adolescents. Am J Psychiatry 146:1061–1062, 1989

Henggeler SW, Clingempeel WG, Brondino MJ, et al: Four-year follow-up of Multisystemic Therapy with substance-abusing and substance-dependent juvenile offenders. J Am Acad Child Adolesc Psychiatry 41:868–874, 2002

Hughes CW, Emslie GJ, Crismon L, et al: The Texas Children's Medication Algorithm Project: report of the Texas Consensus Conference Panel on Medication Treatment of Childhood Major Depressive Disorder. J Am Acad Child Adolesc Psychiatry 38:1442–1454, 1999

Kagan J, Reznick JS, Snidman N: Biological bases of childhood shyness. Science 240:167–171, 1988

Kandel DB: Stages in adolescent involvement in drug use. Science 190: 912–914, 1975

Kovacs M: The Children's Depression Inventory (CDI). Psychopharmacol Bull 21:995–998, 1985

Kovacs M: The course of childhood-onset depressive disorders. Psychiatric Annals 26:326–330, 1996

Lewinsohn PM, Clarke GN, Seeley JR, et al: Major depression in community adolescents: age at onset, episode duration, and time to recurrence. J Am Acad Child Adolesc Psychiatry 33:809–818, 1994

Lewinsohn PM, Klein DN, Seeley JR: Bipolar disorders in a community sample of older adolescents: prevalence, phenomenology, comorbidity, and course. J Am Acad Child Adolesc Psychiatry 34:454–463, 1995

MacMillan HL, Fleming JE, Streiner DL, et al: Childhood abuse and lifetime psychopathology in a community sample. Am J Psychiatry 158:1878–1883, 2001

March JS, Leonard HL, Swedo SE: Neuropsychiatry of obsessive-compulsive disorder in children and adolescents. Compr Ther 21:507–512, 1995

March JS, Parker JD, Sullivan K, et al: The Multidimensional Anxiety Scale for Children (MASC): factor structure, reliability, and validity. J Am Acad Child Adolesc Psychiatry 36:554–565, 1997

McCloskey LA, Walker M: Posttraumatic stress in children exposed to family violence and single-event trauma. J Am Acad Child Adolesc Psychiatry 39:108–115, 2000

McKenna K, Gordon CT, Lenane M, et al: Looking for childhood-onset schizophrenia: the first 71 cases screened. J Am Acad Child Adolesc Psychiatry 33:636–644, 1994

Mehler P: Diagnosis and care of patients with anorexia nervosa in primary care settings. Ann Intern Med 134:1048–1059, 2001

Mellin LM, Irwin CE, Scully S: Prevalence of disordered eating in girls: a survey of middle-class children. J Am Diet Assoc 92:851–853, 1992

Minuchin S, Rosman BL, Baker L: Psychosomatic Families: Anorexia Nervosa in Context. Cambridge, MA, Harvard University Press, 1978

Mufson L, Weissman MM, Moreau D, et al: Efficacy of interpersonal psychotherapy for depressed adolescents. Arch Gen Psychiatry 56:573–579, 1999

Ollendick TH: Reliability and validity of the Revised Fear Survey Schedule for Children (FSSC-R). Behav Res Ther 21:685–692, 1983

Palla B, Litt IF: Medical complications of eating disorders in adolescents. Pediatrics 81:613–623, 1988

Pleak PR, Meyer-Bahlburg HF, O'Brien JD, et al: Cross-gender behavior and psychopathology in boy psychiatric outpatients. J Am Acad Child Adolesc Psychiatry 28:385–393, 1989

Pynoos RS, Frederick C, Nader K, et al: Life threat and posttraumatic stress in school-age children. Arch Gen Psychiatry 44:1057–1063, 1987

Research Units on Pediatric Psychopharmacology Anxiety Study Group: The Pediatric Anxiety Rating Scale (PARS): development and psychometric properties. J Am Acad Child Adolesc Psychiatry 41:1061–1069, 2002

Rosario-Campos MC, Leckman JF, Mercadante MT, et al: Adults with early onset obsessive-compulsive disorder. Am J Psychiatry 158:1899–1903, 2001

Rynn MA, Siqueland L, Rickets K: Placebo-controlled trial of sertraline in the treatment of children with generalized anxiety disorder. Am J Psychiatry 158:2008–2014, 2001

Scahill L, Riddle MA, McSwiggin-Harden M, et al: Children's Yale-Brown Obsessive-Compulsive Scale: reliability and validity. J Am Acad Child Adolesc Psychiatry 36:844–852, 1997

Schwartz RC, Barrett MJ, Saba G: Family therapy for bulimia, in Handbook of Psychotherapy for Anorexia Nervosa and Bulimia. Edited by Garner DM, Garfinkel PE. New York, Guilford, 1985, pp 280–307

Schwartz RH, Wirtz PW: Potential substance abuse: detection among adolescent patients: using the Drug and Alcohol Problem (DAP) Quick Screen, a 30-item questionnaire. Clin Pediatr (Phila) 29:38–43, 1990

Sonis WA, Yellin AM, Garfinkel BD, et al: The antidepressant effect of light in seasonal affective disorder of childhood and adolescence. Psychopharmacol Bull 23:360–364, 1987

Strober M, Carlson G: Bipolar illness in adolescents with major depression: clinical, genetic, and psychopharmacologic investigation. Arch Gen Psychiatry 39:549–555, 1982

Swedo SE, Rapoport JL, Leonard H, et al: Obsessive-compulsive disorder in children and adolescents: clinical phenomenology of 70 consecutive cases. Arch Gen Psychiatry 46:335–341, 1989

Swedo SE, Leonard HL, Garvey M, et al: Pediatric autoimmune neuropsychiatric disorders associated with streptococcal infections: clinical description of the first 50 cases. Am J Psychiatry 155:264–271, 1998

TADS Team: Treatment for Adolescents with Depression Study (TADS): rationale, design, and methods. J Am Acad Child Adolesc Psychiatry 42:531–542, 2003

Tarter RE: Evaluation and treatment of adolescent substance abuse: a decision tree method. Am J Drug Alcohol Abuse 16:1–46, 1990

Terr LC: Childhood psychic trauma, in Basic Handbook of Child Psychiatry, Vol 5. Edited by Call JD, Cohen RL, Harrison SI, et al. New York, Basic Books, 1987, pp 262–272

Theander S: Outcome and prognosis in anorexia nervosa and bulimia: some results of previous investigations, compared with those of a Swedish long-term study. J Psychiatr Res 19:493–508, 1985

Vitiello B, Behar D, Wolfson S, et al: Diagnosis of panic disorder in prepubertal children. J Am Acad Child Adolesc Psychiatry 29:782–784, 1990

Walkup JT, Labellarte MJ, Riddle MA, et al: Fluvoxamine for the treatment of anxiety disorders in children and adolescents. N Engl J Med 344:1279–1285, 2001

Weissman MM, Wolk S, Goldstein RB, et al: Depressed adolescents grown up. JAMA 281:1707–1713, 1999

Windle M, Windle RC: Depressive symptoms and cigarette smoking among middle adolescents: prospective associations and intrapersonal and interpersonal influences. J Consult Clin Psychol 69:215–226, 2001

Wolk SI, Weissman MM: Suicidal behavior in depressed children grown up: preliminary results of a longitudinal study. Psychiatric Annals 26:331–335, 1996

■ ADDITIONAL READING

Eating Disorders

Rome ES, Ammerman S, Rosen DS, et al: Children and adolescents with eating disorders: the state of the art. Pediatrics 111:e98–e108, 2003

Substance-Related Disorders

American Academy of Child and Adolescent Psychiatry: Practice parameters for the assessment and treatment of children and adolescents with substance use disorders. J Am Acad Child Adolesc Psychiatry 36 (10 suppl):140S–156S, 1997

Dias PJ: Adolescent substance abuse assessment in the office. Pediatr Clin N Am 49:269–300, 2002

Estroff TW (ed): Manual of Adolescent Substance Abuse Treatment. Washington, DC, American Psychiatric Press, 2001

Jaffe SL: Adolescent Substance Abuse Intervention Workbook: Taking a First Step. Washington, DC, American Psychiatric Press, 2000 (includes both a workbook for teens and a manual for staff)

Moolchan ET, Ernst M, Henningfield JE: A review of tobacco smoking in adolescents: treatment implications. J Am Acad Child Adolesc Psychiatry 39:682–693, 2000

Weinberg NZ, Rahdert E, Colliver JD, et al: Adolescent substance abuse: a review of the past 10 years. J Am Acad Child Adolesc Psychiatry 37:252–261, 1998

Schizophrenia

American Academy of Child and Adolescent Psychiatry: Practice parameter for the assessment and treatment of children and adolescents with schizophrenia. J Am Acad Child Adolesc Psychiatry 40 (7 suppl):4S–23S, 2001

Mood Disorders

American Academy of Child and Adolescent Psychiatry: Practice parameters for the assessment and treatment of children and adolescents with bipolar disorder. J Am Acad Child Adolesc Psychiatry 36 (10 suppl):157S–176S, 1997

American Academy of Child and Adolescent Psychiatry: Practice parameters for the assessment and treatment of children and adolescents with depressive disorders. J Am Acad Child Adolesc Psychiatry 37 (10 suppl):63S–83S, 1998

Mufson L, Moreau D, Weissman MM, et al: Interpersonal Psychotherapy for Depressed Adolescents. New York, Guilford, 1993

Shaffer D, Waslick BD: The Many Faces of Depression in Children and Adolescents. Washington, DC, American Psychiatric Press, 2002

Wilkes TCR, Belsher G, Rush AJ, et al: Cognitive Therapy for Depressed Adolescents. New York, Guilford, 1994

Anxiety Disorders

American Academy of Child and Adolescent Psychiatry: Practice parameters for the assessment and treatment of children and adolescents with anxiety disorders. J Am Acad Child Adolesc Psychiatry 36 (10 suppl):69S–84S, 1997

American Academy of Child and Adolescent Psychiatry: Practice parameters for the assessment and treatment of children and adolescents with obsessive-compulsive disorder. J Am Acad Child Adolesc Psychiatry 37 (10 suppl):27S–45S, 1998

American Academy of Child and Adolescent Psychiatry: Practice parameters for the assessment and treatment of children and adolescents with posttraumatic stress disorder. J Am Acad Child Adolesc Psychiatry 37 (10 suppl):4S–26S, 1998

March JS (ed): Anxiety Disorders in Children and Adolescents. New York, Guilford, 1995

Ollendick TH, King NJ, Muris P: Fears and phobias in children: phenomenology, epidemiology, and aetiology. Child and Adolescent Mental Health 7:98–106, 2002

Gender Identity Disorder

Zucker KJ: Gender identity disorder in children and adolescents, in Treatments of Psychiatric Disorders, 3rd Edition, Vol 2. Gabbard GO, Editor-in-Chief. Washington, DC, American Psychiatric Press, 2001, pp 2069–2094

Sleep Disorders

Howard BJ, Wong J: Sleep disorders. Pediatrics in Review 22:327–342, 2001

6

DEVELOPMENTAL
DISORDERS

The pervasive developmental disorders (PDDs), including autistic disorder, and specific developmental disorders are coded on DSM-IV-TR (American Psychiatric Association 2000) Axis I. Mental retardation is the only developmental disorder now coded on Axis II.

■ MENTAL RETARDATION

Clinical Description

The DSM-IV-TR diagnosis of mental retardation requires low intelligence (IQ of approximately 70 or below), deficits in adaptive functioning, and onset prior to age 18 years. Adaptive skills include communication, self-care, home living, social skills, community resource use, self-direction, health and safety, functional academics, leisure, and work. Clinical features vary according to the degree of retardation (Table 6–1).

Epidemiology

Prevalence of mental retardation in the United States ranges from 1% to 3%, depending on the definition of adaptive functioning, and is highest among school-age children. All levels of severity of mental retardation are more common in males (overall, about 1.5:1). Mental retardation secondary to biological factors is as common in upper as in lower socioeconomic groups. When the etiology is not

TABLE 6–1.	Clinical features of mental retardation			
	Mild	**Moderate**	**Severe**	**Profound**
IQ	50–55 to about 70	35–40 to 50–55	20–25 to 35–40	Below 20–25
Percentage of mentally retarded population	85	10	4	1
Predominant socioeconomic class	Low	Less low	Even distribution	Even distribution
Academic level achieved by adulthood	6th grade	2nd grade	Below 1st grade	Below 1st grade
Education	Educable	Trainable (self-care)	Simple skills	—
Residence	Community	Sheltered	Mostly living in highly structured and closely supervised settings	Mostly living in highly structured and closely supervised settings
Economic	Makes change	Makes small change	Can use coin machines	Dependent on others for money management
	Holds a job	Usually able to manage pocket money	Can take notes to stores when shopping	
	Budget planning with effort or assistance			

biological, however, lower socioeconomic groups predominate, and the degree of retardation is usually mild.

Comorbidity

Of all mentally retarded children and adolescents, 30%–70% also have a psychiatric disorder. This rate is significantly higher than in youngsters of normal intelligence, in part because neurobiological causes of mental retardation place the child at greater risk of psychiatric disorder. Almost every diagnostic category in psychiatry is represented.

The most common presentation is a constellation of symptoms that includes impulsivity, irritability, hyperactivity, short attention span, and language delay. The prevalence of attention-deficit/hyperactivity disorder (ADHD) in mentally retarded individuals is between 4% and 11%, a rate nearly identical to that in the general population. Symptoms of ADHD can be observed even in nonverbal children. In children with mental retardation, inattention may be a sign of inappropriate classroom placement rather than of a behavior disorder. Frustration may lead to aggressive temper outbursts.

Autism and other PDDs are 100 times more likely to occur in children and adolescents with mental retardation than in nonretarded children. Although 5% of all mentally retarded individuals are autistic, approximately 75% of autistic patients are mentally retarded. Both mental retardation and autism can be caused by congenital rubella syndrome, tuberous sclerosis complex, and phenylketonuria, strengthening the association. Some symptoms seen in autism, including self-injurious behaviors, social isolation, and communication deficits, also may be found in persons with severe mental retardation. Autism is diagnosed when there is evidence of severe social impairment relative to the patient's developmental level. Stereotypic movements, including hand shaking or waving, body rocking, head banging, mouthing of objects, self-biting, picking at skin, or self-hitting, are among the more common psychiatric presentations in mentally retarded individuals with an IQ below 50. The prevalence is inversely related to IQ. Pica, rumination, cluttering, stuttering, and other language and speech disorders occur at higher rates in association with mental retardation.

Depression can be a complication of mental retardation (e.g., in response to extra burdens, poor self-image, and social stigmatization) or simply a coincidence, and occurs at a rate similar to or higher than that in the general population. The disorder is probably underdiagnosed, because greater attention is paid to individuals who are irritable and aggressive than to those manifesting sadness or withdrawal. Depression in verbal, mildly mentally retarded individuals presents with the typical symptoms, although the patient's reports may be more concrete. The diagnosis in moderately or severely retarded youth, however, requires observation in several settings. Occasionally, depression is confirmed only by successful pharmacological or behavioral treatment. Rarely, individuals with mental retardation may have rapid-cycling bipolar mood disorders. Suicidal ideation and behavior among mentally retarded individuals are far more prevalent than commonly thought.

Twenty-five percent of youth with mental retardation have significant symptoms of anxiety. Diagnoses include generalized anxiety disorder, phobias, panic disorder, posttraumatic stress disorder, and obsessive-compulsive disorder. Fears of failing and loss of caregivers are among the environmental factors that increase the vulnerability of persons with mental retardation to anxiety disorders. Mentally retarded patients may not have the cognitive or verbal skills to describe specific cognitive or emotional symptoms, increasing the clinician's reliance on behavioral observation and report of caregivers.

Etiology

Mental retardation results from psychosocial, biological, and environmental factors, usually in combination. In 30%–40% of the cases, despite rigorous medical and environmental investigations, the etiology is unclear. Birth asphyxia, prematurity, and low birth weight are no longer viewed as significant sources of mental retardation, except in extreme cases.

Most mild retardation is idiopathic, associated with sociocultural or psychosocial disadvantage, and familial (i.e., typically seen in the offspring of retarded parents). Intellectual and adaptive deficits are presumed to be determined by the interaction of a polygenic mechanism and social factors (Table 6–2).

Moderate, severe, and profound retardation are less likely to be idiopathic. Mental retardation is associated with more than 200 recognized biological syndromes. Known biomedical etiologies are identified in 25% of all cases of mental retardation and in 60%–90% of cases of severe or profound mental retardation (Table 6–3).

Fragile X syndrome is the most common inherited cause of mental retardation (1 in 1,250 males and 1 in 2,500 females). Characteristic physical stigmata (long face, prominent ears, prominent jaw, and macroorchidism [large testes]) are seen most clearly after puberty. Males present with sleep continuity disorders during the first years of life. Patients may also have a high arched palate; hyperextensible finger joints; soft, velvetlike skin; and flat feet. A review of the medical history may reveal seizures, recurrent infections, hernias, strabismus, or scoliosis.

TABLE 6–2.   **Psychosocial causes of mental retardation**

Poverty	Malnutrition
	Disease and infection
	Inadequate preventive care and medical treatment
	Sociocultural deprivation
Parental factors	Low IQ
	Psychiatric disorders
	Inadequate help-seeking behavior
	Lack of psychosocial stimulation
	Poor parenting skills
	Child abuse and neglect
Lack of community programs	Early identification and diagnosis
	Early intervention and infant stimulation
	Specialized education
	Vocational training and independent living

TABLE 6–3.	**Biological causes of mental retardation**
Genetic	Single gene defects—dominant
	Inborn errors of metabolism—recessive
	Chromosomal abnormalities (e.g., fragile X syndrome, trisomy 21 [Down syndrome])
	Polygenic inheritance
Prenatal	Maternal illness (e.g., diabetes, toxemia)
	Maternal infection passed to fetus (e.g., rubella, cytomegalovirus, toxoplasmosis, syphilis, herpes, human immunodeficiency virus)
	Toxins (e.g., alcohol, tobacco, narcotics, lead, anticonvulsants)
	Brain malformations
	Extreme malnutrition
	Intrauterine growth retardation
Perinatal	Extreme prematurity
	Blood group incompatibility
	Brain trauma
	Cerebrovascular accident
Infancy or childhood	Brain infection (e.g., meningitis, encephalitis)
	Head trauma
	Neurological disease
	Brain tumor
	Hypothyroidism
	Radiation
	Lead intoxication
	Asphyxia
	Severe malnutrition

Among patients with fragile X syndrome, cognitive impairment ranges from learning disabilities with a normal IQ to profound retardation. Fifty percent have borderline IQ or mental retardation. In females (who are partially protected by having two X chromosomes), a "carrier" state is associated with mild mental retardation or specific developmental disorders. The mean IQ drops in proportion to the percentage of cells with the mutation on the active X chromosome. Behavior problems are particularly prominent in males, with 70% meeting diagnostic criteria for ADHD. Anxiety disorders are more common in fragile X syndrome than in any other form of mental retardation. In female fragile X patients, shyness and social anxiety with poor interpersonal rapport, poor eye contact, social isolation, social oddness, and in some cases selective mutism, are prevalent. The behavior can appear schizotypal in nature. Language and speech deficits include poor abstraction, immature syntax, unusual speech rhythm, expressive and receptive language deficits, and articulation problems. Neuropsychological deficits include perseveration, inattention, poor concentration, and mood lability. Social interactions may be impaired by odd communication patterns and mannerisms. Autism is diagnosed in approximately 15% of patients with fragile X syndrome; others have prominent features of pervasive developmental disorder not otherwise specified (PDD NOS) or avoidant personality disorder.

Course and Prognosis

The course of mental retardation can be influenced by active treatment. Medical care should address underlying conditions that can cause brain injury (e.g., shunting for hydrocephalus, diet for phenylketonuria). Associated medical conditions that compromise the child's functioning can be prevented or adequately managed. Such conditions include seizures, otitis media, injury secondary to self-abusive behavior, and deafness and congenital cataracts associated with Down syndrome. Outcome is also influenced by environmental variables, including parental intelligence, psychological resilience, and material resources, as well as community resources and barriers.

More severe levels of mental retardation are diagnosed before the child is school age, particularly when associated with a known phenotype or syndrome. In moderate to mild retardation, diagnosis is uncommon before age 5 years, rises sharply in the early school years, and peaks in the later school years. Higher prevalence during the school years is usually attributed to the adaptive and intellectual demands of school (especially for social interaction and abstract thinking). At all levels of severity, the normal sequence of cognitive developmental stages occurs, but the rate of developmental progress is slow and there is a ceiling on ultimate achievement. Delays in speech and language development may limit ability to express negative affect, leading to impulsive anger and low frustration tolerance. Insufficient financial resources, inappropriate or inadequate educational programming, and prejudices of communities and health care personnel can result in a wide variety of developmental, social, and medical complications. Mental retardation is not necessarily a lifelong affliction. Proper training that addresses clinical needs and uses the patient's strengths can improve the level of functioning. The prognosis in mental retardation may be expected to improve as therapeutic and habilitative interventions become more available.

Evaluation and Differential Diagnosis

Intelligence is routinely measured by standardized tests (refer to Table 2–7 in Chapter 2). For very young children, the Bayley Scales of Infant Development or the Denver Developmental Screening Test may be used to estimate level of cognitive development.

Adaptive functioning may be judged by many means, including standardized instruments for assessing social maturity and adaptive skills. The Vineland Adaptive Behavior Scales (see Table 2–7) assess typical performance (not optimal ability) of the "daily activities required for personal and social sufficiency." The information obtained by a semistructured interview of a parent or caregiver yields a multidimensional measure of adaptive behaviors in five "domains": communication, daily living skills, socialization, motor skills, and maladaptive behaviors. Age-dependent expected competency scores of adaptive skills are established for children from infancy to age 18 years at different levels of mental retardation. The American Association on Mental Retardation's Adaptive Behavior Scale (ABS) evaluates adaptive skills from age 3 years to adult and is divided into two sections: developmental and self-help skills and maladaptive behaviors.

Medical evaluation begins with a careful history that includes a review of familial disorders, neurophysiological insults, diseases with progressive deterioration, and seizure disorder. The physical examination should include a neurodevelopmental assessment of functional abilities and impairments and the presence of abnormal neurological signs. Laboratory investigations are particularly important when the mental retardation has no clear etiology. Brain imaging may identify lesions that are surgically correctable or at least explanatory. If seizures are suspected, an electroencephalogram (EEG) is indicated.

Mental retardation requires modifications in the standard psychiatric examination, according to the level of language and cognitive development. These patients suffer from multiple disabilities and medical disorders that affect mood and behavior. Clinical assessment must be comprehensive and based on the patient's presentation in multiple settings. Hyperactivity, aggression, sadness, lack of enthusiasm, excessive anxiety, and formal thought disorder are not primary features of mental retardation and should lead to a full psychiatric evaluation, as should a significant change in mood, behavior, sleep, appetite, or level of adaptive functioning.

The differential diagnosis of mental retardation includes *environmental deprivation, learning disorders, autism and other PDDs, communication disorders, borderline intellectual functioning,* and *severe visual or hearing impairment.*

Treatment

To address the multiple disabilities and complications associated with mental retardation, developmentally sensitive multimodal treatment is optimal. The psychiatrist should coordinate medical and psychiatric evaluations, parental guidance (support, education, behavior management, educational and environmental planning, long-term monitoring, and advocacy), and the standard therapies for concomitant psychiatric disorders. It is important to ensure the safety of the patient and those around him or her. This may include brief periods of physical restraint or the use of medication, but on a limited basis and with the understanding that such emergencies should prompt a reassessment of diagnosis and treatment.

Behavior modification techniques such as removing inappropriate attention; changing deviant communication patterns (e.g., rewarding use of words or sign); consistently applying social, self-care, academic, and vocational expectations; and using environmental contingencies can reduce the frequency and severity of self-injury, stereotypies, pica, and asocial behavior. The behavioral program should be consistent and applied across settings, including home and school. Specialists may provide educational and developmental training to enhance speech and language; motor, cognitive, social, and occupational functioning; and adaptive skills such as toileting, dressing, grooming, and eating.

Developmentally oriented psychotherapeutic interventions may be effective to manage crises or to address long-term psychosocial goals. Therapy can focus on tangible objectives for the patient, including greater independence, recognizing and expressing emotion, dealing with the reactions of others, developing social skills, and handling personal and practical challenges. Group therapy for adolescents and young adults can be useful for social skills training. Family therapy can focus on learning about the disability, emphasizing the patient's strengths, reducing guilt and overprotection, and fostering greater independence.

Although no pharmacological treatments are available for mental retardation per se, the frequency of concurrent Axis I disorders suggests the use of psychotropic medication. Treatment effects are often difficult to assess in developmentally disabled patients. Their impaired verbal skills may complicate the diagnostic process, measurement of efficacy, and detection of adverse effects. Heterogeneity of retarded children leads to variability in treatment effect. Youngsters with structural brain abnormalities often react differently to medications than do children with normal IQ, even when target symptoms are similar. Medications used for medical or neurological disorders associated with mental retardation may have problematic side effects and should be started at lower doses with more gradual increases.

Methylphenidate and dextroamphetamine are effective in the treatment of symptoms of impulsivity, hyperactivity, and inattention in ADHD in mildly to moderately mentally retarded children. Few studies exist on the psychopharmacological treatment of depression in these patients, but selective serotonin reuptake inhibitors (SSRIs), such as fluoxetine (20–40 mg/day), may improve mood, energy level, interest, and motivation with minimal side effects. Cyclic mood disturbances have been treated successfully with lithium, although patients may experience cognitive dulling, gastrointestinal distress, tremor, fatigue, and a worsening of eczema. In these cases, carbamazepine and valproic acid are reasonable alternatives. Mentally retarded patients may present with bouts of aggression and self-destructive behavior that require prompt intervention and have led to the use of medications. These behaviors may be a symptom of a psychiatric disorder such as depression, bipolar disorder, or schizophrenia. Atypical agents are frequently recommended because individuals with mental retardation are more susceptible to tardive dyskinesia and tardive akathisia. Serotonergic agents, lithium, and β-blockers may be successful in the treatment of aggression, stereotypies, self-injury, and compulsive behaviors.

In prepubertal children with fragile X syndrome, orally administered folate reduces the frequency of fragile sites in vivo and may improve behavior and attention.

■ PERVASIVE DEVELOPMENTAL DISORDERS

PDDs are divided into several categories that include autistic disorder (formerly called infantile autism), Asperger's disorder, and PDD NOS (to accommodate atypical or less severe cases). In these disorders, development is not merely delayed but also "atypical" or "deviant." PDD is not simply a collection of delays in specific skills or domains but implies broad disruption of functions.

Autistic Disorder

Clinical Description

The DSM-IV-TR criteria for autistic disorder (Table 6–4) focus on severe impairment, relative to chronological and mental age, with onset by age 3 years, in three key areas: social interaction, communication and play, and interests and activities. Autistic disorder has a wide spectrum of severity.

Social deficits are the most consistent and reliable indication of autism. Younger children fail to seek out peer interactions, whereas older individuals may express an interest in friendships and seek interpersonal experiences but lack the skills to initiate and maintain relationships. Persons with autism show persistent deficits in appreciating the feelings and thoughts of other people and in understanding the process and nuances of social communication. They prefer solitary games and relate to others primarily as "objects" in their play.

Spoken language is either delayed or totally absent, with patients unable to initiate or sustain conversation. Communicative speech and gesturing are limited or difficult to understand because of echolalia, pronoun reversals, and idiosyncratic meanings. Phonological (sound production) and syntactic (grammar) functions may be relatively spared, with more significant impairments of verbal semantics (sociocultural meanings) and pragmatics (rules of interpersonal exchange) and nonverbal aspects of communication. Imaginative and symbolic functions (e.g., use of toys in play) may be dramatically impaired and play is characterized by rituals, stereotypies, motor mannerisms, and preoccupations with parts of objects.

Most individuals with autism have subnormal intelligence, but a few show significant improvements in measured IQ with time or treatment. Poor performance also may be a result of the patient's lack of interest in taking tests. Approximately 80% of autistic patients are mentally retarded. Subtest results are often greatly scattered and inconsistent over time. The patient may have unusual or special capacities (savant skills) in music, drawing, arithmetic, or calendar calculation.

TABLE 6–4. **DSM-IV-TR diagnostic criteria for autistic disorder**

A. A total of six (or more) items from (1), (2), and (3), with at least two from (1), and one each from (2) and (3):

(1) qualitative impairment in social interaction, as manifested by at least two of the following:

(a) marked impairment in the use of multiple nonverbal behaviors such as eye-to-eye gaze, facial expression, body postures, and gestures to regulate social interaction

(b) failure to develop peer relationships appropriate to developmental level

(c) a lack of spontaneous seeking to share enjoyment, interests, or achievements with other people (e.g., by a lack of showing, bringing, or pointing out objects of interest)

(d) lack of social or emotional reciprocity

(2) qualitative impairments in communication as manifested by at least one of the following:

(a) delay in, or total lack of, the development of spoken language (not accompanied by an attempt to compensate through alternative modes of communication such as gesture or mime)

(b) in individuals with adequate speech, marked impairment in the ability to initiate or sustain a conversation with others

(c) stereotyped and repetitive use of language or idiosyncratic language

(d) lack of varied, spontaneous make-believe play or social imitative play appropriate to developmental level

(3) restricted repetitive and stereotyped patterns of behavior, interests, and activities, as manifested by at least one of the following:

(a) encompassing preoccupation with one or more stereotyped and restricted patterns of interest that is abnormal either in intensity or focus

(b) apparently inflexible adherence to specific, nonfunctional routines or rituals

(c) stereotyped and repetitive motor mannerisms (e.g., hand or finger flapping or twisting, or complex whole-body movements)

(d) persistent preoccupation with parts of objects

TABLE 6–4.	DSM-IV-TR diagnostic criteria for autistic disorder *(continued)*

B. Delays or abnormal functioning in at least one of the following areas, with onset prior to age 3 years: (1) social interaction, (2) language as used in social communication, or (3) symbolic or imaginative play.

C. The disturbance is not better accounted for by Rett's disorder or childhood disintegrative disorder.

Epidemiology

Estimated prevalence of autism, based on strict DSM-IV-TR criteria, is 4.8 per 10,000 in the United States general population (Fombonne 1998). Broader autism spectrum disorders may occur at a rate of 20 per 10,000. There is a male predominance of 4–5 to 1. Girls who are affected tend to be severely retarded. Early reports of an association between upper socioeconomic class and the disorder are not valid and were related to sampling biases.

Etiology

Autism is a strongly genetic condition. The etiology of autism spectrum disorders is likely to involve multiple genes, which makes the identification of specific factors more difficult. The prevalence of autism in siblings is 4.5%. Autism is 215 times more frequent among siblings born after an autistic child than in the general population (Ritvo et al. 1989). Monozygotic twins have a higher rate of concordance than dizygotic twins, but it is not 100%, thus implicating early environmental biological insults as well. There is no evidence that psychosocial factors or parenting patterns cause autistic disorder.

A specific medical cause of autism can be identified in some individuals, most often in those with profound or severe mental retardation. The association with postnatal neurological infections, congenital rubella, phenylketonuria, cerebral palsy, Down syndrome, and neurofibromatosis is not greater than chance. Perhaps 5% have fragile X syndrome, and there is strong association with tuberous sclerosis. Seizure disorders appear in 35%–50% of patients by age 20 years, more commonly in the presence of concurrent mental retardation.

Brain-imaging studies demonstrate a wide range of abnormalities but no consistent or diagnostic pattern. Computed tomography scans show changes (ventricular enlargement, left temporal abnormalities, abnormal symmetry). Magnetic resonance imaging shows developmental hypoplasia of two discrete areas in the cerebellum (Courchesne et al. 1988) and forebrain morphological abnormalities (Gaffney et al. 1989).

Various autoimmune disorders are overrepresented. Forty percent of autistic patients appear to have specific autoantibodies to serotonin-1A receptors (which are not present in brain-damaged or nonautistic patients) (Todd and Ciaranello 1985). An elevation in peripheral levels of serotonin has also been noted, affecting potentiation at synapses and possibly playing a role in the development of the central nervous system. Neurochemical studies are not, however, diagnostic. Despite considerable attention in the lay press, there is no evidence that links the mumps, measles, and rubella (MMR) vaccine to autism.

Course and Prognosis

Autistic disorder is often apparent in early infancy, and parents may seek a pediatric opinion during the first year (often suspecting deafness). In some patients, the full disorder does not appear until after age 3 years. An initial period of seemingly normal development may be followed by developmental arrest or by regression with loss of previously developed abilities.

Children with autism usually make gradual but erratic improvement, particularly during the school-age years. Occasionally patients make rapid unexplained developmental progress. Medical illness and environmental stress may precipitate regression, which may include more compulsive and self-abusive behaviors, occasionally requiring pharmacological intervention. Adolescents may experience either continued development or behavioral deterioration. Seizure disorders are more likely to appear during adolescence.

Educational and supportive services have a marked beneficial effect. Even more severely autistic persons can learn some adaptive skills. For the less severely impaired, treatment may lead to social skills and adaptations that permit employment and independent or group home living. Predictors of good adaptive outcome include higher IQ, better language skills (especially the ability to communicate verbally by age 5 years), greater social skills, and later appearance of symptoms.

As adults, many autistic individuals continue to improve gradually but retain clinical evidence of residual organic brain damage. Depending on the severity of the autistic disorder, perhaps 2%–15% achieve a nonretarded level of cognitive and adaptive function, with 33% able to function independently as adults. Adults remain socially aloof, however, and often oppositional. Expressive and receptive language may appear normal, but deficits in social communication and empathy persist.

Evaluation

The evaluation of the child with suspected autistic disorder should be a collaborative process. Early developmental and medical histories are important. As part of the psychiatric evaluation, a workup of autistic disorder includes assessment of language, cognition, social skills, and adaptive functioning. Neuropsychological and speech and language specialty testing can document abnormalities in abstract and pragmatic language, encoding of complex information, attentional skills, and executive functions. Neurological examination is used to detect possible inborn metabolic, structural, or degenerative diseases or seizures. An EEG (for seizure disorder or developmental regression) and chromosome analysis (for fragile X) may be advised. Audiological examination for possible deafness and examinations for other sensory deficits may be done. Patients with a tendency to mouth materials are at greater risk for lead intoxication. A psychologist experienced with these difficult youngsters must evaluate intellectual potential. Standardized diagnostic checklists (e.g., the Childhood Autism Rating Scale [CARS]) are based on clinical observation and parental recall of early behavior.

Differential Diagnosis

Autism should be differentiated from other *PDDs. Rett's disorder* occurs predominantly in females and includes deceleration of head growth, marked mental retardation, hand-washing stereotypies, and loss of purposeful motor skills. *Asperger's disorder* does not cause delays in language development, cognitive development, age-appropriate self-help skills, or adaptive behavior. The child develops intense but unusual interests and loses social skills. *Childhood disintegrative disorder* has a characteristic pattern of developmental regression beginning at age 2 years. Differential diagnosis also includes congenital *deafness* (but deaf children typically learn an alternative lip or sign language, lose their isolative behaviors, and develop sensitive expressive communication), congenital *blindness* (but blind children relate socially), *developmental expressive and receptive language disorders* (but these children are typically more sociable, communicate well in gestures, and do not have stereotypic and repetitive behavioral patterns), and juvenile-onset *schizophrenia* (distinguished by hallucinations, delusions, and thought disorder). Children with pure *mental retardation* have a more even pattern of delays and do not have bizarre behaviors or deficits in social relatedness. The differential diagnosis is particularly difficult in children with severe to profound mental retardation. In very young children, *reactive attachment disorder* may be a consideration, but these cases are typically characterized by severe neglect. In *selective mutism* the patient is able to speak in some situations. *Degenerative neurological diseases* may resemble PDD.

Children or adults with autistic disorder may have comorbid mood or anxiety disorders or symptoms of overactivity, inattention, and impulsivity (the diagnosis of ADHD is excluded in the presence of PDD).

Treatment

Patients fortunate enough to have early access to rigorous multimodal treatment show significant improvement. The milieu should be highly structured and should include special education, speech and language instruction, vocational training (for adolescents), and teaching of adaptive skills. Behavior therapy reduces unwanted symptoms; promotes speech, social interaction, and assertiveness; increases self-reliance and self-care skills; and facilitates exploration. Parent guidance is critical, both to provide education and to deal with emotional reactions such as guilt or denial. Parents can contribute to the child's learning of language and self-care and adaptive skills, arrange for special education and for adjunctive services, and make long-term plans for the child. Training in behavior management skills is essential for a tolerable home environment and for maximizing the child's potential.

Acute hospitalization or longer-term residential treatment may be needed. Long-term follow-up is required, including periodic reassessment for the possible appearance of seizures or mood or anxiety disorders.

Psychotropic medications may be used to control behavior or to treat coexisting psychiatric disorders. Low doses of nonsedating neuroleptics, in conjunction with a highly structured treatment program, may help control behavioral symptoms, reduce excessive activity levels, and enhance the effect of behavior therapy. Neuroleptics are the most frequently studied medications in well-controlled trials and may be used in cases of severe aggression, interpersonal withdrawal with paranoid or delusional thoughts, and stereotypies. Controlled studies of atypical neuroleptics such as risperidone demonstrate clinical effectiveness with more benign side effect profile. The risk of tardive dyskinesia may be higher in these patients because of the length of treatment and perhaps biological vulnerability.

Psychostimulant medication may decrease symptoms of impulsivity, overactivity, and distractibility, although treatment results are inconsistent. In some patients, rituals and stereotypies are exacerbated because of dopamine agonist effects. SSRIs such as fluvox-amine are sometimes effective in reducing obsessive-compulsive behaviors. Fluoxetine (20–40 mg/day) can relieve depressive symptoms in adolescents with autism. Clomipramine decreases the frequency of some self-abusive behaviors. The α_2-adrenergic receptor agonist clonidine has been effective in double-blind reports and case studies examining behavioral control, but tolerance often develops with prolonged use. Naltrexone (an opiate-receptor blocking agent) has little effect on the social and cognitive symptoms of autism, but occasionally decreases the frequency of self-injurious behavior, hyperactivity, and ritualistic behaviors. Buspirone and β-blockers have been suggested to address aggression in persons with autism.

This chronic and often severe disorder can lead to parental desperation, unrealistic endorsements, and nonscientific pursuits of unconventional treatments. The field is plagued by unsubstantiated treatments that are at best ineffective and at worst divert time, energy, and resources from conventional treatments, or even have toxic effects (Herbert et al. 2002).

Asperger's Disorder

Asperger's disorder is characterized by deficits in social interaction and repetitive, restricted, and stereotyped behavior and interests but not by mental retardation or impaired language.

■ SPECIFIC DEVELOPMENTAL DISORDERS

In each of the specific developmental disorders (Table 6–5), there is a discrepancy between potential and actual acquisition of skills and knowledge, although there is controversy regarding the emphasis on impairment relative to IQ.

Epidemiology

Estimated prevalence of each of the specific developmental disorders in elementary school–age children ranges from 2% to 10%.

TABLE 6–5.	DSM-IV-TR specific developmental disorders
Learning disorders	Reading disorder
	Mathematics disorder
	Disorder of written expression
Motor skills disorder	Developmental coordination disorder
Communication disorders	Expressive language disorder
	Mixed receptive-expressive language disorder
	Phonological disorder
	Stuttering

About 5% of all school children in the United States are classified as having a learning disorder.

Etiology

Lower socioeconomic classes are overrepresented in the specific developmental disorders. There is a male predominance of 3–4:1. Etiology may vary among the disorders, but is presumably related to cortical deficits secondary to organic damage, delayed maturation, or genetics. Frequent comorbidity among specific developmental disorders suggests that these impairments reflect multiple cerebral dysfunctions. Numerous theories regarding hemisphere development and specialization have been proposed to explain the developmental disorders. Epidemiological studies find specific developmental delays in both right-handed and left-handed individuals, consistent with a complicated polymorphic genetic relationship between laterality and developmental delay.

Family histories in all subtypes of specific developmental disorder show an overrepresentation of reading, speech, and language disorders in the siblings and parents of affected children, although pedigrees are not consistent with a single mode of transmission. First-degree relatives have a 35%–45% risk of having a reading disorder, compared with a 3%–10% rate in the general population (Pennington 1995). The concordance rate in identical twins approaches 100%.

Learning Disorders

Clinical Description

Learning disorders are defined by the delay in expected cognitive development in specific abilities. The child functions below age or grade level. Academic or adaptive impairment is required. The delay is not secondary to a sensory defect or known neurological disorder. Associated symptoms often include impairment of left–right orientation, sound discrimination, and perceptual-motor skills.

Etiology

Maternal smoking during pregnancy, low birth weight, prenatal and perinatal mishaps, overt neurological disorders, and EEG abnormalities appear to be associated with the appearance of developmental reading disorder.

Course and Prognosis

Learning disorders are frequently unrecognized and present instead as school refusal, oppositional defiant disorder, somatoform disorder, or agoraphobia. These patients are embarrassed by their academic difficulties, dislike school, and avoid schoolwork. Diagnoses are typically made in grade school. In later school years, problems involving organizational skills (note taking, time management, and maintenance of books and papers) may be signs of residual cortical deficits, even if basic skills were well remediated. In college and graduate school, individuals may have difficulty learning foreign languages, writing efficiently, or reading fluently.

Axis I disorders are overrepresented in families of patients with learning disorders. Psychological and behavioral complications of learning disorder include low self-esteem, anxiety, demoralization, poor frustration tolerance, lack of enjoyment in learning, passivity or rigidity in new learning situations, truancy, and school dropout. A strong relationship exists between reading disorder and ADHD; some of this is attributable to heredity. The interaction between conduct disorder and learning disorder is likely to be complex and multifactorial. Comorbid depression or anxiety disorders appear to be relatively common, but good epidemiological data are not available.

Over time, mild cases may resolve through persistent remediation, practice, and compensation for deficits, but others retain specific learning deficits as adults. Often, secondary emotional and behavior problems persist beyond the duration or direct relevance of the developmental deficits. Young women with reading disabilities tend to bear children at younger ages, while young men are more likely to be unemployed. Adults may need to make accommodations in their lives and choice of career to cope with residual deficits.

Evaluation and Differential Diagnosis

Because of the high rate of comorbidity, evaluation of learning disorders includes assessment of the full range of abilities (specific academic skills, speech and language, and motor function), cognitive tests (including IQ), and observation of the child's behavior and quality of teaching in the classroom. Testing procedures must be sensitive to the ethnic and cultural background of the patient. Academic delays may develop as a consequence of poor teaching, cultural background, and lack of opportunity. The clinician also must evaluate the child for possible *mental retardation, ADHD, mood disorder* (causing low motivation), *anxiety disorder* (causing reduced attention), and other psychiatric and neurological disorders. Children with *communication disorders* may need tests that use nonverbal measures of intelligence to evaluate learning disorders. Sensory perception tests are needed to rule out impaired *vision* or *hearing.*

Treatment

Because many specialists and teachers may be involved in the education of a child with multiple deficits, multidisciplinary communication is vital, particularly during school transitions. The Individuals with Disabilities Education Act (IDEA), the successor to

U.S. Public Law 94-142, mandates for all children with disabilities the right to a "free appropriate public education," including special education and related services designed to their needs in the least restrictive context possible. In practice, remediation of only basic skills is funded, and deficits must be severe to qualify (e.g., 2 years behind expected level). An Individualized Education Program (IEP) is designed for each child, but the quality of evaluation and treatment services varies. Part-time resource rooms, full-time self-contained classrooms, and mainstream classrooms (with special-education consultants) provide the major part of special education. Specialized schools and residential treatment programs are rarely used due to scarcity and expense.

The IEP includes specific accommodations, including (depending on the type of disorder) use of a calculator, typewriter, or word processor; time-extended tests; individual or small-group tutoring; or self-paced programmed texts or computerized self-instruction. Behavioral techniques are often used to improve motivation, emphasize success, foster enjoyment of new skills, reduce rigidity in learning, and promote application in new situations.

Parents of children with learning disorders should be included in educational planning. Supportive counseling may help them to avoid contributing to a climate of negativity and criticism and to adjust their child's and their own expectations to anticipate slower-than-standard learning but (unlike mental retardation) with no clear ceiling on educational achievement.

Individual psychotherapy may help reduce secondary psychological complications such as low self-esteem, temper tantrums, lack of assertiveness, and inflexibility. Psychopharmacological therapy is not helpful for specific developmental disorders but may be for concurrent disorders.

Motor Skills Disorder: Developmental Coordination Disorder

In this condition there is delayed learning of motor skills that is sufficient to cause functional impairment and is not caused by a known physical disorder. About 6% of children ages 5–11 years have significant impairments of gross or fine motor abilities. ADHD is commonly also present. Remediation is warranted to minimize sequelae such as scapegoating by peers, sports avoidance, academic difficulties (due to slow and illegible handwriting), and vocational impairment.

Communication Disorders

Clinical Description

Communication disorders are defined by delays in specific speech or language abilities that interfere with academic or adaptive functioning and that are not a result of PDD, mental retardation, sensory deficit, or structural or neurological disorder. There is a continuum of increasing severity of impairment from stuttering and phonological disorder, through expressive language disorder, to mixed receptive-expressive language disorder. In mixed receptive-expressive language disorder, both decoding (comprehension) and encoding (expression) are impaired, leading to more severe academic and social disruption than in expressive language disorder alone. A child may have more than one disorder, and multiple cortical deficits are usually observed, particularly in sensory information processing and temporal auditory processing. Nonverbal comprehension may be preserved or impaired to varying degrees, but compensation through spontaneous use of gestural language or nonverbal communication is common.

Epidemiology

Expressive or receptive language disorders are evident in from 1% to 13% of the population. Three percent to 5% have a developmental expressive language disorder, usually with a childhood onset. Mixed expressive language disorder is found in 3% of school-age children (Beitchman and Young 1997). Language disorders are more common in males and in children with psychiatric disorders, mental retardation, or hearing impairment.

Etiology

Many aspects of motor, sensory, and cognitive development must be intact for speech and language to develop normally. By age 5 years, children are expected to speak fluently and to comprehend speech. Adult articulation skills should be present by age 8 years. The range of normal functioning is broad, and development of language and speech skills continues for many years. Development of articulation and vocabulary is highly influenced by the child's environment. Verbal and nonverbal communication skills include word finding (access and retrieval of verbal information), word relationships (semantics), sentence formation (syntax), giving and receiving feedback, following conversational structure and flow, responding to the context, adapting to meanings and external events (pragmatics), responding to one's internal sense of events, and monitoring one's own communicative productions (metalinguistic skills). The development of these skills is a formidable task to achieve in 5 years.

The etiology of deficits is often unknown, but there is strong evidence for the heritability of expressive language disorders, with and without articulation problems. Environmental factors also contribute and may include faulty speech models within the family and lack of stimulation of language. Hearing loss, even if mild, plays a significant role in the etiology of language and speech disorders. During the period of language development, fluctuating hearing capacity or degrees of hearing loss that are considered medically insignificant can persistently diminish verbal IQ and academic performance (Howie 1980). Even mild hearing loss (25–40 decibels) (resulting from chronic otitis media or perforation of the tympanic membrane) may delay development of articulation, expressive and receptive language, reading, and spelling.

Course and Prognosis

Deficits in articulation (speech sound production), expression (oral language production and use), and reception (comprehension) may be observable by age 2–3 years. Delays in speech and language frequently improve during development, so that early delays are not strongly predictive of subsequent psychiatric and learning disorders. Children with mixed receptive-expressive language disorder, however, have a poorer prognosis than those with expressive language disorder alone. Speech and language skills are eventually acquired in most cases, but other characteristics (concomitant psychiatric disorders, neuromotor problems, low IQ) may predict worse outcome.

Complications of speech and language disorders include progressive academic impairment, psychological distress, low self-esteem, anxiety regarding learning, and school dropout. These children may have difficulty maintaining a conversation or expanding on a topic. Problems in social interactions may lead to peer problems and overdependence on family members. When frustrated, the young child may have tantrums or the older child may refuse to speak.

About 50% of children with communication disorders have concomitant Axis I diagnoses, and another 20% have other developmental disorders, especially academic skills disorders (Cantwell and Baker 1987).

Evaluation and Differential Diagnosis

Multidisciplinary assessment is required to evaluate communication disorders. Specialized speech and language evaluation includes articulation, receptive skills (understanding single words, word combinations, and sentences), and expressive language skills (syntactic structures, vocabulary, and social appropriateness). The clinician may observe family characteristics and free speech between parents and child to assess social skills and nonverbal communication (vocalizations, gestures, and gazes). The clinician should obtain hearing acuity evaluation using audiometry or auditory evoked response (which does not require the child's cooperation) and evaluate auditory attention (losing flow of conversation, inability to hear in a crowd, distractibility), discrimination, and memory. Nonverbal measures of IQ (e.g., Leiter International Performance Scale,

Columbia Mental Maturity Scale) are used in cases of suspected language delay.

Differential diagnosis includes *autistic disorder, selective mutism, deafness, mental retardation, medical and neurological disorders,* and *acquired aphasia.* In adolescence, social awkwardness, stereotypies, resistance to change, and low frustration tolerance may approach the severity of autistic disorder, but youngsters with specific communication disorders have better social communication, empathic awareness, and abstraction than do those with autism.

Treatment

Hearing deficits should be addressed whenever possible, and aggressive treatment of otitis media is prudent. Social involvement, imitation, and imaginative play are encouraged to increase verbal, communicative, and symbolic skills. Referral to a speech and language pathologist is essential. Special education should be maintained until symptoms improve. Once a child is "mainstreamed," speech and language therapy and supplemental academic supports may still be required. Psychiatric treatment of concurrent attentional, emotional, or behavior problems and educational management of academic skills disorders may be involved.

Stuttering

Clinical Description

Stuttering, a disruption of speech timing and fluency, is characterized by involuntary and irregular hesitations and blocking and prolongations, repetitions, interjections and substitutions of sounds, syllables, and words. The dysfluency typically worsens during periods of performance anxiety or communicative stress. The symptoms are often absent during singing, reading aloud, talking in unison, or talking to pets or inanimate objects. People who stutter are acutely aware of their symptoms and cannot readily improve their speech by slowing or by focusing attention on their speech rate or rhythm. The disorder compromises academic, occupational, and social functioning.

Epidemiology

The prevalence of stuttering is about 1% in children and slightly less in adolescents. The male-to-female ratio is approximately 3:1.

Etiology

Current etiological theories of stuttering include genetic, neurological, and behavioral factors, probably reflecting several etiological subtypes. Familial transmission is common, with the disorder appearing in about 20%–40% of first-degree relatives (especially males). A strikingly higher concordance in monozygotic than in dizygotic twins suggests a genetic mechanism, perhaps a polygenic model with lower penetrance in females (Pennington 1995).

In rare cases, stutterlike dysfluency can be caused by psychotropic medications (e.g., tricyclic antidepressants, neuroleptics, lithium, alprazolam).

No evidence indicates that anxiety, neurosis, or family dynamics cause stuttering, although anxiety and frustration secondary to stuttering may worsen the dysfluency.

Course and Prognosis

For toddlers, stuttering is usually a transient developmental symptom lasting less than 6 months, but 25% of patients with early onset of stuttering have persistent stuttering beyond age 12 years. Stuttering usually begins at ages 2–4 years but occasionally occurs at ages 5–7 years; it rarely starts during adolescence. Spontaneous improvement occurs in 50%–80% of patients. At the onset of illness, the child is usually unaware of the symptom. The disorder typically waxes and wanes during childhood.

Complications include fearful anticipation, eye blinking, involuntary tension of the jaw and face muscles, tics, and avoidance of problematic words and situations. Negative reactions by family and peers may affect self-image, social skills, and language development and lead to academic impairment, occupational problems, and social withdrawal.

Evaluation and Differential Diagnosis

Evaluation of stuttering includes a full developmental history and neurological and audiological examinations. Referral to a speech and language pathologist for evaluation is indicated in all cases. The therapist should assess the dysfluency in monologue, conversation, play, and mild stress conditions and observe parent–child interactions for communicative stress placed on the child (e.g., rapid questioning, interruptions, repeated corrections, frequent topic shifts). Behavioral assessment documents secondary restrictions in social interactions and activities.

Treatment

Speech therapy involves intensive training of fluent speech skills, the fostering of self-esteem and social assertiveness, and the use of behavior therapy methods, such as modification of environmental and conversational factors that trigger stuttering, relaxation, role-playing, feedback, practice in speaking in different settings (reading aloud, choral reading, alone, in a group, in front of a classroom, on a telephone), and talking with different people (parents, relatives, friends, strangers). Education and counseling of family members are advised.

Psychotherapy generally is not indicated but might be considered for secondary symptoms or associated problems. Antianxiety drugs have minimal value.

■ REFERENCES

American Psychiatric Association: Diagnostic and Statistical Manual of Mental Disorders, 4th Edition, Text Revision. Washington, DC, American Psychiatric Association, 2000

Beitchman JH, Young A: Learning disorders with a special emphasis on reading disorders: a review of the past 10 years. J Am Acad Child Adolesc Psychiatry 36:1020–1032, 1997

Cantwell DP, Baker L: Developmental Speech and Language Disorders. New York, Guilford, 1987

Courchesne E, Yeung-Courchesne R, Press GA, et al: Hypoplasia of cerebellar vermal lobules VI and VII in autism. N Engl J Med 318:1349–1354, 1988

Fombonne E: Epidemiology of autism and related conditions, in Autism and Pervasive Developmental Disorders. Edited by Volkmar FR. Cambridge, UK, Cambridge University Press, 1998, pp 32–63

Gaffney GR, Kuperman S, Tsai LY, et al: Forebrain structure in infantile autism. J Am Acad Child Adolesc Psychiatry 28:534–537, 1989

Herbert JD, Sharp IR, Gaudiano BA: Separating fact from fiction in the etiology and treatment of autism: a scientific review of the evidence. Scientific Review of Mental Health Practice 1:23–43, 2002

Howie VM: Developmental sequelae of chronic otitis media: a review. J Dev Behav Pediatr 1:34–38, 1980

Pennington BF: Genetics of learning disabilities. J Child Neurol 10 (suppl 1):S69–S77, 1995

Ritvo ER, Jorde LB, Mason-Brothers A, et al: The UCLA–University of Utah epidemiologic survey of autism: recurrence risk estimates and genetic counseling. Am J Psychiatry 146:1032–1036, 1989

Todd RD, Ciaranello RD: Demonstration of inter- and intraspecies differences in serotonin binding sites by antibodies from an autistic child. Proc Natl Acad Sci U S A 82:612–616, 1985

■ ADDITIONAL READING

American Academy of Child and Adolescent Psychiatry: Practice parameters for the assessment and treatment of children and adolescents with language and learning disorders. J Am Acad Child Adolesc Psychiatry 37 (10 suppl):46S–62S, 1998

American Academy of Child and Adolescent Psychiatry: Practice parameters for the assessment and treatment of children, adolescents, and adults with mental retardation and comorbid mental disorders. J Am Acad Child Adolesc Psychiatry 38 (12 suppl):5S–31S, 1999

American Academy of Child and Adolescent Psychiatry: Practice parameters for the assessment and treatment of children, adolescents, and adults with autism and other pervasive developmental disorders. J Am Acad Child Adolesc Psychiatry 38 (12 suppl):32S–54S, 1999

King BH, State MW, Shah B, et al: Mental retardation: a review of the past 10 years: part I. J Am Acad Child Adolesc Psychiatry 36:1656–1663, 1997

State MW, King BH, Dykens E: Mental retardation: a review of the past 10 years: part II. J Am Acad Child Adolesc Psychiatry 36:1664–1671, 1997

7

SPECIAL CLINICAL
CIRCUMSTANCES

This chapter covers a wide variety of situations and conditions that are not psychiatric diagnoses but in which psychiatric clinical skills may be useful or even required. Emergencies require expert assessment and prompt intervention. The effects of family transitions or adolescent pregnancy may become apparent in pediatric or school settings. Childhood obesity and physical illness raise psychological issues that can profoundly affect medical treatment. The children of parents with psychiatric disorders are often ignored by systems of care designed for adults.

■ EMERGENCIES

Assessment and Triage

Emergencies present most often in psychiatric, pediatric, or general hospital emergency rooms, but they also occur in other psychiatric and pediatric settings and in schools (Table 7–1). The clinician rapidly assesses the potential for physical danger or acute psychiatric deterioration, evaluates support systems, may initiate treatment, and makes a disposition for further evaluation and treatment. In situations that are potentially dangerous to the youth or to others, a delay in intervention may result in acute exacerbation or increased resistance to treatment or actual harm.

An emergency evaluation must be brief and focused (Table 7–2). The clinician should talk with the child or adolescent and the rele-

---

TABLE 7–1.   **Common psychiatric emergencies in children and adolescents**

Suicidal behavior, threats, or intent
Victim of physical abuse or severe neglect
Victim of sexual abuse or rape
Violent behavior or threats of violence
Delirium or other behavior or mental status changes secondary to medical illness or to prescribed medication
Nonpsychotic hallucinations in young children
    Night terrors
    Acute phobic hallucinations
Psychosis
Acute anxiety reactions, hyperventilation
Acute school refusal
Fire setting
Running away
Substance abuse
Anorexia nervosa or bulimia nervosa
Conversion symptoms

---

vant adults both alone and together. Important collateral information can be gathered by telephone, from as many informants as possible (with appropriate consent). To ensure patient and staff safety and facilitate immediate intervention, the clinician must assess immediately for

- Medical illness or medication side effect
- Head trauma
- Intentional or accidental overdose
- Drug or alcohol intoxication or withdrawal
- Need for physical restraint or containment to prevent aggression or elopement
- Need to prevent a parent from removing the child from the emergency room
- Drugs or weapons carried by or available to the patient

TABLE 7–2.	Outline of emergency history
Demographics	Age
	Residence
	School and current grade
	Financial status
	Primary caregiver
Chief complaint	Who initiated the emergency visit?
	What happened?
	What did the patient intend to do?
	How was the patient discovered?
	How did the patient and others react?
Recent suicide attempts	Overdose of prescribed or over-the-counter medication
	Use of firearms
	Hanging
	Other self-injury
	Presence of alcohol or illicit drugs
History of present illness	Development of symptoms
	Intervention attempts and their results
	Involvement of social agencies
History of emotional or behavior problems	Depression
	Suicide attempts
	Aggression
	Conduct disorder
	Drug or alcohol use
	Psychosis
Adaptive functioning with family, school, and peers	
Stressors in patient and family	
Abbreviated developmental history	Mental retardation
	Regression from previous level of functioning

TABLE 7–2.	Outline of emergency history *(continued)*
Family situation	Family living arrangements
	Other family or adults involved or who could be involved
	Adult stability, competence, relationship with the patient, attitude toward the patient and his or her problems
	Physical abuse, neglect, substance abuse
Family history of psychiatric illness or suicide	
History of medical illness and review of symptoms	

A careful mental status examination is crucial in an emergency situation, with special focus on signs of psychosis, organicity, intoxication, suicidality, poor judgment, or impulsivity. Medical evaluation should be pursued as indicated (Table 7–3). The cause of a sudden change in behavior should be considered organic until proven otherwise. "Medical clearance" in the emergency room does not guarantee the absence of physical disorder as a cause of psychiatric symptoms.

TABLE 7–3.	Emergency medical evaluation

Physical and neurological examination
  Potential causes of organicity
  Evidence of drug ingestion
  Evidence of physical or sexual abuse
  Medical complications of an eating disorder
Laboratory tests according to clinical indications
  Follow-up findings on medical history and physical examination
  Pregnancy test
  Blood and urine drug screen
  Blood alcohol level
  Tests for sexually transmitted diseases

The clinician often has difficulty making a definitive DSM-IV-TR (American Psychiatric Association 2000) diagnosis in a single evaluation in an emergency setting, especially if collateral information is limited. Only a triage decision regarding further evaluation and treatment may be possible. Abbreviated feedback, education, and explanation are appropriate in the emergency setting. When the disposition or treatment is uncertain, the primary issue is safety (Table 7–4). The decision whether to hospitalize a young person is often determined by the ability of supervising adults to tolerate the young person's behavior or to ensure safety.

TABLE 7–4.   **Options for emergency dispositions**

Begin crisis intervention in emergency setting

Send home with outpatient referral or appointment to return to emergency room

Provide other family members with information on outpatient referral or appointment to return to emergency room

Observe in the emergency room

Contact child welfare or protective services for placement outside the home in a shelter or foster home or for supervision in the home

If the patient is medically unstable, hospitalize in pediatric unit (may need constant observation) with psychiatric consultation

Psychiatric hospitalization

Involve juvenile court

Suicide

Suicidal behavior is life threatening in all of its forms and should, therefore, be taken seriously regardless of age or circumstance. In pediatric patients, adults may assume that the intention of the youth's suicidal behavior is not serious and may not seek treatment. Very young children may lack the cognitive and physical skills to act on suicidal ideation, but a preoccupation with self-destructive behavior suggests significant psychiatric disturbance. Even the most blatant "gesture" can prove fatal, especially in a child whose assessment of physical danger may be immature and unrealistic.

The need for accurate and prompt identification of suicidal behaviors is essential given the tendency for these symptoms to recur within days or weeks.

Epidemiology

The Youth Risk Behavior Survey (Grunbaum et al. 2002), conducted by the Centers for Disease Control and Prevention, found that in the past year, 19% of high school students had "seriously considered attempting suicide," nearly 15% made a specific plan to attempt suicide, close to 9% made a suicide attempt, and 2.6% made a medically serious suicide attempt. In prepubertal children, the male-to-female ratio of completed suicide attempts is 3:1; a figure that increases to 5.5:1 in the 15- to 24-year age group. However, the prevalence of suicidal ideation and attempts is higher in females by a ratio of 1.6:1. Males choose more lethal methods of suicide, including firearms and hanging, whereas females resort to overdose, carbon monoxide poisoning, and jumping. Suicide attempts using firearms are particularly lethal, especially when combined with substance use. Approximately 2 million teenagers in the United States attempt suicide each year, and nearly 2,000 die of suicide. The most common means are rifles, shotguns, or handguns (Shaffer and Greenberg 2002). In males, a history of suicidal behavior increases the risk of completed suicide. The association in females is not as strong. Gay, lesbian, and bisexual youth are more likely to become suicidal because they typically experience multiple risk factors including depression, substance abuse, sexual victimization, rejection by family, and bullying by peers. The incidence of suicides in male teenagers increased dramatically from the mid-1960s to the mid-1980s, but has been declining since 1990 (Shaffer and Greenberg 2002). The reason for the decline is unclear, but may be related to improved detection and treatment of adolescent depression.

Course and Prognosis

Psychiatric disorders are a risk factor for serious and recurrent suicidal behavior. Nearly all suicide victims have a psychiatric diagnosis, particularly affective disorder, in boys often comorbid with substance abuse and/or conduct problems. Unfortunately, only one-third of suicide attempters are ever referred to a mental health facility. Additional risk factors include previous noncompliance with psychiatric treatment, social isolation, poor school performance, abuse and neglect, parental psychiatric illness, and family history of completed suicide. Medical illness increases suicide risk, especially central nervous system damage secondary to trauma, seizure, infection, or chemotherapy. Adolescent suicides may be preceded by stressful events, including the loss of a romantic relationship; reprimands in school or at home; or academic, family, or legal difficulties. Access to firearms increases risk.

Evaluation

When evaluating a youth after a suicide attempt, the clinician should obtain a detailed history of the circumstances preceding and following the attempt; symptoms of mood disorder, substance abuse, or impulsive behavior; wishes to die or to influence others at the time of the attempt; whether a friend or family member has committed suicide (looking for "contagion"); and coping skills and supports in the patient and family. Patients may present with a decline in social functioning characterized by isolation, legal problems, school suspensions, and running away from home. The seriousness of the attempt is determined by a consideration of lethality and intention. *Lethality* is a measure of the likelihood of death and is based on method, location, and the likelihood of being found. *Intention* is a description of what the patient wished to happen and is based on information provided by the patient and the interpretation by the clinician. Patients with a previous history of suicide attempts or who use methods other than ingestion and superficial cutting should be considered at higher risk. Assessment of risk factors for subsequent suicide attempts is essential (Table 7–5). Information should be collected from multiple sources including the patient, caregiver, school, and any other individual close to the patient.

TABLE 7–5.   **Risk factors for repeat suicide attempt**

Patient history

Verbalization or threats regarding suicide

Substance abuse

Poor impulse control

A recent loss or other severe stressor

Previous suicide attempt(s)

A friend or family member who has committed suicide

Exposure to recent news stories or movies about suicide

Poor social supports

Victim of physical or sexual abuse

Nature of the attempt

Accidental discovery (versus attempt in view of others or telling others immediately)

Careful plans to avoid discovery

Hanging or gunshot

Family

Wishes to be rid of child or adolescent

Does not take child's problems seriously

Overly angry and punitive

Depression or suicidality in family member

Unwilling or unable to provide support and supervision

Mental status examination

Depression

Hopelessness

Regret at being rescued

Belief that things would be better for self or others if dead

Wish to rejoin a dead loved one

Belief that death is temporary and pleasant

Unwillingness to promise to call before attempting suicide

Psychosis

Intoxication

Treatment

In determining disposition, safety is the first concern. A brief hospitalization may be useful to complete a more detailed assessment and begin treatment, even in youths who deny continuing suicidality. Compliance with outpatient treatment recommendations can be improved if the therapist provides an appointment date and time and contacts the patient and family before the initial visit. Family involvement in treatment planning draws them into the therapy and educates them about psychiatric diagnoses, the lethality of the behavior, and the purposes of treatment. Caretakers should be told directly to lock away potentially lethal medications and to remove firearms from the home (or at least lock them securely, with ammunition stored and locked in a separate location). Although "no-suicide contracts" do not eliminate risk, the discussion can provide insight into the thinking of both patient and caregivers.

Subsequent treatment includes treating primary psychiatric disorders, improving problem solving and stress reduction skills, and stabilizing the home and school environment. A model of dialectical behavior therapy has been developed for suicidal adolescents (A.L. Miller et al. 1997), based on adult models, but has not been systematically tested.

Child Maltreatment

In all psychiatric evaluations, the clinician should retain a high index of suspicion and collect information about the possibility of physical or sexual abuse. All states have laws requiring professionals who suspect child abuse to report it to the designated authorities. Mandated reporting is not confined to *confirmed* abuse. If evidence is sufficient to raise a serious question, the situation must be reported to prompt an official investigation. Clinicians acting in good faith are immune from liability for reporting, but legal penalties are assessed for failing to report. When the clinician suspects abuse, he or she should tell the parents that an investigation will ensue and that helpful services may be available from the child protection agency. Abusive parents are often frightened by their loss of control and remorseful for the injury to the child. They are overwhelmed by stressors and may be relieved to have aid in protecting the child. If the child is in immediate danger, he or she should be admitted to a pediatric service (by means of a court order, if necessary) until the investigation and determination of disposition are complete. In cases of significant abuse in which the parent is the perpetrator or is unable to protect the child, the protective service agency should place the child in an emergency shelter or foster home. At times, security guards or police may be necessary to complete the disposition and keep the parent from absconding with an abused child.

Physical and Emotional Abuse and Neglect

Epidemiology. Reported rates of child and adolescent physical abuse and neglect steadily increased according to National Incidence Studies in 1980, 1986, and 1993. Reported rates of emotional neglect are likely to be underestimates because child protection agencies are primarily concerned with the physical safety of children. There are no gender differences until adolescence, when females are more likely to be victims of physical abuse. Fatalities are more likely in younger populations, with more than 75% in children younger than 3 years. Although approximately 1,500 children are fatally abused annually in the United States, the figure is likely an underestimation, given the tendency to report ambiguous deaths as accidental.

Clinical description and etiology. Physical abuse is defined as injury or risk of injury to a child younger than age 18 years as a consequence of being hit with a hand or object or being kicked, shaken, thrown, burned, stabbed, or choked by a parent or parent substitute. Children who are threatened, verbally abused, or given harsh but nonphysical forms or punishment are considered to be emotionally abused. The most common abuser is the child's parent or guardian or the boyfriend of the child's mother. Risk factors for abuse include social isolation of parents, violence between parents, management of behavior problems with corporal punishment, inappropriate expectations for the child's developmental level, caretaker use of alcohol and drugs, and stressors on the family such as unemployment and overcrowding.

Neglect is more difficult to define than abuse, and clarification often requires a pediatric hospitalization with a comprehensive medical, psychiatric, and social evaluation. Neglect may be considered in five categories: 1) medical care neglect, 2) gross safety neglect (lack of supervision), 3) physical neglect (food and shelter), 4) emotional neglect, and 5) educational neglect (the latter two types are not recognized by all states). Emotional neglect applies when the patient is not given adequate attention and affection or is exposed to traumatic and inappropriate behaviors. Poverty contributes even more powerfully to neglect than to abuse. Many neglecting parents have never experienced or witnessed appropriate parenting. Some are mentally retarded, and others abuse drugs or alcohol or have mental illness.

Evaluation.   Physicians should have a high index of suspicion for abuse when evaluating an injured child whose presentation is atypical. The history may yield clues such as delayed seeking of medical care, an explanation that does not fit the injury or the child's developmental level, and frequently changing stories. Injuries characteristic of abuse include, but are not limited to

- Multiple injuries in various stages of healing
- Bruises in the pattern of fingers or belts
- Burns, especially from cigarettes or scalding by water
- Spiral bone fractures
- Head and eye injuries
- Ruptured viscera

Evaluation of suspected abuse or neglect includes a complete physical examination (with radiological studies as indicated) and private interviews with the parents; the child (if old enough to talk) or adolescent; and other persons, such as siblings, babysitters, relatives, and neighbors. Youth may hide abuse because of fears that peers or family members will respond negatively (e.g., blame the victim). Although corporal punishment of children by parents (and, in many states, by teachers or principals) is still accepted by many cultural groups in the United States, any injury inflicted by a hard object or by burning, shaking, or throwing should be considered abuse, as should prolonged or severe spanking.

Effects.   Abused and neglected children are at risk for cognitive deficits, neurological impairment, blindness, physical disability, or even death. Psychological sequelae vary widely in severity and nature, commonly including low self-esteem, difficulty trusting others, impaired social relationships, increased impulsivity and irritability, anhedonia, poor school performance, and self-destructive activities including suicide and a variety of risk-taking behaviors. Posttraumatic stress disorder or reactive attachment disorder may ensue. Abuse victims may have depressive, anxiety, oppositional defiant, conduct, or attention-deficit/hyperactivity disorders or substance abuse.

Interventions.   The initial goal of treatment is to prevent the recurrence of abuse. Interventions include hotlines and self-help groups (organized by Parents Anonymous) that are useful for motivated but socially isolated parents who have difficulty controlling their angry responses toward their children.

Victims need interventions for abuse related symptoms, as well as psychiatric evaluation with multimodal treatment as indicated. Day hospital programs provide a safe and nurturing environment to begin abuse specific interventions. Group play therapy can encourage interaction with peers and avoid the solitary play that frequently develops in maltreated children. Options for pharmacotherapy are limited. Propranolol or clonidine may decrease hyperarousal and hypervigilance associated with posttraumatic stress disorder (PTSD).

Parents at high risk include teenagers, new parents, impoverished single parents, and individuals with histories of substance abuse or cognitive limitations. Perpetrators have high rates of depression, substance abuse, and antisocial behavior requiring assessment and treatment. Education in normal child development and principles of behavior management may be useful. Some parents need concrete assistance with housing, food, and medical care. Therapeutic and supportive services are often best provided in the home, because many families are both poorly motivated and insufficiently organized to make use of traditional outpatient services. Short-term placement of the child in foster care may be necessary while parents regroup and/or obtain psychiatric treatment. Child welfare agencies and family courts should be encouraged to determine rapidly whether parents can be rehabilitated and the children returned or whether proceedings should be initiated to terminate parental rights. Too often a child is placed in a succession of foster homes, punctuated by unsuccessful returns to the parents.

Sexual Abuse and Rape

Epidemiology.   Approximately 120,000 cases of sexual abuse are substantiated by child welfare agencies each year. Although the reported incidence of sexual abuse and rape is increasing with mandatory reporting laws and heightened public awareness, it is still likely to be an underestimate. Females are more likely to be victimized than males by 4–5:1. Most perpetrators are male and usually known to the victim. Although the offenders in most reported abuse cases are fathers or stepfathers, retrospective studies also identify uncles or brothers as frequent perpetrators. Extrafamilial and intrafamilial sexual abuse of boys is less frequently reported and prosecuted, even though the psychological consequences may be debilitating. Recent high-profile cases of sexual molestation of young males may bring more clinical, therapeutic, and legal attention to this problem.

Evaluation.   Sexual abuse varies widely in degree of sexual contact; amount of physical or psychological coercion; single vs. repeated incidents; and whether the abuser is a member of the household, another person known to the child, or a stranger. The child may tell a parent, a friend, or a teacher, or there may be physical evidence such as prepubertal vaginal bleeding; recurrent urinary tract infections; inflammation, bruises, or lacerations of the genitals or anus; venereal disease; or pregnancy. Sudden onset of compulsive masturbation, precocious sexual knowledge or behaviors, oppositional behavior, fears, running away, depression, sleep disturbance, somatic symptoms, or decreased academic performance may raise suspicion.

Rape or sexual abuse by a stranger is usually reported by the victim immediately, although boys are less likely to acknowledge abuse because of a fear of retribution, a desire to appear self-reliant, and the social stigma against homosexual behavior. The child is often seen acutely in the emergency room. Sexual abuse by a relative or family friend is more difficult for children to report, is often discredited by the mother, and may result in a family crisis. In cases of father–daughter incest, the mother may suspect or be aware of the abuse, but fear of the father or a wish to "protect the family" prevent her from taking action. The mother may even tacitly encourage the abuse. In these families, a daughter takes on many aspects of the role of the mother and wife who is less available because of depression or physical illness.

The purposes of the initial evaluation are

- To determine whether abuse is likely to have occurred
- To ensure that the child is protected
- To establish the need for medical and psychological treatment

It is important that the evaluation itself does not further traumatize victims of sexual abuse. A team approach, in which health and mental health care professionals work together with the child protection agency and the legal system, avoids subjecting the child to repeated inquisitions. A complete physical examination is indicated, preferably by a pediatrician or pediatric gynecologist who has experience in evaluating abused children and who can carry out the procedures required for legal evidence. The clinician should interview (together and separately) the child, parents, and siblings. Questions about the specifics of the abuse are best saved for private interviews. For children who have difficulty verbalizing, the opportunity to draw or use puppets may be helpful. The use of anatomically correct dolls is controversial. If the alleged perpetrator is not a member of the immediate family, his or her interrogation is often best left to agency or legal officials. More complete evaluation of psychiatric and developmental status should be deferred for a subsequent interview.

Children rarely make false allegations of sexual abuse, except when prompted by a parent embroiled in a custody dispute, adolescent vindictiveness (e.g., to remove a disliked stepfather), or a wish to disguise the teenager's voluntary sexual activity. When false allegations are suspected, a child and adolescent psychiatrist with special expertise should be consulted.

Effects. Victims of sexual abuse are at increased risk of behavioral and emotional problems, and are overrepresented in clinical psychiatric settings. Rates of psychiatric disorders increase as the children approach school age, probably because they begin to recognize the deviant nature of the abuse. Victims report higher rates of major depression, anxiety disorders, conduct disorder, borderline personality disorder, antisocial personality disorder, paranoia, somatization, and bulimia. A history of sexual abuse increases the likelihood of attempted suicide 2- to 14-fold. Full or partial PTSD is common. Symptoms include fear, startle reactions, reenactment of the trauma, flashbacks, sleep disturbance, and depression. Children and adolescents who are victims of particularly severe or long-lasting abuse may experience dissociative reactions and conversion symptoms. The tendency to reenact the trauma may lead to sexual behavior problems. Among victims, risk factors for emotional and behavior problems include family disruption, economic hardship, preexisting psychiatric diagnosis, and scapegoating of the child for reporting the abuse. Psychological symptoms include suicidality, fears, sleep disorder, low self-esteem, sexual precocity or preoccupation, impaired social adjustment, and subsequent sexual dysfunction as an adult. Promiscuity or, in contrast, a phobic reaction with sexual inhibition may develop.

Medical sequelae include damage to the genitals or rectum, acquired immunodeficiency syndrome (AIDS), and other sexually transmitted diseases, which may lead to pelvic inflammatory disease and infertility.

Interventions.   The child must be protected from both further sexual abuse and the effects of reporting it, especially if the perpetrator is the father or the mother's boyfriend. The child should return home only if the abuser has been removed from and does not have access to the home and if the mother can and will protect the child.

Research on treatment for sexually abused children and adolescents is limited. Sexual abuse is an experience rather than a disorder and the treatment targets symptoms and dynamics. Symptoms resulting from abuse vary based on developmental level, with children more likely to experience anxiety and sleep disorders and adolescents more likely to experiment with drugs and delinquent behavior. Cognitive-behavior therapy has been effective in preschool-age children (Cohen and Mannarino 1997).

Treatment interventions are "abuse-specific" and encourage the expression of abuse-related feelings, correct cognitive distortions regarding the abuse, teach prevention skills, and encourage support from other abuse victims. Specific symptoms may persist, however, and require targeted interventions that may include psychopharmacology. The therapist should select a treatment approach based on the characteristics of the child, the presence of psychiatric symptoms, and the family context. Intermittent treatment may be required for effects of abuse that may not appear for months or years. There is no evidence, however, that psychiatric treatment for victims of abuse who are asymptomatic will function as prophylaxis against future problems.

In incest cases, legal pressure may be required to initiate and maintain treatment of the perpetrator. Therapy models that aim at improving family functioning have not been particularly successful. Many parents (whether perpetrator or spouse) of sexually abused children have been abused themselves, making it difficult for them to deal with their child's situation. These parents may benefit from a support group for adult victims of childhood incest. If alcohol is a precipitating factor, successful treatment of the alcoholism markedly decreases the risk of recidivism.

Out-of-Control Behavior

When a child or an adolescent is brought to an emergency room because his or her behavior is out of control (Table 7–6), the clinician must first use whatever physical means are necessary to ensure the safety of the patient, family, and staff.

Evaluation

If a patient has been aggressive, it is important to determine whether a person or object actually has been harmed or only threatened verbally or with gestures. Detailed description of the aggressive behavior includes: precipitants, warning signs, evidence of an altered mental state, actual damage, need for physical restraint, repetitive behaviors, lethality (including access to firearms), solitary vs. group action, and response to any previous treatment. Cultural factors may affect both the precipitant and the response.

The mental status examination includes an assessment of current anger or violent intent, organic cognitive impairment, paranoia, delusions or hallucinations, and impulsivity.

Patients with mental retardation, neurological disorders, or delayed expressive and receptive language are more likely to communicate distress through aggression and require specific adaptation or the treatment plan. The older and larger the youngster, the more seriously aggression must be taken. If attention-deficit/hyperactivity disorder, conduct disorder, psychosis, mental retardation, or drug abuse cause impulsivity and impaired judgment, a more restrictive environment may be needed.

Children and adolescents with a history of escalating violence and pervasive hostility are most problematic. Occasionally youth will show little guilt or remorse for their actions. The risk of aggressive behavior is increased by neuropsychological dysfunction and exposure to violence following head trauma and/or physical abuse.

TABLE 7–6. **Causes of out-of-control behavior in children and adolescents**

Temper outbursts
   Attention-deficit/hyperactivity disorder
   Oppositional defiant disorder
   Conduct disorder
   Mental retardation

Anxiety-provoked aggression
   Separation anxiety disorder
   Panic disorder
   Obsessive-compulsive disorder
   Acute phobic hallucinations (especially in children ages 2–6 years)

Organic delirium
   Medical illness
      Fever
      Electrolyte imbalance
      Central nervous system infection, tumor, trauma, or vascular
        accident
      Seizures
      Endocrine or autoimmune disorder
      Hypoxia
      Metabolic disorder
   Adverse reaction to prescribed or over-the-counter medication
   Toxic ingestion
   Reaction to illicit substance
      Acute intoxication or toxic reaction
      Flashback
      Withdrawal
      Psychotic reaction to chronic drug use

Schizophrenia

Mania

Abuse or neglect
   Posttraumatic stress disorder

Witnessed violence between caregivers may have a greater emotional effect than actual victimization of the child. In such instances, parents model the choice of aggression as a solution to problems. Family assessment is important because relationships among all family members are affected by violence.

Treatment

In the acute situation, medication is sometimes considered, although children have usually calmed and rarely require medication in the emergency room. Special caution in pharmacotherapy is needed if a medical disorder or drug ingestion is suspected. If necessary, acutely psychotic adolescents can be given a neuroleptic (see Chapter 8). Particular attention should be paid to the safe and appropriate use of seclusion and restraint, if needed. The indications are risk of harm to self or others and the failure of less restrictive interventions to control the patient's behavior.

In considering disposition from the emergency room, the clinician must consider the safety of vulnerable persons in the home (e.g., a baby) and the ability of the adults to supervise. Even if the behavior resolves quickly in the emergency room, these youngsters often have multiple social, psychological, academic, and behavior problems that require psychiatric follow-up. The courts and child protective services are frequently involved in disposition planning.

After safety is ensured, the goal of treatment is to address the underlying cause of out-of-control behavior. Psychiatric hospitalization is not effective in the treatment of severe conduct disorders, placing more emphasis on partial hospitalization, residential treatment, therapeutic school placement, and comprehensive home-based treatment programs. The success of outpatient therapy depends on the patient's and family's cognitive abilities and motivation, the severity of antisocial behavior, and use of a systems/ecological approach. Cognitive-behavioral programs like anger management training encourage greater individual control. Social skills training increases alternatives to aggression, if the environmental contingencies can be managed to encourage their use. Family and, when necessary, the legal system should be involved and actively support the treatment process.

■ FAMILY TRANSITIONS

A substantial number of children spend some part of their life with just one parent, whether due to single motherhood, separation, divorce, or death of a parent. Children in single-parent households typically have more responsibility, not only for chores but also for management, decision making, baby sitting for younger siblings, and emotional support of the parent. As a result, these children may be more independent, competent, and responsible than other children but at the expense of having less freedom, more worries, and less closeness with peers. The parent–child relationship can suffer when children resent the additional responsibility.

Divorce

Effects

Divorce affects nearly all aspects of a child's life. It is a process that begins with marital strain and discord (that may last for years), is punctuated by the marital separation, and leads to dramatic changes in family life. To the child, divorce reflects the failure of a relationship that was to serve as a model of love and commitment. A conflict-ridden intact family is, however, more detrimental to children than a stable one-parent home. In fact, marital discord is a more important risk factor for child maladjustment than actual divorce or conflict following divorce (Buehler et al. 1998). High-intensity marital conflict during childhood is associated with attachment difficulties, externalizing and internalizing symptoms in childhood, and psychological disorders as young adults. Parental violence is even more detrimental to children's adjustment than conflict, and repeated exposure to violence predisposes to PTSD in children. Additionally, rates of child abuse and sibling violence are increased in violent compared with nonviolent high-conflict marriages. Protective factors that have been identified for children in high-conflict marriages include a positive relationship with a caregiver and supportive siblings. In addition, for teenagers, peer relationships and a positive self-concept appear to be helpful. Another influence on the impact of high-conflict parental relationships is the manner in which parents settle their disputes. Unresolved or chronic discord is associated with more difficulties for children. Parental conflict in which each parent criticizes the other to the child and attempts to gain the child's alliance is particularly damaging, whether in an intact family or after divorce. Intense parental conflict may also reflect psychiatric symptoms in one or both adults. Children and adolescents commonly blame themselves for the divorce, view themselves as potential saviors, and harbor fantasies that their parents will reunite.

Reactions to parental divorce may vary with the age and developmental level of the child, and the time since divorce. Infants may react with irritability and sleep and feeding difficulties. Children ages 2–6 years commonly experience separation anxiety and behavioral regression such as clinging or loss of toilet training. Children ages 5–9 years may be anxious, sad, and preoccupied with loss of their intact family and separation from their fathers (or sometimes their mothers), whatever the nature of the prior relationship. Slightly older children may feel shame and anger or complain of somatic symptoms, but have somewhat better coping mechanisms to deal with their feelings. Disruptions in peer relationships and academic learning are common. They may feel powerless, frightened, and intensely angry with one or both parents. They are more likely than younger children to take active sides in ongoing battles between their parents. Adolescents tend to react either with depression, acting out, and emotional and social withdrawal from friends and school or with a developmental spurt, showing unexpected maturity, empathy, and compassion and providing significant help to one or both parents. School social adjustment and academic performance may be negatively affected by divorce.

The relative effects of different custody options are difficult to study, although in one 12-year follow-up study of low-income families with contested custody in divorce who had been randomly assigned to mediation or litigation, mediation resulted in greater continuing involvement with the nonresidential parent without an associated increase in coparenting conflict (Emery et al. 2001). Recent research has found a positive correlation between joint legal custody and children's adjustment; however, parents' psychological well-being and the quality of the parent–child relationship are key variables. Divorcing parents who *request* joint custody are likely to be those who are more able to maintain a parental coalition and active involvement of both parents, despite the dissolution of the marriage. Fathers with joint custody are more likely to remain emotionally involved with and financially supportive of the children. If a judge awards joint custody against the wishes of one or both parents, severe conflict is likely to continue, to the detriment of the child. This is particularly true for infants and toddlers who are often forced into overnight visits at a time when separations may be traumatic. Single-parent custody relationships have been effective, particularly when contact with the noncustodial parent remains an option for the child. Even when the noncustodial parent has been unreliable or has acted violently, the child may continue to request visits. Unfortunately, divorce almost always has a detrimental effect on the relationship between the noncustodial parent and the child. Contacts become primarily social, and these parents rarely are partners in the child's discipline or education. There is evidence, however, for noncustodial fathers that the quality of paternal parenting and the child–father relationship are more important than frequency of contact (Amato and Gilbreth 1999).

Marital separation and divorce create social upheaval for the child. The standard of living typically declines, due to spreading the family income over two households instead of one, inadequate child support, and mothers who may be poorly equipped to enter the job market. When a stay-at-home mother must return to work, children may be traumatized by yet another separation. Reduced income may lead to a move to a more modest neighborhood, with resulting separation from familiar peers, neighbors, and school.

Divorce has phases that require repeated adjustment. Some children do poorly during the first year after divorce, a time that forces change on the parent as well as the child. Many parents, coping with their own anger, grief, depression, anxiety, and loneliness, as well as struggling with the financial settlement and the practicalities of maintaining separate households, are emotionally unavailable to their children and unable to provide consistent routine and discipline. Typically, hostility between parents decreases over time. Long-term adjustment is dependent on the ability of the custodial parent to maintain a functional household, continue the child's relationship with the noncustodial parent, avoid economic disaster, and provide emotional nurturance to the child. Adolescents and young adults may experience delayed effects of divorce as they enter dating, falling in love, and marriage.

Although many boys are more oppositional, defiant, and aggressive following divorce than are girls, these behaviors typically predate the divorce. Preexisting symptoms may be exacerbated by parental separation, however. Boys suffer especially from loss of their father, who provides a male model and firmer discipline. Boys are more likely than girls to be exposed to parental fights, receive more inconsistent and negative discipline from divorced mothers, have mothers who report more stress and depression, and receive less positive support and nurturance from mothers, teachers, and peers after the divorce (Hetherington 1979). Most children of divorced parents eventually must readjust to one or more new families, as one or both of their parents remarry. Remarriage of a custodial mother is associated with increased problems in the mother–daughter relationship but decreased behavioral symptoms in boys (Hetherington et al. 1985). Perhaps this is because stepfathers have stronger relationships with stepsons than with stepdaughters. Young adolescents who have functioned in parental roles often have special difficulty adjusting to a stepparent, who usurps some of their duties and privileges. Awareness of the parent's sexual activity is acutely embarrassing to teenagers.

Although some young adults who have faced divorce as children have significant consequences, the majority have resilient outcomes. Children of divorced families have been reported to have more subsequent behavioral problems, including substance use and difficulties with relationships, than those in intact families, although less so than previously believed. Age of the child, time since divorce, parenting styles, and degree of parental/family conflict likely influence these complex issues of postdivorce adjustment (Hetherington 1999).

Interventions

Education regarding expectable reactions to divorce is useful for parents and children. A support group may reduce feelings of isolation and guilt, especially in communities where divorce is uncommon. Postdivorce groups or workshops based in schools offer services with less stigma. Parents Without Partners, a self-help group with chapters nationwide, offers companionship, advice, and moral support from adult peers, as well as educational programs and role models for children. Brief focused therapy can help children and parents deal with their feelings and aid parents in resolving conflict and establishing new lives. In a controlled trial with white, middle-class families undergoing divorce, a 6-year follow-up of a group and individual prevention program with mothers, with or without their school-age children, found that the adolescents from the intervention groups (compared with controls, who received reading material) had fewer mental disorders and fewer sexual partners. Among those initially at higher risk, the intervention subjects had fewer behavior problems and less substance use (Wolchik et al. 2002). Some states provide court-connected programs that offer or mandate evaluation, counseling, crisis intervention, and make recommendations to the judge regarding custody, visitation rights, and child support. Divorce and custody mediation is available as an effective alternative to the adversarial litigation process. However, in circumstances of abuse, violence, mental limitations or illness, the judicial system is appropriate for protection of children and parents. Children and parents with significant symptoms may require more extensive psychiatric evaluation including individual and/or family therapy. Parental psychiatric problems following divorce are associated with more difficulties for children; therefore, prompt treatment for these adults is critical.

Physical Illness in Parents or Siblings

When a family member is chronically or seriously ill, parental resources in time, money, and emotional energy available to other family members are reduced. In addition, nearly all children have at some time wished that something bad would happen to a parent or sibling. If that person then falls ill, the child may literally believe that he or she caused the illness. This "magical thinking" is normal in young children and appears under stress even at later developmental stages.

To the extent that an ill child receives special treatment, sibling rivalry is exacerbated. This may be overt or concealed by the child's guilt or parental shaming. A child or an adolescent often must take on extra chores to substitute for a parent or sibling. Parents can help by equalizing chores, discipline, privileges, and treats as much as developmental stages and physical condition permit.

Childhood disability and illness have an impact on the whole family system, although there is a paucity of systematic study. The sibling of a disabled child may be teased by peers. Correct information about the disability will facilitate coping. Some siblings of children with severe, chronic disabilities are more likely to have symptoms of aggression, depression, social isolation, and oppositional behavior, although not to a sufficient degree to receive a psychiatric diagnosis (Breslau and Prabucki 1987). Families already stressed (e.g., by financial strain or single parenthood) are at higher risk for emotional or behavioral symptoms.

Death of a Family Member

The death of a family member, particularly a parent or primary caregiver, is a traumatic event for a child that can elicit strong emotional or behavioral responses. Bereaved children often experience depressed mood, sadness, longing for the deceased, appetite changes, irritability, social withdrawal, declining school performance, and sleep disturbances. In the first 2 months after parental death, the effect can be profound and may lead to the development of major depression and suicidal ideation. However, the severity of these symptoms wanes over time, and within a year most children no longer have symptoms (R.A. Weller et al. 1991). In a study of the psychosocial functioning of bereaved children from stable families, the children appeared similar to healthy control subjects and were better than the comparison group of depressed inpatients (Fristad et al. 1993). If the death involves trauma, the expected anger and grief may escalate to intense rage or fantasies of revenge or PTSD symptoms. If the death involves a child, the siblings must face their own grief in the context of their grieving parents' emotional withdrawal. Suicide-bereaved children have to address grief as well as the stigma and anguish surrounding suicide. Suicide-bereaved children experienced more anxiety, anger, and shame than children bereaved from parental death not caused by suicide (Cerel et al. 1999).

The terminal phase of the parental illness may, in fact, be more stressful for the child. During this time, the child is exposed to the physical changes and painful consequences of life-threatening disease. The child also becomes aware of the irreversible nature of the illness and the likelihood of death. Parental illness changes the structure and organization of the family. Family roles and routines change, and family cohesiveness may suffer as the ill parent becomes less available physically and emotionally, and the other parent may be exhausted by caretaking and grief. Terminal phases of illness require more resources for care, which may jeopardize the family's financial stability. When a parent has been ill, the death may mark the end of a tragic and difficult period for the family and begin the process of healing and reorganization.

When a family member dies, the child should be allowed some choice in whether to attend the funeral (if developmentally appropriate). A study by E.B. Weller et al. (1988) showed that attendance at funeral activities did not result in increased psychiatric symptoms 2 months later. Extra support, such as an adult friend or relative, can be helpful through the funeral process, because the surviving parent is often too preoccupied with his or her own grief to be very available to the child. Children can mourn, although they may express their grief in behavior rather than verbally. If the child is especially vulnerable because of a psychiatric disorder or additional stressors, clinical judgment should influence the decision about how to handle the funeral, and extra therapeutic support may be needed.

Parents should explain death in a matter-of-fact, concrete way. Religious explanations should be used only if these are consistent with family beliefs. It is not wise to say that "death is like sleeping" or that "God took a person because He loved him (or her)" because children may then have fears of sleeping or of being taken by God. One could explain that body functions stop working when someone is very old or very sick. The magical thinking and egocentricity that are normal characteristics of children lead them to believe that they may be responsible for the death. They will often be too frightened or guilty to mention this and should be spontaneously reassured that they had nothing to do with the cause of the death.

The child's conceptualization of death plays a role in adjustment. As children mature, they gradually develop an understanding that death is universal and irreversible. Children younger than 2 or 3 years do not understand at all; they are simply made anxious by the separation. At ages 4–5 years, death seems reversible, like sleep or a long journey. Preschoolers believe that dead people can eat, sleep, and play, either in heaven or under the ground, and may view death as reversible, like sleep or a long trip. For 5- to 10-year-olds, death can be personified. A more realistic concept of death develops in children ages 10–11 years. Although by then most understand that death is universal, more than half of fourth graders do not yet clearly understand the irreversibility of death. Elementary school–age children tend to view death as a punishment for bad behavior. Although adolescents cognitively understand the meaning of death, they often do not accept their own mortality.

The longer-term effects of family bereavement depend on how well the surviving parents cope and are able to restore family life functioning. Open and honest expressiveness among mutually supportive family members facilitates this process. If the child's life is further disrupted by economic hardship or changes in school, home, and friends or the child's relationship with the deceased parent had been conflictual, the risk of significant adjustment problems may be increased.

Adoption

Approximately 3% of children and adolescents in the United States are adopted. Adopted children are overrepresented in psychiatric treatment settings, even after controlling for the adolescents' problems and family demographic factors (B.C. Miller et al. 2000). Possible contributing factors to the higher rate of psychiatric referral of adopted children include disruptions in early life, adoptive home problems (such as unrealistic expectations by both the adoptive parents and the child, the parents' negative feelings about the inability to conceive, parental and grandparental favoritism toward natural children, criticism from the extended family, poor communication), and the child's unresolved feelings about being given up for adoption or identity issues. Biological contributions to the higher rate of psychiatric referral may be poor prenatal or perinatal care and genetic contribution from the biological families. The understanding of temperament (see Chapter 2) emphasizes the importance of "goodness of fit" between parent and child. To the extent that there is a genetic contribution to temperament, adopted children may be more likely to be mismatched with one or both parents, increasing the risk of behavior and emotional problems.

Children adopted past infancy are at higher risk for psychiatric problems as a result of the experiences that led to placement for adoption. These children have endured not only the loss of their parent(s) or primary attachment figure, but perhaps also neglect, abuse, and frequent changes of caregiver. Some children adopted after spending their first years in a residential nursery are capable of forming stable affectionate relationships with their adoptive parents, but many show significant social and attentional problems or attachment difficulties.

It is normal for children and adolescents, even those who have not been adopted, to go through stages of questioning whether they are with their "real" parents and whether another set of parents would be better. It is important for adoptive parents not to take these stages too seriously or personally. Although there is not a clear consensus of when the best time is to disclose adoption status, the child's cognitive functioning should be taken into account. The American Academy of Pediatrics recently published a policy statement supporting gay men and lesbians being allowed to adopt their partner's children.

Working Parents

Demographics

The 1998 Census Bureau data revealed that for the first time, families with two working married parents are in the majority. The percentage of working women with an infant doubled from 1976 to 1998. The 2000 Census Bureau data, however, show the percentage of new mothers with children under 1 year of age who were working mothers or looking for employment dropped from 59% to 55%.

Day Care

The effects of day care are difficult to study because of the lack of appropriate control groups. Families in which one parent chooses (or is able) to stay home may be different in many ways from those in which both parents are employed outside of the home. To some degree, outcome depends on the amount of time spent in day care and the quality of the day care setting, especially the staff-to-child ratio and the stability of caregivers. Early, extensive, and continuous day care is associated with less harmonious parent–child relations and increased child aggression and noncompliance (Belsky 2001). Other important variables are the mother's feelings about working and about her job, maternal stress, family financial status, the presence of the father, stability in the home, the quality of the child's attachment, and the child's temperament.

Children's responses to day care vary. Some studies have found that children (especially boys) who have been in group day care are more social, assertive, and aggressive. In contrast, some children may become anxious. Children are not more likely to become primarily attached to the day care provider than to the parent. Investigators have suggested that children in out-of-home care before age 6 months are more likely to show a higher degree of disobedience and resistance to adult directions at age 2 years. On many other measures, however, children who have been in day care since infancy score as well as or better than home-reared children. For families with severely limited parenting skills and other resources, even less-than-optimal day care may represent a positive alternative, especially if the mother can use the opportunity to advance herself educationally or vocationally.

After-School Care

Even after children reach school age, families without a parent at home during the day must arrange child care before and after school, during school holidays, and when the child is ill. Although some innovative school-based programs are available, many parents have few alternatives, even if they can afford them. Some children who are unsupervised after school ("latchkey children") are at increased risk for conduct disorder or emotional problems. Outcome may depend on the child's level of maturity, judgment, and behavior control; the presence of peers in the self-care situation (a risk factor); financial and social stressors on the family; and the family's ability to provide supervision at a distance. Young persons with a psychiatric disorder require more structure and supervision.

■ ADOLESCENT PREGNANCY

Demographics

In 2000, 9% of women 15–19 years of age in the United States became pregnant. Slightly more than half of the pregnancies result in a live birth, one-third have induced abortions, and the remainder have miscarriages or stillbirths (Darroch 2001). Rates are higher among those who are from disadvantaged backgrounds, of African American or Hispanic ethnicity, married, have much older male partners, and live in southern states. The vast majority of pregnancies to unmarried teenagers are unplanned and most are unwanted. Teenagers who are pregnant at age 15 years or younger are twice as likely as women age 22 years or older to have a second child within 2 years. Recent declines in the adolescent pregnancy rate are probably due to decreasing rates of sexual activity, higher rates of condom use, and the availability of longer-acting hormonal contraceptives.

Adolescents who are good students, more educationally ambitious, of higher socioeconomic status, less religious, and who have parents and friends who are more accepting of abortion are more likely to choose abortion. Teenagers tend to complicate the abortion decision by waiting until late in the first trimester when physical risk and expense are higher. Adoption rates have declined as the social stigma on single parenting has decreased, especially in certain socioeconomic subgroups. Teenagers who choose adoption tend to have the support of parents and boyfriends and are more likely to be white, religious, suburban, and of a higher socioeconomic class. Delays in deciding how to deal with an unplanned pregnancy can increase risk for the baby by postponing prenatal care.

The Mother

Adolescents who become pregnant are not a uniform group; they differ by race, socioeconomic status, and age (Furstenberg et al. 1989). In studies controlled for academic aptitude and financial status, teenage mothers are less likely to complete high school, less likely to achieve a stable and well-paying job, more likely to be dependent on public assistance, and less likely to enter a stable marriage than their peers. In addition, teenage mothers are more likely to have anemia and hypertension. Interestingly, those who are able to finish high school, avoid another pregnancy in their teens, and marry do not show negative effects at long-term follow-up when compared with peers who delayed their first pregnancy.

The Child

Lack of adequate prenatal care is a risk factor for prematurity, low birth weight, and neonatal mortality, especially for mothers younger than age 15 years. Children of teenage mothers have higher postneonatal mortality rates and more illnesses and injuries and are at increased risk for sudden infant death syndrome (McAnarney and Hendee 1989). The second child born to an adolescent mother is at risk for low birth weight and prematurity at levels twice as high as in mothers age 20 years or older.

Children, especially sons, of teenage parents appear to be at a developmental disadvantage and may be at higher risk for emotional problems, hyperactivity, aggression, school failure, and incarceration. The daughters of adolescent mothers are more likely to become pregnant before age 18 years than offspring of mothers in their 20s. Relative contributions of poor prenatal care, genetic factors, parental limited education, and poor parenting because of immaturity, financial stresses, and living in disadvantaged neighborhoods with low-quality schools are difficult to tease out.

Interventions

Once an adolescent becomes pregnant, supportive and nonjudgmental therapy for the young woman and her family, along with practical and educational assistance, may facilitate making an informed decision among adoption, abortion, and raising the child. Young mothers are most satisfied with the outcome of their pregnancy when they receive parental support for their decision. Adolescents may not be able to anticipate or understand the consequences of the pregnancy and so require continued support. For teenage mothers raising a child, outreach programs offering prenatal care, child care, parenting training, assistance in completing high school, further academic or vocational training, and enrichment programs such as Head Start for the children can positively affect long-term outcome.

Even a negative pregnancy test provides an opportunity for medical and psychosocial intervention, because these adolescents are likely to become pregnant and are more likely than their peers to have multiple partners. Screening for sexually transmitted diseases, provision of effective contraception, and education regarding "safe sex" and the psychosocial impact of pregnancy should follow a pregnancy test (or completed pregnancy) in all adolescents, whether positive or negative.

■ OBESITY

Clinical Description

Obesity, or medically significant overweight, caused by excess body fat, is coded on DSM-IV-TR Axis III. Body mass index (BMI; weight in kg/height in m²) is the most appropriate measure to screen for childhood obesity and can be adjusted based on age and gender. A BMI greater than the 95th percentile is considered a cutoff for obesity. BMI correlates with levels of hypercholesterolemia, hypertension, and risk for cardiovascular disease, all complications of childhood obesity. When measuring BMI, the clinician must also consider the percentage of body fat. Children who are overweight due to increased muscle mass rather than fat are not at higher medical risk.

Epidemiology

The prevalence of childhood obesity is increasing dramatically, and has even been called an epidemic. Rates are increasing even faster among Hispanic and African American children than in non-Hispanic White children.

Etiology

Genetic, medical, and family environmental factors contribute to the development of obesity. Parental obesity increases the risk three-fold. Infants with low birth weight or who were born of diabetic mothers are more likely to develop obesity. On normal growth curves, children do not increase their BMI between the ages of 1 and 6 years. Children with such an increase are more likely to become persistently obese. Girls are more likely to become obese during adolescence because body fat typically increases, in contrast to males who lose body fat as adolescents. There is little evidence that metabolic rates differ significantly between obese children and those of normal weight. Genetic factors may influence weight gain, but do not explain the dramatic increase in childhood obesity over the past 30 years. During this period, physical activity decreased while intake of fat and refined sugar rose. The home environment of obese children tends to be less supportive, with higher incidence of physical and sexual abuse than in the homes of nonobese children.

Course and Prognosis

Obesity in middle childhood (especially if it persists through adolescence) predicts adult obesity more accurately than does obesity in infancy.

Childhood obesity can result in medical complications including a doubling of the rate of cardiovascular disease and tripling of the risk for diabetes. Severe liver disease with hepatitis and fibrosis may result. Obstructive sleep apnea as a consequence of weight gain can lead to nighttime hypoxemia, cardiac arrhythmias, and right heart failure. Obesity carries a social stigma as well. Children have more difficulty making and keeping friends, negatively affecting levels of self-esteem. Occasionally the fear of fatness can lead to the development of eating disorders, particularly bulimia.

Evaluation and Differential Diagnosis

A complete pediatric examination is indicated to rule out rare specific chromosomal (e.g., Klinefelter's syndrome, Prader-Willi syndrome) or endocrine (e.g., hypothyroidism, Cushing's disease) causes of obesity. The clinician must also understand the eating habits and activity level of the entire family and determine how each caregiver perceives the problem. There should be unanimity among family members because the patient will otherwise receive mixed messages that will undermine treatment.

Treatment

Multimodal treatment of obesity combines cognitive-behavioral modification in a group setting, balanced diet, and exercise, in collaboration with the pediatrician. Traditional psychotherapy is not effective in the treatment of obesity per se. Contingency management is useful in the treatment of obesity in younger children: a chart is used to record points earned for self-monitoring, control of eating, and exercise that may be exchanged for rewards or negotiated backup reinforcers. Adolescents are taught to keep a detailed diary, including food intake and events and feelings proceeding eating. They learn self-reinforcement (making positive statements about themselves when they resist temptation) and coping strategies. "Cognitive restructuring" eliminates negative and self-defeating statements about eating and weight. The youngster who is not an active partner can easily cheat. The most difficult problem is long-term maintenance of appropriate weight. Cognitive-behavioral modification includes "relapse prevention" techniques to learn to identify high-risk situations, use coping strategies such as problem solving and assertiveness, and avoid turning a small slip into a catastrophic lapse.

Nutritional education is essential for both parents and children. The "Traffic Light Diet" (Epstein and Wing 1987) identifies foods as green (to be consumed freely), yellow (to be eaten with caution), and red (to be avoided entirely). A weight-reduction diet must be nutritionally adequate. Extreme diets may have more serious consequences in developing children than in adults.

Family involvement in the treatment of obesity is essential, because parents control access to food, at least in younger children, and dispense most rewards and punishments. If both parent and child are obese, treatment of the child's obesity is more likely to succeed if the parent is treated simultaneously *and* loses weight. Interestingly, the child's maintenance of weight loss does not seem to depend on the parent's maintenance. Modeling is apparently important in initial weight loss, but contingent reinforcement and child self-regulation are important in maintenance. For adolescents, separate treatment of the parent may be more effective.

Exercise increases calorie expenditure, increases basal metabolism rate (avoiding the decrease that otherwise accompanies calorie restriction), suppresses appetite, and reduces the medical complications of obesity. Sensible diet plus incorporating increased physical activity into everyday routines, or "lifestyle exercise," are more effective in maintaining weight loss than more intensive aerobic exercise programs, which have lower long-term adherence.

■ PHYSICALLY ILL CHILDREN AND ADOLESCENTS

Developmental Factors in Reaction to Acute Illness, Hospitalization, and Surgery

The emotional response to illness is dependent on the child's stage of development, the amount of discomfort, the type of treatment and its side effects, the practical limitations that result from the illness, premorbid psychiatric problems in the patient, and the child's level of understanding. Parents affect the child's reaction through their own coping mechanisms and the support they provide. Physicians can usually predict the most stressful times in the course of an illness and should take these opportunities to provide additional emotional support. Innovations such as parental rooming-in, unlimited parental visiting, permitting parents to be present while the child is sedated preoperatively, and outpatient surgery to avoid hospital admissions have reduced emotional aftereffects. The use of primary nurses and child development specialists in the hospital has also facilitated children's adjustment. Preparation, individualized to coping style and developmental level, may be done via talks explaining procedures, visits, books, puppet shows, and films.

Infancy

Hospitalized infants younger than 6 months are most upset by the change in the usual routine. It is helpful to have the parents do as much of the caregiving as possible and to arrange for consistent nurses. For the older infant who has formed strong differential attachments, separation is traumatic, and stranger anxiety adds to the infant's distress. Infants respond to the emotional reactions of the primary caregivers. An anxious, tense mother will be less able to soothe and comfort her child than one who is calmer and in better control. The infant's immature cognitive development exacerbates the problem because explanations are of no use. Infants do not recognize that they have an illness or disability and simply respond to discomfort by crying or becoming irritable. Fortunately, most pediatric hospital settings not only permit but also encourage parents to "live in" while their infant is hospitalized. In the absence of an attachment figure, the baby's physical agitation, refusal to eat, and inability to sleep may have serious medical consequences.

Early Childhood

Hospitalized children ages 1–3 years may react to separation from their parents by rejecting parents when they visit, being aggressive toward medical staff, regressing in bowel and bladder control, and/ or refusing to eat. If parents are absent, children may develop depression, sleep disturbance, diarrhea, or vomiting. Maximizing parental presence and providing the child with familiar items from home, especially the child's favorite toy or blanket (transitional object), are helpful. Developmentally, this is a time of increasing exploration and autonomy. Unfortunately, toddlers frequently attempt to master their environment by becoming more oppositional. Parents must exert consistent and reasonable control without encouraging dependent and passive behavior in the child.

For children ages 3–5 years, separation from parents by hospitalization is difficult, even for a child who is comfortably able to separate in other circumstances. Anesthesia and surgery are especially frightening because of normal developmental fears of bodily injury. Children believe that illness and painful treatments are punishment for real or fantasized misbehavior. When possible, preparation by simple explanations and a visit to the hospital may help. Frequent presence of a parent is important. When understandably anxious parents attempt to protect the child's health by limiting the child's activities, including delaying school enrollment, an unintended consequence may be to increase passivity, dependence, and fearfulness in the child.

School Age

Children ages 6–12 years usually tolerate acute illness and hospitalization relatively well, especially when they are prepared, their parents visit daily for substantial periods, and the child's preceding development was on course. They may still have irrational explanations of illness (e.g., that they are being punished or that their parents were unable to protect them). Peer relationships become paramount during this period, and comparisons of physical appearance and capabilities are likely. Medically ill children become aware of their differences and limitations; occasionally their friendships are affected. School attendance and participation are major developmental tasks of childhood; medically ill children have more academic problems than their non–medically ill peers. These problems may be caused by the effects of the illness and its treatment, decreased expectations in the classroom, school absences, or psychosocial stressors. Reactions often include regression or oppositional behavior.

Adolescence

Adolescents have more realistic fears regarding the outcome of illness, such as changes in appearance or inability to continue favorite activities. An injury may make impossible a planned career (e.g., sports, the military). Loss of autonomy and privacy are especially painful for adolescents. The adolescent should be given some control over treatment to avoid struggles between the patient and the caregiver and to convey that the adolescent's opinions are important. Occasionally, noncompliance can be an expression of suicidal ideation, particularly when the consequences are life threatening. Physical appearance and sexuality emerge as priorities during adolescence, and patients with sequelae of illness, injury, or treatment need additional reassurance.

Chronic Illness

The Child's Reaction

Chronic illness can lead to interference with academic, social, and recreational development. Autonomy and control of the child's own body are jeopardized, and self-esteem may be lowered. Especially in adolescence, peers have little tolerance for differences in appearance or behavior. Children and adolescents with chronic illness without disability are twice as likely as control children to have a psychiatric disorder. Those with disability as well as chronic illness are even more likely to have emotional and attention-deficit disorders, social isolation, and school performance problems. The nature of the disability does not appear to be significant unless it involves the central nervous system. Central nervous system disorders are even more likely to have psychiatric sequelae. Episodic illness is more stressful than persistent medical disorders because of the unpredictability of the problem and the need to respond to sudden changes in physical condition. Psychiatric distress may present as an increase in dependent, fearful behavior; an escalation in risk-taking or acting-out behaviors; or, in older children and adolescents, a tendency to become angry, hostile, and isolative. Somatoform disorders are another manifestation of psychiatric illness. Headaches, recurrent abdominal pain, limb pain, chest pain, or fatigue that are affected by psychological factors interact with symptoms of medical disorders and may be difficult to distinguish. The combination can lead to increased physical disability. Catastrophic injury and devastating illness can lead to symptoms of PTSD in both the pediatric patient and the caregiver. Support should be provided to the child, parent, and medical staff. Psychiatric disorder is not inevitable in chronically ill children and adolescents. Fewer than one-third of those with chronic illness have mental health problems or difficulties with social or school adjustment (Cadman et al. 1987).

The Parents' Reaction

The most critical factor in the child's ability to cope with chronic illness is the response of the family. Medical illness in a child tends to exaggerate all the strengths and weaknesses of the family. At the time of diagnosis, the parents must go through a period of mourning with stages similar to those following a death: anger, denial, grief, and resignation. Medical problems in a child may be viewed by the parent (and others) as a negative reflection on the parent. Parents feel guilty, especially for genetic diseases or pregnancy complications. The psychological status of parents is strongly related to their perception of the child's illness. Physicians must, therefore, attend to the parent's understanding of the disorder and all of its implications. Realistic additional caregiving and financial burdens may stress parents beyond their ability to cope. Chronic illness increases the strain on a marriage but does not appear to increase the rate of divorce. The parents' anger, resentment, guilt, and/or denial may interfere with their ability to communicate with each other and to work with the pediatric team. Parents may distance themselves from the child, become overly close or intrusive, or alternate between the two. Mothers of children with chronic illness are at increased risk for depression.

The Terminally Ill Child or Adolescent

When a young person is dying, parents or medical personnel may make misguided attempts to "protect" the child. These are perceived as in the best interests of the child but more often relate to the difficulties adults have with a child's death. Although young patients may not fully understand their clinical situation, children are astute observers of emotions in their parents, nurses, and doctors. If the child is not dealt with honestly, his or her imagination can be even worse than the reality. Children understand the permanence of death by age 10 or 11 years, although they may not understand the relationship between it and the biological aspects of their illness. Parents or physicians may need to tell children about their terminal illness in stages, as understanding progresses and the child is able to cope with the knowledge. Children are often more concerned about immediate details of treatment and its effect on them than about ultimate survival. The child or adolescent should be given the opportunity, but not be forced, to talk about disease, disability, or death. Drawing, painting, or doll play may be useful symbolic outlets and means of communication.

The terminal phase of an illness leads to a recapitulation in parents of the feelings of denial, anger, grief, depression, and guilt that followed the initial diagnosis. Discussions about death between parent and child should be encouraged as a way to prepare the child, answer his or her questions and fears, and say good-bye. If a child is terminally ill for a long time, anticipatory mourning may be completed, and the parents gradually detach, leaving the child no emotional place in the family. Similarly, physicians may inadvertently avoid the child and family when aggressive treatment is no longer an option and the medical team is resigned to the patient's death. Alternatively, if a child who is expected to die recovers, parents often experience a "Damocles syndrome," living in constant fear of disease exacerbation and death.

The Child or Adolescent With AIDS

Children infected with human immunodeficiency virus (HIV) have even more difficulties than the typical chronically and terminally ill child. These young people may be feared and stigmatized by peers, teachers, other adults in the community, potential foster parents, and, too often, health care personnel. Poverty is common, and parenting may be poor. The psychiatric effects of the disease itself are often added to associated factors that put the child at risk, including an HIV-infected mother who may be dying or dead, a chronic medical illness requiring transfusion (e.g., hemophilia), or adolescent behavior problems that led to indiscriminate intercourse and/or injection drug use. The sequelae of central nervous system infection by the virus (delayed development, cognitive impairment, and organic mood and behavior disorders) add to the burden of illness. Counseling HIV-positive adolescents regarding sexual behavior and their plans for the future is essential.

Adherence to Treatment

Lack of adherence to or compliance with medical procedures and regimens can be a major problem in the care of children and adolescents. Attention to and remediation of each patient's specific causes of noncompliance are essential for optimal medical management. Factors in the child and parent, family dynamics, the nature of the treatment, and the relationship between the child and family and the medical team can all contribute to poor adherence. Severe noncompliance may warrant a full psychiatric evaluation and treatment of individual psychiatric disorders and/or family dysfunction.

Compliance is facilitated by giving the child or adolescent as much responsibility for the treatment as possible, gradually increasing responsibility as interest, understanding, and behavior control improve. The child should participate in decision making and be offered as many choices as possible. Explanations can be targeted to the child's ability to understand. The normal compulsiveness of children ages 6–12 years can be harnessed to develop a habit of charting or record keeping related to the treatment. If children or adolescents are able to develop their own relationships with medical personnel, compliance may be facilitated by avoiding the struggles for independence inherent in the parent–child relationship. Adults should minimize power struggles and, whenever possible, negotiate and solve problems with the young person. At times, a child's noncompliance signals a parent's ambivalence or even opposition to treatment.

Treatment

Psychotherapy

Supportive individual, family, and/or group education and psychotherapy are often valuable for the patient and parents. Instruction in social problem-solving and coping skills may be beneficial.

Support Groups

Support groups for children and adolescents and for parents, both separately and as families, may be enormously helpful. These groups provide emotional support and inform the patient and the family about challenges the disease is likely to present. Chronically ill children may benefit from disease-specific camps and recreation programs with medical supervision, which permit them more normal activities and provide a respite for parents.

Pharmacotherapy

Indications for the use of pharmacotherapy in medically ill children and adolescents do not differ from those in routine psychiatric cases. Drug choice and management decisions are, however, affected by the illness and should be made in conjunction with the pediatric specialist. Disorders that are the direct consequence of medical illness, including delirium and organic affective states, respond well to aggressive pharmacological interventions. Situational and anticipatory anxiety related to medical procedures may benefit from hydroxyzine, diazepam, or alprazolam. Treatable depression should be actively sought, because depression is not an inevitable response to illness and may dramatically impede recovery.

Behavior Modification

Techniques such as behavior contracting with contingency management and self-monitoring with self-reinforcement are invaluable in improving medical and behavioral compliance. Children who refuse or are unable to swallow oral medication can be taught to take pills using instruction, modeling, contingent rewards, and a behavior-shaping protocol that involves successively larger candies or placebos (Pelco et al. 1987).

Cognitive-behavioral techniques can be used to ameliorate a variety of chronic physical symptoms and symptom-related behaviors. For example, in treating headache, the antecedents and consequences of pain are determined (by keeping a pain diary, if the child is old enough), and attempts are made to modify events and situations that precipitate or positively reinforce pain. The clinician works with the patient, parents, teachers, pediatrician, and significant others to emphasize functioning normally despite pain as well as stress management techniques. Reductions in pain and pain-related behaviors give patients a sense of control and mastery and a return to age-appropriate activities. *Stress inoculation* helps to prevent anxiety in children before medical and dental procedures and reduces anxiety, pain, or discomfort connected to repeated procedures such as chemotherapy injections, bone marrow aspirations, and spinal taps in chronically ill children. Stress inoculation consists of multicomponent cognitive-behavioral approaches, including education, modeling procedures, systematic desensitization, hypnosis, contingency management, imagery, and breathing exercises.

Hypnosis is readily used in children, who are generally more hypnotizable than adults. Different techniques are appropriate for children of different ages. Hypnosis is used in treating physical symptoms with a psychological component or managing severe physical symptoms (pain, nausea) associated with a medical disorder or treatment.

Relaxation training for children and adolescents is used to manage pain in pediatric migraine, juvenile rheumatoid arthritis, and hemophilia. These techniques can result in decreased subjective experience of pain, reduced need for analgesics, and even improved mood, self-esteem, and physical and social functioning. Relaxation techniques are also used in treating asthma or cystic fibrosis in patients who hyperventilate.

■ CHILDREN OF PSYCHIATRICALLY ILL PARENTS

Risks and Resilience

Children of mentally ill parents are at increased risk for psychiatric disturbance, due to both genetic factors and the effect of mental illness on parenting skills and family environment. Child outcome may be affected by parental marital discord with conflict over child rearing and an inability to provide adequate support in the face of life challenges. Parents may be less affectionate, particularly when struggling with depression, leading to impairment that can extend across generations. Poor decision making may result in inadequate supervision and exposure to danger. Occasionally the parent's psychiatric illness involves the child (e.g., a delusion about the child).

Family disruption may lead to divorce or placement of the child outside of the home. The risk of psychopathology in the child is related to the severity and chronicity of psychiatric illness in the parent. Both assortative mating and a contagion effect may result in two parents with a mental disorder, increasing the likelihood that their offspring will suffer a psychiatric illness.

Children are particularly distressed when their parents are admitted to a psychiatric hospital. Younger children show sleep disturbance, decreased appetite, attention-seeking behavior, separation anxiety, crying (especially at bedtime), and social withdrawal. Adolescents are more able to verbalize their fears, guilt, and concerns about themselves and their parents.

Children whose parents have an affective disorder have an increased (but by no means inevitable) incidence of depressive symptoms and nonspecific behavior and emotional disturbance. Children with an affectively ill parent have a 40% chance of suffering a depressive episode by age 20 and a 60% chance by age 25 years (Beardslee et al. 1998). These children are more likely to experience a variety of internalizing symptoms including recurrent feelings of guilt, interpersonal problems, and difficulties with attachment. Children of schizophrenic parents are more likely to have abnormalities in attention and information processing, even before overt symptoms emerge. Children of patients with anxiety disorders have a markedly increased risk for an anxiety disorder themselves, as well as for symptoms such as fears and worries, school difficulties, somatic complaints, and social isolation (Turner et al. 1987). Having a parent with a personality disorder seems to increase a child's risk for conduct disorder.

A significant minority of children of alcoholic parents have increased behavior problems, especially conduct problems, hyperactivity, impulsivity, hypersensitivity to stimuli, poor self-control, inattention, and emotional symptoms such as anxiety and depression (Bennett et al. 1988; Weinburg 1997). Prenatal alcohol exposure is among the most common nongenetic cause of mental retardation and can contribute to the development of learning and language disabilities. Children of alcohol abusers are more likely to develop alcohol problems themselves, and the disinhibition associated with substance use places them at greater risk for suicide, accidents, unplanned pregnancy, HIV exposure, and school failure. Probable mediating factors include the presence of consistent caregivers in a healthy and secure environment, a stable family with few disruptions and adequate economic support, and the absence of physical or emotional neglect and abuse.

Some "invulnerable" or "resilient" children not only resist and cope with unusual stress but also thrive and succeed despite adversity. Protective factors include a cohesive and emotionally supportive family environment; and external support systems, such as caring extended family members, other adults, and/or institutional supports (e.g., school or community agencies). These children have a strong commitment to extracurricular activities and interpersonal relationships and tend to be confident and self-reliant. They are realistic in their assessment of the family and its limitations, and understand their own coping style when dealing with parental psychiatric illness.

Adolescence is a particularly high-risk period for the development of major depression in the offspring of parents with affective disorder. Successful adaptation in these adolescents is characterized by close, confiding relationships; persistence and success in school and work; and involvement in activities. They are able to separate themselves, cognitively and emotionally, from their parent and their parent's illness, while often functioning as caregivers in the family. Coping skills include accurate cognitive appraisal of the stress to be dealt with, realistic assessment of their responsibilities and powers, and an understanding of the parent's illness (especially that they are not responsible for their parent's depression).

Interventions

Parents can promote resilient traits in their children and moderate the emotional consequences of their psychiatric illness. Communication between spouses and among family members improves the level of understanding and reduces guilt and emotional upset. Children should be referred to appropriate support groups. Individual strengths in the child should be encouraged and nurtured. When parents are receiving psychiatric treatment, the clinician should be alert to possible effects of the illness on the children. Parental psychiatric hospitalization is particularly stressful. There should be at least one family session near the time of admission to explain the need for hospitalization and the anticipated treatment course. Optimally, a member of the treatment team interviews each child to assess developmental level, school performance, peer relationships, coping skills for dealing with and understanding parental illness, and the possible presence of psychiatric symptoms. Efforts can be made to enrich and strengthen the child's support system. Placement with a relative or in foster care may be necessary until the parent can resume child-care responsibilities.

■ REFERENCES

Amato PR, Gilbreth JG: Nonresident fathers and children's well-being: a meta analysis. J Marriage Fam 61:557–573, 1999

American Psychiatric Association: Diagnostic and Statistical Manual of Mental Disorders, 4th Edition, Text Revision. Washington, DC, American Psychiatric Association, 2000

Beardslee WR, Versage EM, Gladstone TRG: Children of affectively ill parents: a review of the past 10 years. J Am Acad Child Adolesc Psychiatry 37:1134–1141, 1998

Belsky J: Emanuel Miller Lecture: developmental risks (still) associated with early child care. J Child Psychol Psychiatry 42:845–859, 2001

Bennett LA, Wolin SJ, Reiss D: Cognitive, behavioral, and emotional problems among school-age children of alcoholic parents. Am J Psychiatry 145:185–190, 1988

Breslau N, Prabucki K: Siblings of disabled children: effects of chronic stress in the family. Arch Gen Psychiatry 44:1040–1046, 1987

Buehler C, Krishnakumar A, Stone G, et al: Interparental conflict styles and youth problem behaviors: a two-sample replication study. J Marriage Fam 60:119–132, 1998

Cadman D, Boyle M, Szatmari P, et al: Chronic illness, disability, and mental and social well-being: findings of the Ontario Child Health Study. Pediatrics 79:805–813, 1987

Cerel J, Fristad MA, Weller EB, et al: Suicide-bereaved children and adolescents: a controlled longitudinal examination. J Am Acad Child Adolesc Psychiatry 38:672–679, 1999

Cohen JA, Mannarino AP: A treatment study for sexually abused preschool children: outcome during a one-year follow-up. J Am Acad Child Adolesc Psychiatry 36:1228–1235, 1997

Darroch JE: Adolescent pregnancy trends and demographics. Curr Womens Health Rep 1:102–110, 2001

Emery RE, Laumann-Billings L, Waldron MC, et al: Child custody mediation and litigation: custody, contact, and coparenting 12 years after initial dispute resolution. J Consult Clin Psychol 69:323–332, 2001

Epstein LH, Wing RR: Behavioral treatment of childhood obesity. Psychol Bull 101:331–342, 1987

Fristad MA, Jedel R, Weller RA, et al: Psychosocial functioning in children after the death of a parent. Am J Psychiatry 150:511–513, 1993

Furstenberg FF, Brooks-Gunn J, Chase-Lansdale L: Teenaged pregnancy and childbearing. Am Psychol 44:313–320, 1989

Grunbaum JA, Kann L, Kinchen SA, et al: Youth risk behavior surveillance—United States, 2001. MMWR Surveill Summ 51(4):1–62, 2002

Hetherington EM: Divorce: a child's perspective. Am Psychol 34:851–858, 1979

Hetherington EM (ed): Coping With Divorce, Single Parenting, and Remarriage: A Risk and Resiliency Perspective. Mahwah, NJ, Lawrence Erlbaum, 1999

Hetherington EM, Cox M, Cox R: Long term effects of divorce and remarriage on the adjustment of children. J Am Acad Child Adolesc Psychiatry 24:518–530, 1985

McAnarney ER, Hendee WR: Adolescent pregnancy and its consequences. JAMA 262:74–82, 1989

Miller AL, Rathus JH, Linehan MM, et al: Dialectical behavior therapy adapted for suicidal adolescents. Journal of Practical Psychology and Behavioral Health 3:78–86, 1997

Miller BC, Fan X, Grotevant HD, et al: Adopted adolescents' overrepresentation in mental health counseling: adoptees' problems or parents' lower threshold for referral? J Am Acad Child Adolesc Psychiatry 39:1504–1511, 2000

Pelco LE, Kissel RC, Parrish JM, et al: Behavioral management of oral medication administration difficulties among children: a review of literature with case illustrations. J Dev Behav Pediatr 8:90–96, 1987

Shaffer D, Greenberg T: Suicide and suicidal behavior in children and adolescents, in The Many Faces of Depression in Children and Adolescents. Edited by Shaffer D, Waslick BD. Washington, DC, American Psychiatric Publishing, 2002, pp 129–178

Turner SM, Beidel DC, Costello A: Psychopathology in the offspring of anxiety disorder patients. J Consult Clin Psychol 55:229–235, 1987

Weinberg NZ: Cognitive and behavioral deficits associated with parental alcohol use. J Am Acad Child and Adolesc Psychiatry 36:1177–1186, 1997

Weller EB, Weller RA, Fristad MA, et al: Should children attend their parent's funeral? J Am Acad Child Adolesc Psychiatry 27:559–562, 1988

Weller RA, Weller E, Fristad MA, et al: Depression in recently bereaved prepubertal children. Am J Psychiatry 148:1536–1540, 1991

Wolchik SA, Sandler IN, Millsap RE, et al: Six-year follow-up of preventive interventions for children of divorce: a randomized controlled trial. JAMA 288:1874–1881, 2002

■ ADDITIONAL READING

American Academy of Child and Adolescent Psychiatry: Practice parameters for forensic evaluation of children and adolescents who may have been physically or sexually abused. J Am Acad Child Adolesc Psychiatry 36:423–442, 1997

American Academy of Child and Adolescent Psychiatry: Practice parameter for the assessment and treatment of children and adolescents with suicidal behavior. J Am Acad Child Adolesc Psychiatry 40 (7 suppl):24S–51S, 2001

Gould MS, Greenberg T, Velting DM, et al: Youth suicide risk and preventive interventions: a review of the past 10 years. J Am Acad Child Adolesc Psychiatry 42:386–405, 2003

Kelly JB: Children's adjustment in conflicted marriage and divorce: a decade review of research. J Am Acad Child Adolesc Psychiatry 39:963–973, 2000

Putnam FW: 10-year research update review: child sexual abuse. J Am Acad Child Adolesc Psychiatry 42:269–278, 2003

Robinson JE: Emergencies I, in Manual of Clinical Child and Adolescent Psychiatry, Revised Edition. Edited by Robson KS. Washington, DC, American Psychiatric Press, 1994, pp 251–282

Sauzier M: Emergencies II: sexual abuse and rape in childhood, in Manual of Clinical Child and Adolescent Psychiatry, Revised Edition. Edited by Robson KS. Washington, DC, American Psychiatric Press, 1994, pp 283–314

8

PSYCHOPHARMACOLOGY

■ SPECIAL ISSUES FOR CHILDREN AND ADOLESCENTS

General Principles

In the treatment of psychiatric disturbances in children and adolescents, psychopharmacology may be a key part of a multimodal treatment plan, the primary intervention, or an adjunct to other forms of treatment. The clinician must educate the family regarding the disorder, its overall treatment, and the child's needs at each developmental stage. The clinician also must consider the meaning of the prescription and administration of a drug to the child, the family, and the child's teachers and peer group.

The clinical practice of pediatric psychopharmacology is impeded by the relative lack of double-blind randomized placebo-controlled trials. Many medications that appeared to be effective in anecdotal reports, case series, and open trials were not shown to be more effective than placebo in double-blind studies. In evaluating the medical literature on drug effects, it is important to distinguish between *statistically* significant and *clinically* significant effects: to know whether the target symptoms are reduced to near-normal levels or merely changed and to determine the clinical meaning of the change. Because groups are heterogeneous, some patients' conditions may improve and others may worsen, resulting in nonsignificant group data. Alternatively, statistically significant group changes may translate into only modest improvement in individual patient functioning and may not be worth the effort, expense, and potential risk of the treatment.

Simultaneous use of more than one medication ("polypharmacy") should be cautious and judicious, due to the increased risk of significant side effects, toxic drug interactions, and difficulty assessing effectiveness.

Developmental Toxicity

The interactions between drug treatment and physical, cognitive, social, and emotional development may produce unique or especially severe side effects. All psychotropic medications have the potential for cognitive toxicity. Because some drug treatments last for years, there is a risk of chronic and cumulative effects. Cognitive blunting can impair developing academic skills, social skills, and self-esteem even before physical side effects are observed, especially in young children. Young patients may have behavioral toxicity (i.e., the worsening of preexisting behaviors or affective states or the development of new symptoms). Behavioral toxicity typically abates after dose adjustments or change of drug.

Indications and Dosage

Once a drug is approved for any indication, the U.S. Food and Drug Administration (FDA) regulates only the company's advertising of the drug, not the prescribing behavior of physicians. Because in the past, pharmaceutical companies have had little incentive to test drugs in children, the majority of psychopharmacological agents and indications (and most drugs used in pediatrics as well) lack pediatric labeling and are "unapproved" or "off-label" for children. As a result, the FDA guidelines as published in the *Physicians' Desk Reference* (PDR) cannot be relied on for appropriate indications, age ranges, or doses for children. Although lack of approval for an age group or a disorder does not imply improper or illegal use, it is prudent to inform the family of these labeling issues, as well as of evidence in the literature for safe and effective use. The physician should make clinical judgments based on the medical literature rather than the PDR.

Dosage may be determined by titration using efficacy and side effects, within guidelines based on age, weight, or blood levels, or by extrapolation from adult doses. Although it is ideal for pediatric drug doses to be derived from data on children, these dosage studies are rare. A useful general principle for dosing is "start low and go slow."

The age-dependent processes of drug absorption, distribution, protein binding, metabolism, and elimination influence optimal dose size and schedule. Young children absorb some drugs more rapidly than do adults, leading to higher peak levels. Age-related factors that may influence distribution include uptake by actively growing tissue and proportional size of organs and tissue masses. Proportion of fat (which serves as a reservoir for lipid-soluble compounds) increases during the first year of life, followed by a gradual loss until (in girls) the prepubertal increase (Briant 1978). The higher the proportion of fat, the lower the total body water content. In children, drugs such as lithium (which are primarily distributed in body water) have a proportionally larger volume of distribution and therefore a lower concentration. By age 1 year, glomerular filtration rate and renal tubular secretion mechanisms reach adult levels. Hepatic enzyme activity develops early, and the rate of drug metabolism is then related to liver size. Relative to body weight, the liver of a toddler is 40%–50% greater, and that of a 6-year-old is 30% greater, than the liver of an adult. Compared with adults or older adolescents, young children generally require a larger dosage per kilogram of body weight of drugs that are primarily metabolized by the liver (Briant 1978). They may also require divided doses to minimize fluctuations in blood level. Near the time of puberty, the rate of hepatic drug transformation often decreases abruptly toward adult levels, requiring more careful monitoring (Jatlow 1987). The pubertal increase in gonadal hormones may be contributory (Ryan et al. 1986). Compared with adults, children tend to have less protein binding of drugs, leaving a greater proportion of the drug biologically active.

Outcome

Assessing the risk-benefit ratio, especially for long-term treatment, is particularly complicated in children and adolescents. Many scientific unknowns persist regarding drug effects during development. Evaluation is complicated by a variety of nonpharmacological effects, including nonspecific therapeutic effects of evaluation and treatment, expectancy in the patient, parent, or teacher, changes in the environment, and the natural course of the disorder (e.g., the waxing and waning of symptoms in Tourette's disorder).

The clinician must specify target symptoms and obtain affective, behavioral, and physical baseline and posttreatment data. Treatment effects can be assessed by interviews of and rating scales for the patient, the parent, and other caregivers (e.g., teachers, inpatient nurses); direct observation in the office, waiting room, or classroom; physical examination; and, as appropriate, specific cognitive tests to measure attention or learning or laboratory tests. The clinician must actively seek both therapeutic and adverse effects because many young patients will not report them spontaneously, and parents may not notice.

The interactions between treatment and the environment raise complex issues for children and adolescents. To assess medication effects in a child or adolescent, the clinician must evaluate and monitor the adult and peer environments as well as the patient. It is important to know what a clinical change and the therapeutic contacts mean to the patient and to family members. For example, a positive drug effect in a child patient may be clouded by a parent's or sibling's negative reaction to the change.

The adults (parents, teachers, or staff in an inpatient unit or residential treatment setting) who care for children may misinterpret the youngster's response to the environment as indicating a need for medication or an improvement that is a result of medication. Some of these adults mistakenly seek to use psychotropic medication alone to control or eliminate a child's troublesome behavior, instead of investigating the family or institutional dynamics that may be provoking and maintaining such behavior or implementing more time-consuming, difficult, and expensive therapeutic or behavioral management strategies or changes in living situation.

Adherence to Treatment

Effective treatment requires a therapeutic alliance and the cooperation of the patient, parents, school personnel, and often other caregivers. Compliance with a treatment regimen can be reduced by factors such as lack of perceived need for treatment, failure to understand the disorder, carelessness, lack of money, misunderstanding of instructions, or refusal to cooperate. Overly complex schedules of drug administration may make accurate administration nearly impossible. Media attention to alleged inappropriate use of medications, especially Ritalin and Prozac, has made some families and teachers highly resistant to pharmacotherapy.

Some children cannot or will not swallow pills. Some drugs are available in elixir form or can be dissolved in juice. Problems with this method of administration may include unpleasant taste, chemical interaction resulting in precipitation of the medication, and inaccurate dosing. Some drugs come in capsules that can be opened and the contents "sprinkled" into applesauce. A behavior modification program to shape pill-swallowing behavior is available on the web at http://www.aboutourkids.org/articles/pillswallowing.html.

Ethical Issues

The careful physician attempts to balance the risks of medication, the risks of the untreated disorder, and the expected benefits of medication relative to other treatments. It is generally preferable to accumulate substantial clinical experience with a new drug in adults before it is used with children and young adolescents.

Consent for pharmacotherapy in children is a complex issue (Popper 1987) that can be made even more difficult if the parents or guardians are in conflict (e.g., in angry divorces or with children in the custody of child welfare). Informed consent is best considered an ongoing process rather than a single event. "Assent" to medication use is considered possible to obtain from a patient older than

7 years (Popper 1987). Formal consent forms are less useful than a documented discussion of therapeutic options with potential risks and benefits. Published information sheets for parents, youth, and teachers are available to supplement discussions with the physician about specific medications (Dulcan and Lizarralde 2002).

■ STIMULANTS

The number of available stimulant preparations (Table 8–1) has increased dramatically. They include a variety of forms of methylphenidate and amphetamine. Magnesium pemoline (Cylert) is very rarely used, because of the risk of potentially life-threatening chemical hepatitis and the monitoring of liver functions that is therefore needed.

Indications and Efficacy

The most well-established indication for stimulants is in the treatment of *ADHD*. (Most studies in the literature used the older terms attention-deficit disorder [ADD] or hyperactivity.) Stimulants retain their efficacy in adolescents (and adults) with symptoms of ADHD. In preschool children, stimulant efficacy is more variable, and the rate of side effects is higher, especially sadness, irritability, clinging, insomnia, and anorexia. Stimulants can improve attention and reduce excessive distractibility in patients with all three subtypes of ADHD. Many children whose symptoms respond positively to stimulants, however, continue to have deficits such as specific learning disabilities and gaps in knowledge and skills caused by inattention, poor social skills, and family problems. Intensive behavior modification may add to stimulant efficacy or permit the use of a lower dose of medication, but it is often difficult to implement and sustain behavioral treatment and to transfer improvements from one setting to another. The National Institute of Mental Health (NIMH) Multimodal Treatment of ADHD (MTA) study showed that optimally titrated methylphenidate was more effective for core ADHD symptoms than intensive behavioral ther-

TABLE 8–1. Stimulant preparations

Drug	Formulation	Doses
Methylphenidate		
Generic		5, 10, 20, SR20
Methylin		5, 10,[a] 20[a]
Methylin ER (6–8 hours)	Wax matrix	10, 20
Ritalin		5, 10, 20
Ritalin SR (6–8 hours)	Wax matrix	20
Metadate ER (6–8 hours)	Wax matrix	20
Ritalin LA (8–10 hours)[c]	Capsule with microbeads SA:LA ratio=50:50	20, 30, 40
Metadate CD (8 hours)[c]	Capsule Diffucap with beads Comes in 30-pill blister pack SA:LA ratio=30:70	20
Concerta (12 hours)	Oros (osmotic controlled-release tablet) SA:LA ratio=4:14	18, 27, 36, 54
MethyPatch	Transdermal system	18 mg Oros=5 mg SA bid or tid or 20 mg SR Not yet available
Dexmethylphenidate		
Focalin	Only dextro isomer	2.5, 5, 10

TABLE 8–1. Stimulant preparations *(continued)*

Drug	Formulation	Doses
Dextroamphetamine		
Generic		5, 10
DextroStat		5,[a] 10[b]
Dexedrine		5
Dexedrine Spansule (6–8 hours)	Capsule with particles	5, 10, 15
Mixed salts of amphetamine		
Adderall		5,[b] 7.5,[b] 10,[b] 12.5,[b] 20,[b] 30[b]
Adderall XR (12 hours)[c]	Capsule with beads SA:LA ratio=50:50	5, 10, 15, 20, 25, 30

Note. LA=long-acting; SA=short-acting.
[a]Scored.
[b]Double-scored.
[c]May be sprinkled.

apy, that optimal methylphenidate treatment plus behavioral treatment was more effective than behavioral treatment alone, and that any of the MTA treatments were more effective than treatment as usual in the community (largely stimulants, but at lower doses, fewer doses per day, shorter duration of treatment, and less close monitoring) (MTA Cooperative Group 1999).

When *conduct disorder* or *oppositional defiant disorder* co-exists with ADHD, stimulant medication can reduce defiance, negativism, and verbal and physical aggression. In children and adolescents with *mental retardation,* stimulants are effective in treating ADHD target symptoms. Stimulants also reduce symptoms of inattention, impulsivity, and overactivity in some children with *pervasive developmental disorders.*

Boys and adults, with or without ADHD, have similar cognitive and behavioral responses to comparable doses of stimulants, except that children report feeling "funny," whereas adults report euphoria (Donnelly and Rapoport 1985). Stimulants act in the brain by binding to the dopamine transporter, thereby increasing the amount of dopamine available in the synapse. Stimulants may preferentially increase neurotransmitter activity at inhibitory synapses and in inhibitory brain areas. Stimulants are absorbed rapidly from the gut and metabolized rapidly. Stimulant medication effects on ADHD occur primarily as the drug is being absorbed and as the plasma concentration is rising.

There are no useful predictors of whether an individual patient with ADHD will respond to a specific medication. Neurological soft signs, electroencephalogram (EEG), or neurochemical measures have not been shown to be useful predictors of response to stimulants (Halperin et al. 1986; Zametkin et al. 1986). Although prior studies were mixed, the NIMH MTA study showed that children who have anxiety comorbid with ADHD do not have a reduced response to stimulants. Most patients with ADHD have some positive response to at least one of the stimulant medications, although a substantial number of children respond to one stimulant but not another (Elia et al. 1991). Stimulant effects on individual target symptoms (Table 8–2), however, vary greatly from child to child and even from one symptom to another in a single patient. A given dose may produce improvement in some areas but no change or worsening in others. Therefore, if one stimulant is ineffective, another should be tried before using another drug class. Methylphenidate is the most commonly used and best-studied stimulant. Amphetamine has a longer duration of action than methylphenidate. Its disadvantages include negative attitudes of pharmacists (including some who are unwilling to stock it), its exclusion from many formularies, and higher potential for abuse. Compared with methylphenidate, amphetamine may have a slightly greater incidence of side effects such as growth retardation, appetite suppression, and compulsive behaviors.

TABLE 8–2.   **Clinical effects of stimulant medications**

Motor effects	Reduce activity to level that fits the context
	Decrease excessive talking, noise, and disruption
	Decrease fidgeting and finger-tapping
	Improve handwriting
	Improve fine motor control
Social effects	Reduce off-task behavior
	Improve ability to play and work independently
	Reduce impulsivity
	Decrease intensity of behavior
	Reduce bossiness
	Reduce verbal and physical aggression
	Improve (but not normalize) peer social status
	Reduce noncompliance and defiance with adults
	Improve parent–child interactions
	Parents and teachers respond with less controlling and more positive behavior
Cognitive effects	Improve effort and attention, especially to boring tasks
	Increase on-task behavior
	Reduce distractibility
	Reduce impulsivity
	Increase quantity and accuracy of academic work

Longer-acting stimulant preparations are appealing for children in whom the duration of action of the standard formulations is very short (2.5–3.0 hours); when severe rebound occurs; or when administering medication every 4 hours (or at school) is inconvenient, inconsistent, stigmatizing, impossible, or insufficiently supervised to prevent diversion of the drug. The older long-acting forms, Ritalin sustained-release (SR) tablets and Dexedrine Spansule capsules, have been joined by several new formulations: Adderall XR (a mixture of amphetamine salts), and the methylphenidate preparations Concerta, Metadate ER, Metadate CD, and Ritalin LA (see Table 8–1). The capsule formulations with beads (Metadate CD, Ritalin LA, and Adderall XR) may be opened and sprinkled onto applesauce for patients who cannot swallow pills. A transdermal long-acting patch formulation of methylphenidate (MethyPatch) is near approval. Dexmethylphenidate (Focalin) contains only the dextro isomer of methylphenidate. Compared with conventional d,l methylphenidate, half the dose of dexmethylphenidate appears to be just as effective, with fewer side effects, and perhaps longer duration.

Although short-term efficacy of stimulants has been clearly demonstrated, it is much more difficult to demonstrate long-term effects. Existing studies have had serious methodological problems (e.g., naturalistic treatment assignment; comorbidity; premature termination of drug; doses too high, too low, or poorly timed; inconsistent adherence to medication; individual variation in response; and insensitive outcome instruments). A long-term prospective randomized controlled trial assigning children with ADHD to stimulant medication or placebo or other treatment is neither ethical nor feasible.

Initiation and Ongoing Treatment

The decision to medicate a child with ADHD is based on the child's inattention, impulsivity, and often hyperactivity that are not due to another treatable cause and that are persistent and severe enough to cause functional impairment at school and usually at home and with peers. For safety reasons, parents must be willing to monitor the medication and to attend appointments with the child. An important part of treatment is education of the child, family, and teacher, including explicitly debunking common myths about stimulant treatment. Stimulants do *not* have a paradoxical sedative action, do *not* lead to drug abuse, and *do* continue to be effective after puberty.

Multiple outcome measures that use more than one source and setting are essential. The clinician obtains baseline data from the school on behavior and academic performance before initiating stimulant medication. The physician should work closely with parents on adjusting the size and timing of doses and obtain frequent reports from teachers and annual academic testing. The Child Attention Problems (CAP) Rating Scale (see Tables 3–3 and 3–4) or the IOWA Conners Scale (see Chapter 3) is useful in gathering weekly data from teachers.

Many experts recommend a systematic stimulant titration using the full range of doses—for example, 5, 10, 15, and 20 mg of methylphenidate (highest dose omitted for very young or small children). Body weight serves only as a rough guide. Doses of amphetamine or dexmethylphenidate (Focalin) are half the milligrams of methylphenidate. A strategy that is still preferred by many clinicians and parents is to start stimulant medication at a low dose and increase by half (if necessary and if pill is scored) or whole pills (within the usual recommended range) every week or two according to response and side effects. By age 3 years, children's absorption, distribution, protein binding, and metabolism of stimulants are similar to those of an adult, although adults have more side effects than do children at the same milligram per kilogram of body weight dose.

The onset of clinical effect for both methylphenidate and amphetamine is within 30 minutes after each dose. A single dose is usually effective for 3–4 hours. Of the immediate-release forms, amphetamine typically has a longer therapeutic duration than methylphenidate. A typical regimen for the immediate-release preparations would be thrice-daily dosing, with medication given after breakfast, after lunch, and after school. Starting with only a morning dose may be useful in assessing drug effect, by comparing morning and afternoon school performance. The need for an after-school dose or for medication on weekends is individually determined by considering target symptoms. A third dose after school has been shown to improve behavior without increasing sleep problems (Kent et al. 1995). Most children with moderate or severe symptoms of ADHD need full coverage, all day and all week. The long-acting formulations may be given once a day, in the morning, with supplementation with immediate release if necessary.

If the initial stimulant drug choice is not effective, or not well tolerated, more than half of nonresponders to methylphenidate or amphetamine respond to the other stimulant.

Medical monitoring includes pulse rate and blood pressure initially and at times of dose change; weight at baseline, during titration, and two to three times a year; and height at baseline and then several times a year. The clinician must look for and inquire about tics at baseline and at every visit. Periodic reevaluation of the need for a dosage increase or decrease or change in timing of administration will optimize improvement.

Although pharmacological tolerance has been reported occasionally, medication administration is often irregular, and lack of adherence should be considered when medication appears to become ineffective. The child should not be responsible for his or her own medication, because these youngsters are impulsive and forgetful at best, and most dislike the idea of taking medication, even when they can verbalize its positive effects and report few if any side effects. They will often avoid, "forget," surreptitiously spit out, or simply refuse to take a dose of medication. Apparent decreased drug effect may be caused by a reaction to a stressful change at home or school, autoinduction of hepatic metabolism (which may require a 10%–20% dosage increase after several months of treatment), lower efficacy of a generic preparation, or abatement of an initial positive placebo effect. If tolerance does occur, another stimulant may be substituted.

The duration of medication treatment is individually determined by whether drug-responsive target symptoms are still present. Treatment may be required through adolescence and into adulthood. If behavioral symptoms are not severe outside of the school setting, the young person may have an annual drug-free trial of at least 2 weeks, or even the whole summer if symptoms are mild. If school behavior and academic performance are stable, a carefully monitored trial off medication during the school year (but *not* at the beginning) will provide data on whether medication is still needed.

Risks and Side Effects

Most side effects are similar for all stimulants (Table 8–3). Giving medication after meals minimizes anorexia. Insomnia may be due to ADHD symptoms, oppositional refusal to go to bed, separation anxiety, or stimulant effect or rebound. Preexisting sleep problems are common in patients with ADHD. Stimulants may either worsen or improve irritable mood. Other than mildly elevated blood pressure, cardiovascular side effects are exceedingly rare. Toxic effects may result if a child chews one of the long-acting forms instead of swallowing it.

The use of stimulants in patients with a personal or family history of tics has been controversial because of concern that new, persistent tics might be precipitated, especially in those children who are at genetic risk. The physician must balance the impairment resulting from tics with that from ADHD symptoms, considering the efficacy and side-effect profile of alternative medications. With appropriate informed consent and careful clinical monitoring, a stimulant (methylphenidate) may remain the first choice. Tics are extremely common in children with ADHD, with or without stimulant medication, and tend to wax and wane. Several studies have demonstrated that few children develop new or worsened tics while on methylphenidate, and many preexisting tics are unchanged or even improve. There is some evidence that amphetamine can increase tic severity, which may persist (Kurlan 2002).

TABLE 8–3. Side effects of stimulant medications

Common side effects (try dose reduction)	Anorexia
	Weight loss
	Irritability (may be worse with amphetamine)
	Abdominal pain
	Headaches
	Easy crying
Less common side effects	Mildly elevated blood pressure
	Insomnia (may be worse with amphetamine)
	Dysphoria (may be worse with amphetamine)
	Social withdrawal
	Impaired cognitive test performance (especially at very high dosages)
	Decrease in expected weight gain
	Rebound overactivity and irritability (try adding small afternoon or evening dose)
	Nervous habits
	Allergic rash, hives, or conjunctivitis
	Transient motor tics (may be worse with amphetamine)
Infrequent side effects	Dizziness
	Nausea
	Anxiety and fearfulness

TABLE 8–3. Side effects of stimulant medications *(continued)*

Rare but potentially serious side effects (usually reversible)	Exacerbation or precipitation of Tourette's disorder (may be worse with amphetamine) Depression Growth retardation Tachycardia Hypertension Psychosis with hallucinations Stereotyped activities or compulsions
Reported with Concerta only	Tablet lodged in throat
Side effects reported with pemoline only	Choreiform movements Dyskinesias Night terrors Lip licking or biting Hepatotoxicity (rare)

Source. Adapted from Efron et al. 1997; Wagner et al. 2001.

Although stimulant-induced growth retardation has been a concern, any decreases in expected weight gain and growth are small and rarely clinically significant. The magnitude may be dose related and appears to be greater with dextroamphetamine than with methylphenidate (Greenhill 1981). Tolerance to this effect has been reported. Medication-free summers (if clinically appropriate) may facilitate height or weight normalization (Klein et al. 1988). Young adults treated in childhood with methylphenidate showed no decrement in final height (Klein and Mannuzza 1988).

Rebound effects such as increased excitability, activity, talkativeness, irritability, and insomnia, beginning 3–15 hours after a dose, may be seen as each dose or the last dose of the day wears off or for up to several days after sudden withdrawal of high daily doses of stimulants. These effects may resemble a worsening of the original symptoms. Management strategies include increasing structure after school, giving a dose of medication in the afternoon that is smaller than the midday dose, using a long-acting formulation, and adding clonidine (Catapres) or guanfacine (Tenex).

Clinically relevant contraindications to the use of stimulant medication are concomitant use of a monoamine oxidase inhibitor (MAOI), schizophrenia or other acute psychosis, glaucoma, or recent stimulant drug abuse. When potential abuse of stimulant medication by the patient, or, more often, by peers or family members is a concern, Concerta may be a good choice, as its once a day administration is easier to supervise, and the physical characteristics of the pill (methylphenidate mixed with an osmotic "sponge") make it impossible to crush and snort or inject.

In the very rare situation in which pemoline is used, the FDA "black box warning" requires that serum alanine aminotransferase (ALT) (formerly SGPT) levels should be determined at baseline, and every 2 weeks thereafter. Pemoline should be discontinued if serum ALT (SGPT) rises to twice the upper limit of normal or if clinical signs and symptoms suggest liver failure. Written informed consent must be obtained on the FDA-approved patient information/consent form prior to starting pemoline. Parents should be instructed to notify the clinician promptly if the child develops vomiting or persistent abdominal distress, nausea, lethargy, or malaise.

No evidence indicates that stimulants as clinically prescribed decrease the seizure threshold.

A cautionary note: The combination of methylphenidate and imipramine has been associated with a syndrome of confusion, affect lability, marked aggression, and severe agitation, which disappears when the medications are stopped (Grob and Coyle 1986). Methylphenidate interferes with hepatic metabolism of imipramine, which results in a longer half-life, elevated blood levels, and a higher risk of cognitive and cardiac side effects.

A selective serotonin reuptake inhibitor (SSRI) may be added to a stimulant for the treatment of comorbid ADHD and depression or anxiety for symptoms remaining after stimulant treatment of the ADHD.

Stimulants are used in combination with clonidine or guanfacine to treat symptoms resistant to a stimulant alone. This is theoretically appealing because of complementary actions and nonoverlapping side-effect profiles. Anecdotal clinical experience supports the usefulness of these two drugs, especially in children with severe ADHD whose symptoms cannot be managed satisfactorily with a stimulant alone. One trial of methylphenidate and clonidine to treat children with ADHD and tics found the combination to be safe and effective (Tourette's Syndrome Study Group 2002). A small controlled trial of methylphenidate and clonidine in youth with ADHD plus aggressive oppositional defiant disorder or conduct disorder suggested safety and efficacy of clonidine alone or in combination with methylphenidate for these indications (Connor et al. 2000). Although there have been reports of sudden death in children who at one time had been taking both methylphenidate and clonidine, the evidence linking the drugs to the deaths is tenuous at best (Wilens and Spencer 1999). Pending further clarification, extra caution has been advised when treating children with cardiac or cardiovascular disease, when combining clonidine with additional medications, or when dosing of medication is inconsistent. There have been no trials of safety or efficacy of guanfacine combined with a stimulant.

■ ATOMOXETINE

Atomoxetine (Strattera), a recently approved nonstimulant medication for the treatment of ADHD, is a potent inhibitor of presynaptic norepinephrine transporters with minimal affinity for other receptors or transporters. Randomized controlled trials have shown efficacy in inattentive and hyperactive–impulsive symptoms of ADHD as reported by parents (Michelson et al. 2001) and teachers. Side effects are generally mild, including sedation, decreased appetite, nausea, vomiting, and dizziness. Taking the medication with food improves tolerability. There are slight increases in blood pressure and pulse, but no QTc prolongation on electrocardiogram (ECG). Atomoxetine may offer the advantages of desipramine without the risk of cardiac side effects or danger in overdose. It is given once a day, or can be divided into two doses (with breakfast and dinner) to reduce side effects. The starting dose is 0.5 mg/kg/day (usually in a single daily dose) for 3 to 4 days; the target dose is 1.2 mg/kg/day. The maximum dose is 1.4 mg/kg/day or 100 mg, whichever is less. The only known drug interaction is with strong CYP2D6 inhibitors or MAOIs.

■ ANTIDEPRESSANTS

Medications called *antidepressants* commonly used for the treatment of children and adolescents are listed in Table 8–4. Paradoxically, more data are available to support the use of these drugs for other pediatric psychiatric disorders than for depression. Although research is advancing, studies in children and adolescents are difficult to do (especially in mood disorders), and extrapolation is still required from data on adults. Remarkably few empirical data on children and adolescents are available to guide therapeutic choices, especially among drugs of the same class. The newest, safest, and most commonly used class of antidepressants is the SSRIs. Studies have not identified differences in efficacy among the SSRIs, so choice is based on side effects, half-life, interactions with other medications, or trial in the individual patient. If a patient does not

TABLE 8-4. Antidepressant medications most often used in children and adolescents

Generic name	Brand name	Typical[a] daily dose <18 years	Indications supported by RCT <18 years
Selective serotonin reuptake inhibitors			
Citalopram	Celexa	20–60 mg	Depression
Fluoxetine	Prozac	5–40 mg	Depression, social phobia, GAD
		10–60 mg	OCD
Fluvoxamine	Luvox	100–200 mg	OCD, social phobia, SAD, GAD
Paroxetine	Paxil	20–50 mg	Depression, OCD
Sertraline	Zoloft	25–250 mg	OCD
		25–200 mg	GAD, depression
Bupropion	Wellbutrin	100–300 mg	ADHD
	Wellbutrin SR		
Tricyclic antidepressants[b]			
Clomipramine	Anafranil	50–200 mg	OCD
Desipramine	Norpramin	1–3 mg/kg	ADHD
	Pertofrane	2–5 mg/kg	ADHD + tics

TABLE 8–4. Antidepressant medications most often used in children and adolescents *(continued)*

Generic name	Brand name	Typical[a] daily dose <18 years	Indications supported by RCT <18 years
Imipramine	Tofranil	2–5 mg/kg	ADHD, SAD
		25–75 mg	Enuresis
Nortriptyline	Pamelor Aventyl	1–4 mg/kg	ADHD

Note. ADHD=attention-deficit/hyperactivity disorder; GAD=generalized anxiety disorder; OCD=obsessive-compulsive disorder; RCT=randomized controlled trial; SAD=separation anxiety disorder.

[a]Starting doses are lower. Within this range, children require lower doses than do adolescents.

[b]Divided doses required for children.

respond well to the first one chosen, a trial with another SSRI would be indicated. Fluoxetine's especially long half-life may be an advantage if missed doses are likely, but side effects or drug–drug interactions can persist for weeks after fluoxetine is discontinued, and fine-tuning of the dose may be difficult. Escitalopram (Lexapro), a newly approved single-isomer preparation of citalopram, has no research in children.

Tricyclic antidepressants (TCAs) are less often used (especially prior to puberty), because of their more frequent and more serious side effects and lack of demonstrated efficacy in depression.

Other drug classes with considerable research in adults have been studied very little in youth. Trazodone (Desyrel) has been used for insomnia and aggression in children, rather than depression. It is very rarely used in boys due to the potentially very damaging side effect of priapism. Venlafaxine (Effexor) is chemically unrelated to other antidepressants. It is a potent inhibitor of serotonin and norepinephrine reuptake and a weak inhibitor of dopamine uptake. Its side effect profile has been problematic in youth. Mirtazapine (Remeron) is a tetracyclic piperazine/azepine. There are no controlled trials of either drug demonstrating efficacy in children or adolescents.

Indications and Efficacy

Depression

Fluoxetine is the only medication with an FDA-approved indication for depression in patients less than 18 years of age. Selection of an antidepressant is influenced by target symptoms, comorbidity, risk of overdose, and family history of disorder and drug response. After a child or adolescent has been asymptomatic for 4–6 months, the clinician may consider slowly tapering the medication. The medication should not be discontinued when the patient is confronting stressful life events. Some clinicians now maintain an antidepressant indefinitely in young patients who have had multiple episodes of unipolar depression.

Two randomized controlled trials have demonstrated efficacy of fluoxetine in children and adolescents and one of paroxetine in adolescents with major depressive disorder (Keller et al. 2001). Rates of placebo response are high, not all patients respond to active drug, and few attain complete remission. Several open trials support effectiveness of the other SSRIs in pediatric depression.

Only one double-blind, placebo-controlled study showed an advantage of imipramine over placebo in depressed children (Preskorn et al. 1987), although open studies are more positive. In adolescents, no double-blind study shows efficacy of TCAs over placebo. Combined with lack of demonstrated efficacy, lethality of TCAs in overdose virtually eliminates the use of these drugs in pediatric depression.

Nefazodone (Serzone) has had one positive randomized controlled trial in adolescents with major depressive disorder (Emslie et al. 2002). Enthusiasm has been dimmed, however, by the FDA "black box" warning due to rare cases of life-threatening liver failure.

MAOIs are used in children and adolescents only in treatment-resistant cases (especially of depression in bipolar disorder) because of the risk of severe reactions to dietary indiscretions or drug interaction, especially in suicidal or impulsive patients. Both the patient and the family must be reliable and responsible, and receive repeated dietary instruction and caution. The most common dietary risks for youth are pepperoni and sausage pizza and chocolate.

Obsessive-Compulsive Disorder

The SSRIs paroxetine, fluvoxamine, fluoxetine, and sertraline, as well as clomipramine, have demonstrated efficacy in the treatment of obsessive-compulsive disorder (OCD) in children (Liebowitz et al. 2002). Significant improvement may not appear for several months. SSRIs are the first-line treatment, because of clomipramine's side-effect profile. Clomipramine and its active metabolite inhibit the neuronal reuptake of both serotonin and norepinephrine, so they may be useful in patients who do not respond to SSRIs.

School Avoidance or Separation Anxiety

Although the results of early studies on the efficacy of imipramine for school avoidance or separation anxiety were mixed, imipramine plus cognitive-behavior therapy (CBT) has been shown to be more efficacious than placebo plus CBT in improving school attendance and decreasing symptoms of depression in school-refusing adolescents with comorbid anxiety and depression (Bernstein et al. 2000). Based on clinical experience, an SSRI may be used if anxiety symptoms are so severe that therapy alone is not sufficient to return the child to school.

Other Anxiety Disorders

A multisite randomized controlled trial by the Research Units on Pediatric Psychopharmacology Anxiety Study Group has demonstrated efficacy of fluvoxamine in children and adolescents with social phobia, separation anxiety disorder, or generalized anxiety disorder (Walkup et al. 2001). Sertraline was efficacious in a randomized controlled trial for generalized anxiety disorder in children and adolescents (Rynn et al. 2001).

The efficacy of fluoxetine in selective mutism is suggested by one small controlled trial (Black and Uhde 1994) and several open trials. Despite the lack of research, SSRIs are sometimes used to treat panic disorder in youth, based on downward extrapolation from adults.

Attention-Deficit/Hyperactivity Disorder

Bupropion may decrease hyperactivity and aggression and perhaps improve cognitive performance of children with ADHD and conduct disorder (Conners et al. 1996). One blind, controlled, crossover study found that the efficacy of bupropion was statistically equal to methylphenidate in reduction of behavioral and cognitive symptoms of ADHD (Barrickman et al. 1995).

TCAs are effective in ADHD, but generally less so than stimulants. They are now third- or fourth-line choices for the treatment of ADHD, used only if other drugs are ineffective or not tolerated (unacceptable side effects or exacerbation of tics) (Riddle et al.

1988) or if a stimulant is at risk of being abused or diverted. Drawbacks include the inconvenience and expense of ECG monitoring, serious potential cardiac side effects (especially in prepubertal children), the danger of accidental or intentional overdose, and troublesome anticholinergic and sedating side effects.

Six cases in children and young adolescents of unexplained sudden death during desipramine treatment (three of which occurred following exercise) have been reported (Varley and McClellan 1997). A causal relationship between the medication and the deaths has not been definitively established. The evidence suggests that treatment with desipramine in usual doses is associated with slightly added risk of sudden death beyond that occurring naturally (Biederman et al. 1995). Desipramine may represent a greater risk than other TCAs. Because of these concerns, most clinicians now prefer nortriptyline or imipramine as the first choice when a TCA is used in the treatment of a prepubertal child.

Pervasive Developmental Disorders

There is some evidence that the SSRIs and clomipramine may be helpful in reducing symptoms of OCD, rituals, and insistence on sameness in some youth with autism and other pervasive developmental disorders.

Tourette's Disorder

Nortriptyline or desipramine (up to 3.5 mg/kg/day) may reduce both tics and the common comorbid symptoms of hyperactivity, impulsivity, and inattention (T. Spencer et al. 2002), although concern about cardiac side effects limits their use, especially in prepubertal children. SSRIs or clomipramine may reduce obsessions and compulsions as well as tics in patients with Tourette's disorder.

Enuresis

Behavioral treatments, which avoid drug side effects and have higher remission rates, are the first choice for enuresis. Medication may be useful on a short-term basis or for special occasions (e.g., overnight camp). All TCAs are equally effective in the treatment of nocturnal enuresis. The mechanism is unclear, but it does not seem to be by altering sleep architecture, by treating depression, or via peripheral anticholinergic activity. In 80% of patients, TCAs reduce the frequency of bed-wetting within the first week. Total remission, however, occurs in relatively few. Wetting returns when the drug is discontinued, but the success rate may be higher if the drug is tapered gradually. DDAVP (desmopressin), an analogue of anti-diuretic hormone administered as a nasal spray or tablets, is as effective as the TCAs with fewer side effects but is more expensive.

Sleep Disorders

TCAs are used occasionally for severe sleep terror disorder or sleepwalking disorder.

Initiation and Ongoing Treatment

Typical therapeutic daily dose ranges are in Table 8–4. The general principle "start low and go slow" applies.

Selective Serotonin Reuptake Inhibitors

SSRIs do not require medical assessment prior to or during treatment. Particularly with anxiety disorders, very low initial doses and slow titration will minimize side effects that could lead to refusal to take medication. A typical starting dose is the lowest dose pill available, or half a pill, if scored. The liquid formulation of fluoxetine may be used for very gradual titration. Fluoxetine is sometimes prescribed on an every-other-day basis because it has a long half-life and active metabolites. A very long-acting form is now available (Prozac Weekly) for patients who may not take medication regularly due to forgetting or resistance.

Bupropion

The clinical history should include an examination for seizures and factors that predispose to seizures (e.g., head trauma, other central nervous system problems, other drugs that lower the seizure threshold, eating disorders). An EEG may be indicated before starting bupropion if an eating disorder or a seizure diathesis is possible. Bupropion is administered in two or three daily doses, beginning with a dose of 37.5 or 50 mg twice a day, with gradual titration over 2 weeks to a usual maximum of 250 mg/day (300–400 mg/day in adolescents). A single dose should not exceed 150 mg. Blood levels do not appear to be useful. An SR formulation is now available that may be given once or twice a day.

Tricyclic Antidepressants

Because of the potential toxicity of TCAs in overdose, clinicians must remind parents to supervise closely the administration of a TCA and to keep the medication in a safe place.

Before initiating treatment with a TCA, the physician obtains a complete medical history and physical examination, including measurement of baseline vital signs and a careful history seeking cardiac symptoms such as chest pain, dyspnea, actual or near syncope, palpitation, and tachycardia. Congenital hearing impairment may signal a genetic syndrome that is associated with cardiac abnormalities and increased risk of sudden death (Ambrosini et al. 1995). The physician should review the family history for possible contraindications to TCA use, such as arrhythmias (especially long QT syndrome), unexplained fainting, conduction defects, cardiomyopathy, early-onset cardiovascular disease, or sudden death. An initial ECG is essential to establish a baseline and to detect preexisting Wolff-Parkinson-White syndrome, which could result in death. Serial ECGs after each dose increase of 50–100 mg/day (at least 48 hours after the increase) are recommended when the dose is greater than 2.5 mg/kg/day of imipramine or 1.0 mg/kg/day of nortriptyline. The ECG is monitored periodically after a stable dose is reached. Blood pressure and pulse rate should be measured initially and when the dosage is increased. Because TCAs lower the seizure threshold, if the history suggests head trauma or seizures, an EEG is indicated before starting treatment.

Treatment should be initiated with a small dose of the TCA and gradually increased (Table 8–5 shows titration parameters). Plasma levels vary widely at a given daily dose. Some experts believe that plasma-level monitoring may help determine optimum dose (if a laboratory that measures TCA levels reliably is available) (Preskorn et al. 1988a), but this is controversial. Medication cannot be safely titrated by plasma level, because no known level exists below which toxicity can be assured not to occur. Plasma level determinations are recommended in patients whose symptoms do not respond to usual doses (possibly low levels) or those who have severe side effects at usual doses (possibly very high levels). Unexplained withdrawal symptoms may indicate missed doses. Because TCA-induced cardiac conduction changes are predictable, an ECG may be useful in monitoring regularity of administration.

Prepubertal children likely need a higher weight-corrected dosage of imipramine than do adults and are prone to rapid dramatic swings in blood levels from toxic to ineffective (Sallee et al. 1986; Winsberg et al. 1974). Therefore, they should take three (or two for nortriptyline) divided daily doses to produce more stable levels and prevent daily withdrawal symptoms (Ryan 1992). Older adolescents may be given a single daily dose.

Attention-deficit/hyperactivity disorder. Medication doses used for ADHD are typically lower than those used for depression, and therapeutic effect is seen more quickly. Nortriptyline is started at 10 or 25 mg/day and may be increased as tolerated until clinical effect or 4.5 mg/kg/day (divided into two doses) is reached. The serum level (50–150 ng/mL) may relate to therapeutic response (Geller et al. 1986). Imipramine (or desipramine) is begun at 25 mg/day and increased in 25-mg increments once or twice weekly (divided into three daily doses in prepubertal children). Plasma levels do not predict efficacy.

Obsessive-compulsive disorder. Response to medication may be delayed for 8 or even 12 weeks after reaching the expected therapeutic dose. Therefore, the physician should wait at least 10–12 weeks before changing drugs, adding an augmenting drug, or using

TABLE 8–5.	Guidelines for use of tricyclic antidepressants in children and adolescents

Limits to titration: reduce dose or discontinue drug if reached

	Children	Adolescents
P-R interval (seconds)	0.2	0.2
QRS interval (seconds)	0.12 130% of baseline	0.12 130% of baseline
QTc interval (seconds)	0.46	0.46
Resting heart rate (beats/minute)	110–130	110–120
Chronic blood pressure (mm Hg)	120/80	140/90
Clinical	Palpitations	
	Syncope or near-syncope	

Source. Gutgesell et al. 1999; Wilens et al. 1996.

a high-dose strategy. Early in treatment, some patients have an exacerbation of OCD symptoms or report feeling agitated or "jittery." This phenomenon usually subsides after a few weeks. Treatment typically is required for years. Relapse is common when medication is stopped.

In OCD unresponsive to SSRIs, a starting dose of clomipramine 25 mg/day has been recommended, with increases of 25–50 mg/day every 4–7 days. The maximum recommended dose is 3 mg/kg/day, up to 200 mg/day, although 50 mg/day (or 1 mg/kg/day) may be sufficient.

Separation anxiety.   Family therapy, consultation with school personnel, and behavioral treatment should be used before and with medication to treat separation anxiety. Typical starting doses of imipramine are low (e.g., for children ages 6–8 years, 10 mg at bedtime; for older children, 25 mg at bedtime). The dose may be increased by 10–50 mg/week, depending on the child's age. Clinical experience suggests that symptoms in some children respond to a low dose, whereas others may require doses in the antidepressant range. Response may take as long as 6–8 weeks. Medication is continued for at least another 8 weeks and then gradually withdrawn.

Enuresis.   Before starting medication, the clinician should obtain a baseline measurement of wet and dry nights, with use of daily charting to monitor progress. Much lower dosages are needed than for the treatment of depression. Medication is given at bedtime. Maximum dose of imipramine is 2.5 mg/kg/day. Tolerance may develop, requiring an increased dosage. TCAs lose their effect entirely in some children. If medication is used chronically, a drug-free trial should be done at least every 6 months, because enuresis has a high spontaneous remission rate.

Depression.   For imipramine and desipramine, the starting dosage is 1.5 mg/kg/day, which may be increased every 4 days by 1 mg/kg/day to a maximum dosage of 5 mg/kg/day or 200 mg/day, whichever is smaller. Nortriptyline may have fewer side effects and a more precise therapeutic window of 60–150 ng/mL. It has a longer half-life than imipramine and may be given twice a day in children. Milligram per kilogram dosages for nortriptyline are about one-third of those for imipramine, and variation in metabolism is greater (Geller et al. 1986).

Risks and Side Effects

All antidepressants can precipitate hypomania or mania.

Selective Serotonin Reuptake Inhibitors

Somatic side effects (anorexia, weight loss, weight gain, headaches, upset stomach, nausea, vomiting, tremor, drowsiness) are relatively mild and usually short-lived. Behavioral complications of several different types may occur (Walkup and Labellarte 2001). Behavioral activation or increased activity level is common, perhaps related in part to akathisia. Symptoms of more problematic behavioral toxicity include restlessness, insomnia, social disinhibition, and agitation. Bipolar switching or manic reaction is less common, and includes changes in mood, behavior, and impulse control. Suicidal ideation, self-destructive behavior, aggression, and psychotic symptoms have been reported to coincide with treatment, although children with these symptoms typically had preexisting risk factors. Some patients develop apathy or an amotivational syndrome after weeks or months of SSRI treatment, consisting of emotional blunting, inertia, passivity, and loss of interest and energy. This can superficially resemble sedation or worsening of depression, and parents and patients may not recognize the problem. A small decrease in dose may be helpful. Pediatric clinicians are not used to considering sexual side effects, but the sexual dysfunction commonly associated with SSRIs may be distressing for adolescent boys. Bleeding or bruising is very rare but possible (Lake et al. 2000).

Because SSRIs inhibit the cytochrome P450 isoenzymes, there is considerable potential for adverse drug interactions. Serotonin syndrome is a very rare, potentially fatal reaction to addition or increase in dose of a serotonergic agent (most often in combination with another prescribed or over-the-counter medication or an herbal remedy) characterized by extreme restlessness and agitation; fever; motor symptoms of myoclonic jerking, severe hyperreflexia, clonus, and fasiculations; and gastrointestinal symptoms of nausea, vomiting, and diarrhea. Seizures, severe hypotension, ventricular tachycardia and disseminated intravascular coagulation can occur in severe cases.

Withdrawal symptoms, including dizziness, headache, nausea, vomiting, diarrhea, tics, insomnia, irritability, lethargy, anorexia, and dysphoria, may occur after sudden discontinuation of the drug. This may be less of a problem with fluoxetine, due to its very long half-life, and more likely with paroxetine and fluvoxamine.

Bupropion

Allergic reactions to bupropion, including rash, urticaria, and rare serum sickness, are relatively common. Other side effects include agitation, insomnia, fatigue, nausea, anorexia, dry mouth, dizziness, and "spaciness" (Conners et al. 1996; Barrickman et al. 1995).

Bupropion may exacerbate tics (T. Spencer et al. 1993). Seizures are possible in patients with an eating disorder or if a single dose exceeds 150 mg or the daily dose exceeds 450 mg. Rapid dose increase may result in psychotic symptoms.

Tricyclic Antidepressants

The physician should be alert to the risk of potentially lethal intentional overdose or accidental poisoning, not only by the patient but also other family members, especially young children.

TCAs have a quinidinelike effect that slows cardiac conduction time and repolarization. At dosages of greater than 3 mg/kg/day of imipramine, children and adolescents may develop an increased pulse rate, a lengthened P-R interval that may progress to a first-degree atrioventricular heart block, and occasionally widening of the QRS complex. Prolongation of the QTc interval may be a sensitive indicator of cardiac effect (Table 8–5). In children and adolescents, desipramine in dosages up to 6 mg/kg/day produces small but statistically significant ECG changes (intraventricular conduction defects) but not clinically evident cardiac symptoms or blood pressure changes (Biederman et al. 1989). The tendency of prepubertal children to have wider swings in blood levels may place them at higher risk for serious cardiac conduction changes. Approximately 5% of the population has a genetic defect in TCA metabolism that causes them to be "slow hydroxylators," increasing risk for toxicity.

Anticholinergic side effects are common, although most are transient and respond to a decrease in dosage. Drowsiness and dizziness may occur at initiation of treatment, and typically diminish with time. Dry mouth (which may lead to increased dental caries with long-term use) can usually be managed with sugarless gum or increased water intake. Drying of bronchial secretions may be especially problematic for asthmatic patients. Constipation is common, and may be eased by a regular toileting schedule, a high-fiber diet, and increased liquid intake. In the occasional situation in which a stool softener is needed, Colace (docusate sodium; 200 mg at bedtime) can be used. TCA-induced tremor may respond to decreased dosage. Urinary retention, narrow-angle glaucoma, blurred vision, syncope, and increased diastolic blood pressure are rare in children and adolescents. Other reported side effects include nightmares, abdominal pain, chest pain, headache, anorexia, weight loss, and transient rashes. TCAs may lower the seizure threshold, with worsening of preexisting EEG abnormalities, and occasionally lead to a seizure. Side effects with a probable allergic mechanism include worsening of eczema and rare thrombocytopenia.

Symptoms of behavioral toxicity include irritability, worsening of psychosis, agitation, anger, aggression, forgetfulness, and confusion. In the treatment of depression, transient increased crying and expressed sadness are sometimes seen in previously withdrawn children. In children with tics, TCAs may either exacerbate or reduce motor symptoms. Central nervous system toxicity can appear as irritability, psychotic symptoms, agitation, anger, aggression, nightmares, forgetfulness, or confusion, especially at plasma levels of imipramine plus desipramine greater than 450 ng/mL. A drug blood level may be required to differentiate toxicity from a worsening of the original depression (Preskorn et al. 1988b).

Sudden cessation of moderate or higher dosages of TCAs results in a flulike anticholinergic withdrawal syndrome with nausea, cramps, vomiting, headaches, and muscle pains. Behavioral manifestations may include social withdrawal, hyperactivity, depression, agitation, and insomnia. TCAs should therefore be tapered over a 2- to 3-week period rather than being abruptly discontinued.

■ LITHIUM CARBONATE

Indications and Efficacy

Mood Disorder

Lithium may be considered in the treatment of bipolar affective disorder, mixed or manic, and for prophylaxis of bipolar disorder in children and adolescents who have a documented history of recurrent episodes. It is effective for acute stabilization in many adolescents with mania, although adjunctive antipsychotic medication or a benzodiazepine (e.g., lorazepam) is often required. Lithium may be efficacious for children of bipolar depressed parents who have behavior disorders without an apparent affective disorder or for children and adolescents who have behavior disorders accompanied by mood swings. Children and adolescents with mania tend to have a less dramatic response to lithium than do adults. Mania in children with preadolescent onset tends to have a poorer response to lithium than does adolescent-onset mania (Strober et al. 1988).

Aggression

One study of youth with severe aggression, especially with impulsivity and explosive affect, showed lithium to be equal or superior to haloperidol in reducing aggression, hostility, and tantrums, with fewer side effects, but results of other studies have been mixed. Positive response may be more likely in patients with mood symptoms, a family history of mood disorders, lithium-responsive relatives, or a history of brain injury. Lithium also may be useful in mentally retarded youths with severe aggression directed toward themselves or others.

Initiation and Ongoing Treatment

Lithium should not be prescribed unless the family is willing and able to consistently administer multiple daily doses and obtain lithium blood levels. In addition to the usual medical history and physical examination, complete blood count (CBC) with differential, electrolytes, thyroid function studies, blood urea nitrogen (BUN), and creatinine should be determined before lithium is started. A urinalysis and ECG also should be obtained. An EEG may be indicated. Adolescent girls should have a pregnancy test if clinically indicated.

Lithium carbonate (Lithostat, Eskalith) is the most commonly used formulation because of its reliable serum levels and reasonable cost. Controlled-release lithium (Lithobid, 300 mg, or Eskalith CR,

450 mg) may be used, especially in younger children. Because these formulations are not cleared as rapidly as regular lithium, twice-daily administration is sufficient, and more steady blood levels are achieved. No systematic studies have been done in children to compare the efficacy and side effects of different dosing schedules.

In prepubertal children, traditional practice is to start lithium at 300 mg/day for several weeks and slowly increase it to 900 mg/day. Usual child and adolescent therapeutic doses range from 900 to 1,200 mg/day, although daily doses of up to 2,000 mg may be required. Therapeutic levels can be safely attained in a much shorter time by using a weight-based dosage guide (Weller et al. 1986). Also, published nomograms can be used to calculate dosages based on blood levels after single test doses (Alessi et al. 1994; Geller and Fetner 1989). The higher glomerular filtration rate in children compared with adults usually requires a higher milligram-per-kilogram dose before puberty.

Lithium's half-life could permit once-a-day dosing in adolescents. However, because children have more rapid lithium clearance than do adults, multiple divided doses may be necessary to maintain therapeutic levels. In addition, some patients have gastrointestinal distress when they take the entire daily dose at bedtime. Lithium is therefore usually given two or three times a day with meals, even though divided doses have the disadvantage of potentially decreasing adherence to the prescribed regimen.

Therapeutic levels in children are generally similar to those in adults: 0.6–1.2 mEq/L. Under usual circumstances, levels should not exceed 1.4 mEq/L. Peak serum levels will occur within 1–2 hours after ingestion. Steady-state serum levels are achieved after 5 days. To measure the serum level, blood should be drawn 8–12 hours after the last evening dose and before the first morning dose. Levels are obtained once or twice weekly during the initial dosage adjustment and monthly thereafter.

A psychiatric evaluation is needed at least once a month to ensure that the lithium is tolerated well and to monitor compliance. The clinician should periodically check BUN, creatinine, and creatinine clearance because lithium may alter kidney function. A thyroid-stimulating hormone (TSH) test should be obtained every 4–6 months. The clinician must be alert to possible clinical signs of hypothyroidism that could be mistaken for fatigue or a retarded depression.

No studies have addressed the issue of how long to continue lithium. A naturalistic study (Strober et al. 1990) found that adolescents who discontinued lithium were three times more likely to relapse compared with those who continued taking the medication. Most relapses occurred within the first year after cessation of treatment. Once lithium is started, it seems advisable to continue administration for at least 6 months, and preferably a year. If studies of lithium termination in adults are applicable to children, an even longer duration of treatment might be considered. Experience in adult patients with worsening of cycling and decreased response to treatment following intermittent lithium use suggests special caution regarding discontinuation of mood stabilizers. Lithium should be discontinued by gradual tapering. The clinician should closely follow up the patient after lithium is discontinued and should monitor the patient for signs of relapse to mania or for symptoms of depression so that episodes can be treated early.

Risks and Side Effects

Lithium is well tolerated by many children and adolescents, but children younger than 7 years are more prone to side effects, especially at higher lithium doses and serum levels (Hagino et al. 1995). The most common side effects in children (tremor, weight gain, headache, nausea, diarrhea) rarely require discontinuation of lithium. Polydipsia and polyuria may cause enuresis and prevent attainment of a therapeutic level. Lithium may produce goiter and/or hypothyroidism, which may have more significant consequences in developing children than in adults. Lithium effects on blood glucose level are controversial, but reactive hypoglycemia is possible. Acne may be induced or aggravated. Isotretinoin should not be used to treat acne in sexually active girls because of teratogenicity. Lithium carbonate is deposited in bones and has been found to mobilize calcium from bones in adults, but whether there is any significant effect on growing children is unknown. Lithium has not been reported to interfere with bone growth. Hypokalemia is a very rare side effect that can be managed by dietary supplementation (e.g., two bananas, two large carrots, two cups of skim milk, half of a honeydew melon, or an avocado daily), which is preferable to taking potassium tablets that taste bad and can further irritate the gastrointestinal tract. Because of its teratogenic potential, lithium is relatively contraindicated in sexually active girls.

Toxicity is closely related to serum levels, and the therapeutic margin is narrow. The patient and the family should be told to call the doctor immediately if the patient develops a febrile or gastrointestinal illness, uses rigorous dieting to lose weight, or takes diuretics or nonsteroidal anti-inflammatory agents (often taken by adolescent girls to relieve menstrual distress). Lithium should be stopped while a patient has fever, vomiting, or diarrhea. Vigorous exercise in hot weather can lead to lithium toxicity, and parents should be cautioned to make sure the patient drinks enough water. Erratic consumption of large amounts of salty snack foods may cause wide fluctuations in lithium blood levels.

■ ANTIPSYCHOTICS

Naming of this category of drugs is awkward, because many of the indications are for nonpsychotic conditions. There are two groups of these medications. The older *typical* antipsychotics, also known as *neuroleptics* or *major tranquilizers*, include chlorpromazine (Thorazine), fluphenazine (Prolixin), haloperidol (Haldol), perphenazine (Trilafon), pimozide (Orap), thiothixene (Navane), and trifluoperazine (Stelazine). Newer medications are called *atypical* because they have less risk of tardive dyskinesia and other extrapyramidal side effects due to their serotonergic antagonism, as well as antidopaminergic activity. The traditional neuroleptics are all dopamine antagonists. The most commonly used atypicals are risperidone (Risperdal), olanzapine (Zyprexa), and quetiapine (Seroquel). The atypical clozapine (Clozaril) is rarely used because of potentially fatal agranulocytosis and cardiomyopathy, as well as a greater risk of seizures. A newer atypical, ziprasidone (Geodon), carries a risk of cardiac arrhythmias, limiting its usefulness. The recently approved atypical aripiprazole (Abilify) promises less weight gain, minimal extrapyramidal symptoms, and no increase in QTc, but there are no published data in children.

Indications and Efficacy

In most circumstances, an atypical would be used as the first-line drug, rather than a typical antipsychotic. Thorazine may be useful as a prn medication, however, if sedation is needed, and thiothixene may be used if atypicals result in extreme weight gain. There are as yet no intramuscular or depot formulations of atypicals (except for ziprasidone, which has cardiac side effects), so if those formulations are needed, haloperidol, fluphenazine, or another typical neuroleptic would be indicated.

Schizophrenia

Several typical neuroleptics appear to have modest efficacy in schizophrenic children and adolescents (Campbell et al. 1999). In general, however, young schizophrenic patients are less responsive to pharmacotherapy than are adults and continue to have substantial impairment, even if the more florid symptoms abate. No evidence suggests superior efficacy of one traditional neuroleptic over another. Concerns about the development of tardive dyskinesia with long-term use of the typical neuroleptics and the prominence of negative symptoms in young schizophrenic patients suggest preference for the atypicals risperidone, olanzapine, or quetiapine as initial treatment. Several open trials are positive for the atypicals, and two small double-blind trials found atypicals superior to haloperidol. Atypicals may improve negative as well as positive symptoms. A small number of patients do not respond sufficiently to any of the atypicals and require haloperidol as a sole or adjunctive antipsychotic medication.

Neuroleptic resistance is common in young schizophrenic patients, although a child who has not responded to one neuroleptic may respond to another. If the response is insufficient after a 6-week trial at adequate doses (and assured compliance), another neuroleptic (usually in a different class) should be tried. Common therapeutic errors leading to the perception of neuroleptic resistance include incorrect diagnosis, subtherapeutic or excessive medication doses, premature changes in medication before efficacy can appear, failure to monitor target symptoms or ensure patient compliance, hasty or irrational polypharmacy, and failure to provide psychosocial therapies (McClellan and Werry 1992).

Developmental Disorders

Drugs such as haloperidol or trifluoperazine may result in behavioral improvement. In doses of 0.5–4.0 mg/day, haloperidol significantly reduced hyperactivity, stereotypy, and withdrawal, without adversely affecting cognitive performance. In addition, haloperidol improved discrimination learning and language acquisition when used in combination with positive reinforcement and behavioral interventions (Campbell et al. 1982).

Due to the more benign side-effect profile, atypicals have largely replaced typical neuroleptics, with the possible exception of treatment-resistant stereotypies. Open trials suggest that very low doses of atypicals can reduce aggression, anxiety, agitation, irritability, and obsessional behaviors and increase social awareness and attention in children and adolescents with autistic disorder, Asperger's disorder, and mental retardation. Hypoactive autistic children do not generally respond well to typical antipsychotics.

Recent multisite randomized controlled trials have shown positive results for risperidone in reducing severely disruptive behaviors in children with subaverage intelligence quotient (Aman et al. 2002; Snyder et al. 2002). Positive effects were maintained in a 1-year open follow-up (Turgay et al. 2002). Risperidone was shown in a randomized controlled trial to reduce severe tantrums, irritability, aggression, and self-injurious behavior (but not the core symptoms of autism) in children with autistic disorder (Research Units on Pediatric Psychopharmacology Autism Network 2002).

Mania

Olanzapine, risperidone, and quetiapine may be useful as adjuncts in the treatment of acute mania.

Tourette's Disorder

Efficacy is often difficult to evaluate in Tourette's disorder because of the natural waxing and waning of symptoms. Concern about possible tardive dyskinesia from typical neuroleptics makes risperidone a more frequent choice for both aggressive symptoms and tics. If risperidone leads to excessive weight gain or is ineffective, both haloperidol and pimozide reduce tics, but discontinuation may lead to severe withdrawal exacerbation of symptoms for up to several months, and other side effects may be intolerable.

Aggressive Conduct Disorder Unresponsive to Other Interventions

Studies of hospitalized severely aggressive children ages 6–12 years have found that several typical neuroleptics are effective compared with placebo in reducing aggression, hostility, negativism, and explosiveness. The risk of cognitive dulling and tardive dyskinesia place typical neuroleptics low on the list of medication options for aggression, however. Chlorpromazine leads to unacceptable sedation at relatively low doses.

A small randomized controlled trial found low doses of risperidone to be more effective than placebo in reducing some measures of aggression in youths with conduct disorder (Findling et al. 2000).

Other Disorders

These medications, increasingly the atypicals, are used in crisis situations to decrease severe agitation, explosiveness, and aggression seen in hospitalized youth with various disorders, although systematic efficacy data are lacking.

Initiation and Ongoing Treatment

Before initiating neuroleptic medication, the physician should obtain a complete physical examination. A CBC with differential and liver profile are needed at baseline and at regular intervals. Much closer monitoring is required when using clozapine. The clinician should carefully examine each patient for abnormal movements with a scale such as the Abnormal Involuntary Movement Scale (AIMS) before administering a neuroleptic and periodically thereafter (Munetz and Benjamin 1988). Especially in children with autistic disorder or Tourette's disorder, it may be difficult to distinguish medication-induced movements of tardive dyskinesia or withdrawal dyskinesias from those characteristic of the disorder itself. The clinician should explain the risk of movement disorders to parents and patients (as appropriate) before starting treatment and at intervals thereafter. Weight should be followed closely, with nutritional counseling and attempts to increase exercise implemented as early as possible. An ECG should be considered before starting any of the atypicals or thioridazine.

An EEG is needed before clozapine treatment because of the potential for seizures and EEG abnormalities. Detailed informed consent is especially crucial for this drug (Towbin et al. 1994).

Doses must be titrated with careful attention to reduction in target symptoms and to side effects. Age, weight, and severity of symptoms do not provide clear dose guidelines. Antipsychotic drugs are highly lipophilic. Chlorpromazine has been shown to have a lower plasma concentration in children than in adults after the same weight-adjusted dose (Rivera-Calimlim et al. 1979). However, the magnitude of the difference exceeds that expected from the small proportional excess of adipose tissue in children compared with adults. This is probably because of children's increased efficiency of hepatic biotransformation (Jatlow 1987). Developmental changes in protein binding may be influential as well.

The initial dose should be very low, with gradual increments no more than once or twice a week. Loading doses or rapid titration do not accelerate clinical improvement but do increase side effects and decrease compliance. Children metabolize these drugs more rapidly than adults do but also require lower plasma levels for efficacy (Teicher and Glod 1990). Although a single daily dose (usually at bedtime) is generally preferred for maintenance, divided doses may be used during titration to minimize side effects and permit finer dose adjustments. Neuroleptics should be maintained at the lowest effective dose. Regular monitoring for efficacy and side effects is required. A standard protocol should be followed for clozapine (Towbin et al. 1994).

Olanzapine is available as a disk (Zyprexa ZYDIS Orally Disintegrating Tablet) that dissolves rapidly in the mouth, a useful formulation when quick action is needed or when pill swallowing is difficult or resisted. Risperidone and several of the typical neuroleptics are available as a liquid formulation.

If a typical neuroleptic is to be used, one of the higher-potency drugs, such as haloperidol, fluphenazine, trifluoperazine, or perphenazine may be best, unless sedation is required. The lower-potency compounds (e.g., chlorpromazine and thioridazine [Mellaril]) are best avoided because of sedation, cognitive dulling, and memory deficits that can interfere with learning in school and in treatment programs. Thioridazine is now very rarely used because it prolongs the cardiac QTc interval.

Schizophrenia

Treatment is started with risperidone, olanzapine, or quetiapine. If response is insufficient, another of those three drugs may be tried. Clozapine is considered only after failed treatment with two or three of the other atypicals as well as one of the typical neuroleptics. Usual starting doses for children are 0.5 mg of risperidone bid, olanzapine 5 mg at bedtime, or quetiapine 25 mg bid. For haloperidol, daily doses for children are 0.25–6.0 mg. Older adolescents with schizophrenia may require doses of neuroleptics in the adult range. Young adolescents fall in between, and doses must be empirically determined. Even less is known about optimal doses of the atypical antipsychotics.

Full efficacy may not appear for several months (as long as 6 months for risperidone). Positive symptoms (delusions and hallucinations) tend to decline first, followed by cognitive symptoms (thought disorder) and, very slowly, negative symptoms (apathy, anergy, withdrawal). To monitor outcome, parent and teacher reports are essential, in addition to self-reports from adolescents. Standardized clinician rating scales, such as the Positive and Negative Syndrome Scale for Schizophrenia, derived from the Children's Psychiatric Rating Scale, are sensitive to neuroleptic-induced improvement in children (E.K. Spencer et al. 1994).

Current practice for adults with schizophrenia is to continue neuroleptic treatment indefinitely; however, firm recommendations regarding children are lacking because of the difficulty in making a definitive diagnosis and the possibility of developmental toxicity. Neuroleptics should be discontinued by gradual tapering to prevent rebound symptoms.

Pervasive Developmental Disorders

Unless serious side effects require immediate discontinuation, a trial of sufficient length is necessary to determine whether the drug is efficacious. If the drug appears to be helpful, it should be continued for at least several months. At 3- to 6-month intervals, the drug should be discontinued so that the child may be observed for withdrawal dyskinesias and to determine if the drug is still necessary. Some children may have physical withdrawal symptoms or a rebound phenomenon consisting of worsening of behavior for up to 8 weeks after drug discontinuation.

Tourette's Disorder

Because Tourette's disorder is chronic and not usually an emergency, clinicians can carefully monitor patients for several months before starting medication. This is especially useful because of the natural waxing and waning of symptoms, and the tendency to present at times of peak symptoms. A baseline of symptoms is established, and psychological and educational interventions can be implemented. The dose of risperidone is typically 0.25 mg once or twice a day, with gradual titration to 6 mg/day if needed and tolerated.

Acute Psychosis or Severe Agitation

In a crisis, chlorpromazine (0.5–2.0 mg/kg) or haloperidol (0.01–0.05 mg/kg) can be given orally every 1–2 hours until symptoms are controlled or side effects appear. The physician must closely monitor patients to observe particularly for hypotension or acute dystonia. The total daily dose is then used for routine short-term management.

Risks and Side Effects

Children and adolescents are more prone to side effects from antipsychotic drugs than are adults. The most common and problematic side effect of the atypicals is excessive weight gain, perhaps greatest with olanzapine. In a few cases, excessive weight gain is associated with liver abnormalities or onset of diabetes mellitus. Elevations in prolactin may cause galactorrhea and breast tenderness in both males and females and amenorrhea in adolescent girls. Sedation and cognitive dulling may interfere with learning in school and compound negative symptoms. Among the atypicals, clinical impressions suggest that risperidone is more likely to cause extrapyramidal symptoms (EPS) and elevated prolactin levels, but is less sedating. Excessive weight gain is common. Olanzapine often causes elevated prolactin. Quetiapine is more sedating, but causes less EPS and prolactin elevation, and perhaps less weight gain. Although ziprasidone causes less weight gain, it has been associated with cardiac QTc prolongation. Aripiprazole, a recently approved atypical, appears to be weight neutral. Clozapine is associated with blood dyscrasias and seizures.

Acute extrapyramidal side effects (EPS), including dystonic reactions, parkinsonian tremor and rigidity, drooling, and akathisia, are common. Laryngeal dystonia is potentially fatal. Acute dystonia may be treated with oral or intramuscular diphenhydramine (25 or 50 mg) or benztropine (0.5–2.0 mg). When medication is initiated in an outpatient, the clinician should instruct a responsible adult to watch for a dystonic reaction and provide a supply of medication to give to the patient if needed. Adolescent boys seem to be more vulnerable to acute dystonic reactions than adult patients are, so the physician may be more inclined to use prophylactic antiparkinsonian medication. Clinical experience suggests that children do not respond well to anticholinergics, and reduction of neuroleptic dose is therefore preferable. For treatment or prevention of parkinsonian symptoms, adolescents may be given benztropine (1–2 mg/day) in divided doses. Chronic parkinsonian symptoms are often drastically underrecognized by clinicians (Richardson et al. 1991). The neuromuscular consequences may impair performance of age-appropriate activities, and the subjective effects may lead to noncompliance with medication. Although risperidone's side-effect profile is more benign than that of other neuroleptics, children appear to be more sensitive than adults to developing EPS while taking this drug (Mandoki 1995). Very gradual titration of dose may ameliorate this problem.

Akathisia may be especially difficult to identify in very young patients or those with limited verbal ability. It may be misinterpreted as anxiety or agitation and mistakenly exacerbated with an increase in neuroleptic dose. Clonazepam (Klonopin, 0.5 mg/day) may reduce neuroleptic-induced akathisia (Kutcher et al. 1987) in adolescents.

Tardive dyskinesia or withdrawal dyskinesias are frequent in children treated with typical neuroleptics (Campbell et al. 1997; Kumra et al. 1998). Most withdrawal dyskinesias are transient. Very rarely, potentially irreversible tardive dyskinesia has been documented in children and adolescents after as brief a period of treatment as 5 months. Other withdrawal-emergent symptoms include nausea, vomiting, loss of appetite, diaphoresis, and hyperactivity. Various behavioral withdrawal symptoms may appear up to several weeks after neuroleptic discontinuation and persist for as long as 8 weeks (Gualtieri et al. 1984). These must be distinguished from a return of symptoms of the original disorder. A prolonged drug-free trial may be indicated, if possible, to ascertain whether neuroleptics are truly needed. Although this is less of a problem with the atypicals, withdrawal dyskinesia has been reported after risperidone discontinuation.

Neuroleptic malignant syndrome (NMS), a potentially fatal side effect, is manifested by hyperthermia, muscle rigidity, autonomic hyperactivity, and changes in consciousness (Silva et al. 1999). It has been reported to be associated with the atypicals, as well. Adolescents may present with serious medical complications or may have NMS without fever (Hynes and Vickar 1996). NMS is treated by discontinuation of the neuroleptic and use of aggressive supportive measures. The use of specific medications to treat NMS has not been studied in adolescents, although case reports suggest the use of bromocriptine or L-dopa.

Abnormal laboratory findings are less often reported in children than in adults, but the clinician should be alert to the possibility, especially of agranulocytosis or hepatic dysfunction. If an acute febrile illness or easy bruising occurs, medication should be withheld and a CBC with differential and liver enzymes should be obtained. Children may be at greater risk for neuroleptic-induced seizures than are adults, because of their immature nervous systems and the very high prevalence of abnormal EEG findings in seriously disturbed children (Teicher and Glod 1990). If excessive thirst or urination or weight loss occur, blood glucose should be measured for possible diabetes.

Of particular concern is behavioral toxicity, manifested as worsening of preexisting symptoms or development of new symptoms such as hyper- or hypoactivity, irritability, apathy, withdrawal, stereotypies, tics, or hallucinations.

Anticholinergic side effects, such as hypotension, dry mouth, constipation, nasal congestion, blurred vision, and urinary retention, are unusual in children. Chlorpromazine and thioridazine increase the risk of sunburn. Thioridazine is associated with pigmentary retinopathy, retrograde ejaculation, abdominal pain, and enuresis.

When used for treatment of nonpsychotic disorders, haloperidol, pimozide, and risperidone have been reported to cause separation anxiety and school avoidance (Hanna et al. 1999).

Side effects are a significant problem in the long-term use of haloperidol for Tourette's disorder. Frequent complaints include lethargy, feeling like a "zombie," dysphoria, personality changes, weight gain, parkinsonian symptoms, akathisia, and intellectual dulling. Some side effects of pimozide are similar to those of haloperidol but seem to be less severe. However, pimozide causes ECG changes in up to 25% of patients, including T-wave inversion, U waves, QTc prolongation, and bradycardia, although these appear to be less significant than originally thought.

■ MINOR TRANQUILIZERS, SEDATIVES, AND HYPNOTICS

Indications and Efficacy

Anxiety

Benzodiazepines have been effective in the treatment of anxiety disorders in children, although controlled trials are limited by small sample sizes, low doses, short duration, and high placebo response rates. Open-label studies suggest that benzodiazepine response is greater for physical symptoms than the psychological symptoms of anxiety. Alprazolam (Xanax) has been helpful in children with separation, avoidant, and overanxious disorders and in pediatric oncology patients who have anticipatory and acute situational anxiety associated with bone marrow aspirations and spinal taps (Gualtieri et al. 1984; Pfefferbaum et al. 1987). Clonazepam (2 mg/day) may be helpful for some children with separation anxiety disorder (Graae et al. 1994), but stronger evidence exists for its effectiveness in the treatment of panic disorder, generalized anxiety, and school and social anxiety.

Buspirone (BuSpar, 15–30 mg/day) may be useful in the treatment of generalized anxiety disorder in adolescents (Popper 1993) and a variety of anxiety "symptoms" in children and adolescents (in case reports and open-label studies).

Sleep Disorders

Diazepam (Valium) or clonazepam (Klonopin) may be used for severe night terrors, persistent true insomnia, or somnambulism.

Initiation and Ongoing Treatment

Infants and children absorb benzodiazepines faster and metabolize them more quickly than adults do (Gualtieri et al. 1984). Younger children require more frequent dosing. The usual daily dose ranges for children and adolescents are lorazepam (Ativan, 0.25–6.00 mg), diazepam (1–20 mg), and alprazolam (0.25–4.00 mg). Prescriptions should be written for weeks rather than months because of the potential for dependence. Minor tranquilizers, sedatives, and hypnotics should be discontinued by gradual tapering to avoid withdrawal symptoms that include seizures, anxiety, malaise, irritability, headache, sweating, gastrointestinal distress, insomnia, or muscle tension. Physicians should also be aware of potential nonprescribed use of benzodiazepines, in which family members give these medications to adolescents or the adolescent uses them for the purpose of intoxication.

Buspirone is typically administered in doses of 0.2–0.6 mg/kg/day divided into three doses per day. The starting dose for prepubertal children is 2.5–5.0 mg/day, increasing 2.5 mg every 3–4 days to a maximum of 20 mg/day. Adolescents start at 5–10 mg/day, increasing 5–10 mg every 3–4 days to a maximum of 60 mg/day. Therapeutic effects may not be seen for as long as 2–4 weeks, and the medication should be discontinued if there is no therapeutic effect at a maximal dose after 6 weeks.

Risks and Side Effects

In addition to the risks of substance abuse and physical or psychological dependence with the benzodiazepines, possible side effects of minor tranquilizers, sedatives, and hypnotics include sedation, ataxia, diplopia, tremor, confusion, emotional lability, and worsening of psychosis. Paradoxical or disinhibition reactions may occur, manifested by acute excitation, irritability, increased anxiety, hallucinations, increased aggression and hostility, rage reactions, insomnia, euphoria, and/or incoordination (Campbell et al. 1985). Although buspirone may produce insomnia, dizziness, anxiety, nausea, headache, restlessness, agitation, depression, and confusion in adults, limited studies in children have reported few side effects. Buspirone can be discontinued rapidly over a 4-day period.

■ ANTICONVULSANTS

Indications and Efficacy

Patients experiencing severe impulsive aggression with emotional lability and irritability may warrant a trial of an anticonvulsant. These medications may be particularly effective in the treatment of mixed states and rapid-cycling bipolar disorder (Evans et al. 1987). Based on extrapolation from adults and several open trials, carbamazepine (Tegretol) and valproic acid (Depakene, Depakote) are used to treat juvenile bipolar disorder (especially if nonresponsive to lithium), but no randomized controlled trials have been done in children or adolescents.

Initiation and Ongoing Treatment

Before initiating anticonvulsants, the physician should measure hemoglobin, hematocrit, white blood cell count, platelets, and liver function and then repeat every month for 4 months (more often if counts are low), then every 3–6 months or if a rash, sore throat, bleeding gums, easy bruising, malaise, or fever occurs. The clinician should routinely monitor plasma levels because children metabolize the drug more rapidly than adults do. Autoinduction of hepatic enzymes may require a dose increase to maintain blood levels.

Valproic Acid

There is no relationship between blood levels of valproic acid and therapeutic effect. However, serum concentrations of greater than 45 µg/mL are recommended for the treatment of manic behavior. Oral doses for adolescents begin at 15 mg/kg/day divided into two doses per day. In severe mania, a loading dose of 20 mg/kg/day will produce a more rapid response. Doses can subsequently be increased every 3 days by 10 mg/kg/day to a maximum dose of 60 mg/kg/day.

Carbamazepine

The initial dose of carbamazepine for pediatric patients is 100 mg/day. It can be increased by 100–200 mg/day at weekly intervals. Young patients are typically maintained on 10–20 mg/kg/day divided into two or three doses per day. Blood levels are drawn 2–4 days after achieving a steady-state plasma concentration. Plasma concentrations of 4–14 µg/mL are adequate for an anticonvulsant effect, but levels for psychiatric effect are unknown.

Risks and Side Effects

Caution is indicated in the use of anticonvulsants in sexually active girls because of teratogenicity. Side effects of carbamazepine include nausea, vomiting, vertigo, ataxia, drowsiness, diplopia, nystagmus, tics, muscle cramps, decreased thyroid function, immune thrombocytopenia, dysregulation of serum lipid status, rare blood dyscrasias, hepatitis, renal impairment (Evans et al. 1987), urinary incontinence, hair loss, motor and vocal tics, exacerbation of seizures, rash, and interstitial pneumonitis. Reversible dose-related leukopenia may occur early in the course of treatment. Adverse behavioral reactions, such as mania, extreme irritability, agitation, insomnia, obsessive thinking, hallucinations, delirium, psychosis, paranoia, hyperactivity, and aggression, are particularly important to watch for; they may be seen during the first 1–4 weeks of treatment and may be more frequent in children than in adults (Evans et al. 1987).

Adverse effects of valproic acid include gastrointestinal symptoms, liver toxicity (mainly seen in children younger than 3 years who are taking multiple anticonvulsants), occasional blood dyscrasias, and very rare pancreatitis. Clinicians should monitor patients for the presence of nausea, vomiting, easy bruising, lethargy, malaise, or persistent abdominal distress. Any liver toxicity usually resolves within weeks of discontinuing the drug. Persistent abdominal pain requires checking serum amylase for pancreatitis. The causal link between valproic acid and polycystic ovaries is controversial.

Phenobarbital (administered for the treatment of seizures) often has psychiatric side effects, such as impaired memory and attention, hyperactivity, irritability, aggression, and depressed mood.

The physician should be familiar with the multiple interactions between anticonvulsants and psychotropic (and other) drugs.

■ ANTIHISTAMINES

Indications and Efficacy

Diphenhydramine (Benadryl) or hydroxyzine (Atarax, Vistaril) may be used for severe initial insomnia that has not responded to psychological interventions. This strategy should be used only for a short time to interrupt a dysfunctional sleep cycle or to manage a brief crisis. Antihistamines are prescribed for the treatment of agitation or distress, although no controlled studies exist. Diphenhydramine may be used to treat acute dystonic reactions secondary to neuroleptics. Antihistamines have no known anxiolytic action.

Initiation and Ongoing Treatment

For insomnia, children younger than 6 years can begin taking 12.5 mg of diphenhydramine elixir at bedtime, with a 6-mg increase every 2–3 days as needed. For children ages 6–12 years, 25 mg is given initially and may be increased to 50–75 mg. Adolescents may be given 50 mg to start, with 25- to 50-mg increments until the desired effect is achieved. The half-lives of these medications may be as long as 13 hours.

Risks and Side Effects

The most common side effects of antihistamines are dizziness and oversedation. Occasionally incoordination, blurred vision, dry mouth, nausea, abdominal pain, and agitation are seen. At high doses, the seizure threshold is lowered. Leukopenia and agranulocytosis are extremely rare. Antihistamines have been reported to cause acute dystonic reactions and possibly, with chronic administration, tardive dyskinesia. They should not be used for asthmatic patients (because they dry mucous membranes) or in the presence of glaucoma or bladder neck obstruction (because of anticholinergic effects). Antihistamines can cause behavioral and cognitive disinhibition, although not usually aggression.

■ ANTIPARKINSONIAN AGENTS

Antiparkinsonian drugs are used to treat EPS of neuroleptics in adolescents (rarely in children). The anticholinergic drug benztropine (Cogentin, 0.5–2.0 mg/day) or diphenhydramine (25–50 mg/day) are most often used, usually in divided doses. Because prepubertal children usually do not respond well to anticholinergics, the neuroleptic dose is typically decreased instead.

■ CLONIDINE AND GUANFACINE

Clonidine and guanfacine hydrochloride are α-adrenergic agonists approved for the treatment of hypertension. Guanfacine has a longer half-life than clonidine and is considered to be a more effective treatment for inattention. Children who cannot tolerate the sedative side effects of clonidine or who experience rebound effects on tics, sleep, or ADHD symptoms may respond well to guanfacine.

Indications and Efficacy

Tourette's Disorder

The efficacy of clonidine for Tourette's disorder per se has been controversial. However, a recent randomized controlled trial in children with both chronic tics (including Tourette's disorder) and ADHD showed efficacy of clonidine in reducing both tics and impulsivity and hyperactivity (Tourette's Syndrome Study Group 2002). A small randomized controlled trial in children with Tourette's disorder found clonidine and risperidone equally effective in reducing tics (Gaffney et al. 2002). A modest randomized controlled trial of children with tic disorders and ADHD showed that guanfacine significantly improved (compared with placebo) teacher and clinician ratings of ADHD symptoms, decreased errors on a continuous performance test (placebo subjects increased errors), and decreased tic severity by 31% (compared with 0% on placebo) (Scahill et al. 2001).

Attention-Deficit/Hyperactivity Disorder

Clonidine improves frustration tolerance and compliance and reduces emotional outbursts in ADHD but does not improve attention (see above). It may be used at bedtime to decrease ADHD overarousal or oppositional behavior or to ameliorate insomnia caused by stimulant effect or rebound. Ritalin and clonidine are sometimes given in combination for difficult-to-treat ADHD. In a randomized controlled trial, the combination improved teacher report most (compared to placebo) (Tourette's Syndrome Study Group 2002). A small randomized controlled trial comparing methylphenidate, clonidine, and methylphenidate plus clonidine in children with ADHD plus aggressive oppositional or conduct symptoms found that all three treatments were associated with significant improvement in attention, impulsivity, and oppositional and conduct symptoms on parent and teacher rating scales and laboratory measures, with few differences among groups (Connor et al. 2000).

Other Symptoms

Clonidine may be effective in the management of aggressive behavior, impulsivity, oppositional behaviors, self-injurious behavior, and symptoms of agitation that accompany posttraumatic stress disorder.

Initiation and Ongoing Treatment

Before initiating clonidine, the physician should take a cardiovascular history and obtain a physical examination (including blood pressure and pulse rate measurements); ECG may be advisable for very young children, although The American Heart Association states that ECG monitoring is not necessary for children on clonidine. Vital signs should be taken with the patient lying and standing. The physician should determine the fasting glucose level in patients with a family history of diabetes. Clonidine is contraindicated in patients with a history of syncope, bradycardia, or heart block.

Clonidine is initiated at a low dose of 0.05 mg/day (one-half pill) at bedtime, and titrated gradually over 2–4 weeks to 0.15–0.40 mg/day (0.003–0.01 mg/kg/day) in three or four divided doses. This minimizes side effects, particularly sedation. The medication should be continued for 2–8 weeks at a maximal dose before determining treatment success (Pliszka et al. 2000). A transdermal skin patch improves compliance and reduces toxic and rebound effects on blood vessels and blood pressure. The transdermal form lasts only 4–5 days in children compared with 7 days in adults; the patch may be cut to adjust dosage (Hunt 1987).

Onset of therapeutic action is delayed 2–4 weeks. The maximal therapeutic effect of a given dose may not be reached for several months. Clonidine should be discontinued by gradual tapering to avoid a withdrawal syndrome consisting of increased blood pressure and pulse rate, and a possible severe ventricular tachyarrhythmia (Popper 2000).

Guanfacine is started at 0.5 mg/day (one-half tablet) and then gradually increased by 0.5 mg every 3–4 days to a maximum dose of 4 mg. One milligram of guanfacine is equivalent to 0.1 mg of clonidine. These α-adrenergic agonists can replace each other by gradually increasing one and tapering the other.

Risks and Side Effects

The most troublesome side effect of clonidine is sedation, which is most prominent early in treatment and generally decreases after several weeks. Patients may experience rebound hyperactivity and irritability. The most serious side effects are cardiovascular and include hypotension, bradycardia, rebound tachycardia and hypertension, and asymptomatic ECG conduction changes. Clonidine can further complicate depression and dysphoria. Less common side effects include headache, abdominal pain, weight gain, rash, and decreased glucose tolerance. The skin patch often causes a local hypersensitivity reaction. Although fatalities and serious side effects have been reported in children who had received clonidine plus methylphenidate, all cases were complicated and causality is not at all clear. A recent randomized controlled trial using the combination found no cardiac side effects (see section on Stimulants). Guanfacine has a longer half-life and fewer and milder side effects (primarily irritability and sedation) and less rebound than clonidine. Surprisingly, guanfacine used for the treatment of ADHD has little effect on vital signs.

■ PROPRANOLOL

Indications and Efficacy

The β-adrenergic blocker propranolol (Inderal) may be useful in patients with otherwise uncontrollable rage reactions and impulsive aggression, especially those with evidence of organicity (Williams et al. 1982). Anecdotal reports suggest that propranolol (in divided doses up to 2.5 mg/kg/day) reduces agitation and hyperarousal in children and adolescents with posttraumatic stress disorder. Propranolol, as well as newer β-blockers that are longer acting and have fewer central effects, may reduce aggression and increase socialization in persons with autistic disorder or mental retardation.

Initiation and Ongoing Treatment

β-Blockers are relatively contraindicated in patients with asthma, diabetes, bradycardia, heart block, heart failure, or hypothyroidism. An ECG is recommended if clinically indicated. The physician should obtain a fasting glucose level and a glucose tolerance test in patients with a family history of diabetes.

In children and adolescents, the initial dosage of propranolol is 10–20 mg three times a day, to be increased every 3–4 days by 10–20 mg/day. The physician should monitor pulse rate (maintain above 50) and blood pressure (minimum 80/50 mm Hg). Dosage is titrated to clinical effect or side effects. A standard daily dose is 10–120 mg for children and 20–300 mg for adolescents (2–8 mg/kg/day) divided into three doses a day. Maximum improvement at a particular dosage may not be seen for up to 8 weeks (Yudofsky et al. 1987). β-Blockers should be discontinued by gradual tapering to avoid rebound hypertension and tachycardia.

Risks and Side Effects

Side effects of propranolol include bronchoconstriction, bradycardia, and hypotension. Unlike previously thought, there is no increased risk of depression and minimal risk of fatigue or sedation. Propranolol significantly increases blood levels of neuroleptics such as chlorpromazine and thioridazine.

■ REFERENCES

Alessi N, Naylor MW, Ghaziuddin M, et al: Update on lithium carbonate therapy in children and adolescents. J Am Acad Child Adolesc Psychiatry 33:291–304, 1994

Aman MG, Smedt GD, Derivan A, et al: Double-blind, placebo-controlled study of risperidone for the treatment of disruptive behaviors in children with subaverage intelligence. Am J Psychiatry 159:1337–1346, 2002

Ambrosini PJ, Emslie GJ, Greenhill LL, et al: Selecting a sequence of anti-depressants for treating depression in youth. Journal of Child and Adolescent Psychopharmacology 5:233–240, 1995

Barrickman LL, Perry PJ, Allen AJ, et al: Bupropion versus methylphenidate in the treatment of attention-deficit hyperactivity disorder. J Am Acad Child Adolesc Psychiatry 34:649–657, 1995

Bernstein GA, Borchardt CM, Perwien AR, et al: Imipramine plus cognitive-behavioral therapy in the treatment of school refusal. J Am Acad Child Adolesc Psychiatry 39:276–283, 2000

Biederman J, Baldessarini RJ, Wright V, et al: A double-blind placebo controlled study of desipramine in the treatment of ADD, II: serum drug levels and cardiovascular findings. J Am Acad Child Adolesc Psychiatry 28:903–911, 1989

Biederman J, Thisted RA, Greenhill LL, et al: Estimation of the association between desipramine and the risk for sudden death in 5- to 14-year old children. J Clin Psychiatry 56:87–93, 1995

Black B, Uhde TW: Treatment of elective mutism with fluoxetine: a double-blind, placebo-controlled study. J Am Acad Adolesc Psychiatry 33:1000–1006, 1994

Briant RH: An introduction to clinical pharmacology, in Pediatric Psychopharmacology: The Use of Behavior Modifying Drugs in Children. Edited by Werry JS. New York, Brunner/Mazel, 1978, pp 3–28

Campbell M, Anderson LT, Small AM, et al: The effects of haloperidol on learning and behavior in autistic children. J Autism Dev Disord 12:167–175, 1982

Campbell M, Green WH, Deutsch SI: Child and Adolescent Psychopharmacology. Beverly Hills, CA, Sage, 1985

Campbell M, Armenteros JL, Malone RP, et al: Neuroleptic-related dyskinesias in autistic children: a prospective, longitudinal study. J Am Acad Child Adolesc Psychiatry 36:835–843, 1997

Campbell M, Rapoport JL, Simpson GM: Antipsychotics in children and adolescents. J Am Acad Child Adolesc Psychiatry 38:537–545, 1999

Conners CK, Casat CD, Gualtieri CT, et al: Bupropion hydrochloride in attention deficit disorder with hyperactivity. J Am Acad Child Adolesc Psychiatry 35:1314–1321, 1996

Connor DF, Barkley RA, Davis HT: A pilot study of methylphenidate, clonidine, or the combination in ADHD comorbid with aggressive oppositional defiant or conduct disorder. Clin Pediatr 39:15–25, 2000

Donnelly M, Rapoport JL: Attention deficit disorders, in Diagnosis and Psychopharmacology of Childhood and Adolescent Disorders. Edited by Weiner JM. New York, Wiley, 1985, pp 178–197

Dulcan MK, Lizarralde C (eds): Helping Parents, Youth, and Teachers Understand Medications for Behavioral and Emotional Problems: A Resource Book of Medication Information Handouts, 2nd Edition. Washington, DC, American Psychiatric Publishing, 2002

Efron D, Jarman F, Barker M: Side effects of methylphenidate and dextroamphetamine in children with attention deficit hyperactivity disorder: a double-blind, crossover trial. Pediatrics 100:662–666, 1997

Elia J, Borcherding BG, Rapoport JL, et al: Methylphenidate and dextroamphetamine treatments of hyperactivity: are there true nonresponders? Psychiatry Res 36:141–155, 1991

Emslie GJ, Findling RL, Rynn MA, et al: Efficacy and safety of nefazodone in the treatment of adolescents with major depressive disorder. Presented at NCDEU, June 2002

Evans RW, Clay TH, Gualtieri CT: Carbamazepine in pediatric psychiatry. J Am Acad Child Adolesc Psychiatry 26:2–8, 1987

Findling R, McNamara NK, Branicky LA, et al: A double-blind pilot study of risperidone in the treatment of conduct disorder. J Am Acad Child Adolesc Psychiatry 39:509–516, 2000

Gaffney GR, Perry PJ, Lund BC, et al: Risperidone versus clonidine in the treatment of children and adolescents with Tourette's syndrome. J Am Acad Child Adolesc Psychiatry 41:330–336, 2002

Geller B, Fetner HH: Children's 24-hour serum lithium level after a single dose predicts initial dose and steady state plasma levels (letter). J Clin Psychopharmacol 9:155, 1989

Geller B, Cooper TB, Chestnut BS: Preliminary data on the relationship between nortriptyline plasma level and response in depressed children. Am J Psychiatry 143:1283–1286, 1986

Graae F, Milner J, Rizzotto L, et al: Clonazepam in childhood anxiety disorders. J Am Acad Child Adolesc Psychiatry 33:372–376, 1994

Greenhill LL: Stimulant-related growth inhibition in children: a review, in Strategic Interventions for Hyperactive Children. Edited by Gittleman M. New York, ME Sharpe, 1981, pp 39–63

Grob CS, Coyle JT: Suspected adverse methylphenidate–imipramine interactions in children. J Dev Behav Pediatr 7:265–267, 1986

Gualtieri CT, Quade D, Hicks RE, et al: Tardive dyskinesia and other clinical consequences of neuroleptic treatment in children and adolescents. Am J Psychiatry 141:20–23, 1984

Gutgesell H, Atkins D, Barst, R, et al: AHA scientific statement: cardiovascular monitoring of children and adolescents receiving psychotropic drugs. J Am Acad Child Adolesc Psychiatry 38:1047–1050, 1999

Hagino OR, Weller EB, Weller RA, et al: Untoward effects of lithium treatment in children aged four through six years. J Am Acad Child Adolesc Psychiatry 34:1584–1590, 1995

Halperin JM, Gittelman R, Katz S: Relationship between stimulant effect, electroencephalogram, and clinical neurological findings in hyperactive children. J Am Acad Child Adolesc Psychiatry 25:820–825, 1986

Hanna GL, Fluent TE, Fischer DJ: Case report: Separation anxiety in children and adolescents treated with risperidone. J Child Adolesc Psychopharmacol 9:277–283, 1999

Hunt RD: Treatment effects of oral and transdermal clonidine in relation to methylphenidate—an open pilot study in ADHD. Psychopharmacol Bull 23:111–114, 1987

Hynes AF, Vickar EL: Case study: neuroleptic malignant syndrome without pyrexia. J Am Acad Child Adolesc Psychiatry 35:959–962, 1996

Jatlow PI: Psychotropic drug disposition during development, in Psychiatric Pharmacosciences of Children and Adolescents. Edited by Popper C. Washington, DC, American Psychiatric Press, 1987, pp 27–44

Keller MB, Ryan ND, Strober M, et al: Efficacy of paroxetine in the treatment of adolescent major depression: a randomized, controlled trial. J Am Acad Child Adolesc Psychiatry 40:762–772, 2001

Kent JD, Bladfer JC, Koplewicz HS, et al: Effects of late-afternoon methylphenidate administration on behavior and sleep in attention-deficit hyperactivity disorder. Pediatrics 96:320–325, 1995

Klein RG, Landa B, Mattes JA, et al: Methylphenidate and growth in hyperactive children. Arch Gen Psychiatry 45:1127–1130, 1988

Klein RG, Mannuzza S: Hyperactive boys almost grown up, III: methylphenidate effects on ultimate height. Arch Gen Psychiatry 45:1131–1134, 1988

Kumra S, Jacobsen LK, Lenane M, et al: Case series: spectrum of neuroleptic-induced movement disorders and extrapyramidal side effects in childhood-onset schizophrenia. J Am Acad Child Adolesc Psychiatry 37:221–227, 1998

Kurlan R: Methylphenidate to treat ADHD is not contraindicated in children with tics. Mov Disord 17:5–6, 2002

Kutcher SP, MacKenzie S, Galarraga W, et al: Clonazepam treatment of adolescents with neuroleptic-induced akathisia. Am J Psychiatry 144:823–824, 1987

Lake MB, Birmaher B, Wassick S, et al: Case report: bleeding and selective serotonin reuptake inhibitors in childhood and adolescence. J Child Adolesc Psychopharmacol 10:35–38, 2000

Liebowitz MR, Turner SM, Piacentini J, et al: Fluoxetine in children and adolescents with OCD: a placebo-controlled trial. J Am Acad Child Adolesc Psychiatry 41:1431–1438, 2002

Mandoki MW: Risperidone treatment of children and adolescents: increased risk of extrapyramidal side effects? Journal of Child and Adolescent Psychopharmacology 5:49–67, 1995

McClellan JM, Werry JS: Schizophrenia. Psychiatr Clin North Am 15:131–148, 1992

Michelson D, Faries D, Wernicke J, et al: Atomoxetine in the treatment of children and adolescents with attention-deficit/hyperactivity disorder: a randomized, placebo-controlled, dose-response study. Pediatrics 108:E83, 2001

MTA Cooperative Group: 14-month randomized clinical trial of treatment strategies for attention deficit hyperactivity disorder. Arch Gen Psychiatry 56:1073–1086, 1999

Munetz MR, Benjamin S: How to examine patients using the Abnormal Involuntary Movement Scale. Hosp Community Psychiatry 39:1172–1177, 1988

Pfefferbaum B, Overall JE, Boren HA, et al: Alprazolam in the treatment of anticipatory and acute situational anxiety in children with cancer. J Am Acad Child Adolesc Psychiatry 26:532–535, 1987

Pliszka SR, Greenhill LL, Crismon ML, et al: The Texas Children's Medication Algorithm Project: report of the Texas Consensus Conference Panel on medication treatment of childhood attention-deficit/hyperactivity disorder, part II: tactics. J Am Acad Child Adolesc Psychiatry 39:920–927, 2000

Popper CW: Medical unknowns and ethical consent, in Psychiatric Pharmacosciences of Children and Adolescents. Edited by Popper C. Washington, DC, American Psychiatric Press, 1987, pp 127–161

Popper CW: Psychopharmacologic treatment of anxiety disorders in adolescents and children. J Clin Psychiatry 54:52–63, 1993

Popper CW: Pharmacologic alternatives to psychostimulants for the treatment of attention-deficit/hyperactivity disorder. Child and Adolescent Clinics of North America 9:605–646, 2000

Preskorn SH, Weller E, Hughes CW, et al: Depression in prepubertal children: dexamethasone nonsuppression predicts differential response to imipramine vs. placebo. Psychopharmacol Bull 23:128–133, 1987

Preskorn SH, Weller E, Jerkovich G, et al: Depression in children: concentration-dependent CNS toxicity of tricyclic antidepressants. Psychopharmacol Bull 24:140–142, 1988a

Preskorn SH, Weller EB, Hughes CW, et al: Relationship of plasma imipramine levels to CNS toxicity in children (letter). Am J Psychiatry 145: 897, 1988b

Research Units on Pediatric Psychopharmacology Autism Network: Risperidone in children with autism and serious behavioral problems. N Engl J Med 347:314–321, 2002

Richardson MA, Haugland G, Craig TJ: Neuroleptic use, parkinsonian symptoms, tardive dyskinesia, and associated factors in child and adolescent psychiatric patients. Am J Psychiatry 148:1322–1328, 1991

Riddle MA, Hardin MT, Cho SC, et al: Desipramine treatment of boys with attention-deficit hyperactivity disorder and tics: preliminary clinical experience. J Am Acad Child Adolesc Psychiatry 27:811–814, 1988

Rivera-Calimlim L, Griesbach PH, Perlmutter R: Plasma chlorpromazine concentrations in children with behavioral disorders and mental illness. Clin Pharmacol Ther 26:114–121, 1979

Ryan ND: The pharmacologic treatment of child and adolescent depression. Psychiatr Clin North Am 15:29–40, 1992

Ryan ND, Puig-Antioch J, Cooper T, et al: Imipramine in adolescent major depression: plasma level and clinical response. Acta Psychiatr Scand 73:275–288, 1986

Rynn MA, Siqueland L, Rickels K: Placebo-controlled trial of sertraline in the treatment of children with generalized anxiety disorder. Am J Psychiatry 158:2008–2014, 2001

Sallee F, Stiller R, Perel J, et al: Targeting imipramine dose in children with depression. Clin Pharmacol Ther 40:8–13, 1986

Scahill L, Chappell PB, Kim YS, et al: A placebo-controlled study of guanfacine in the treatment of children with tic disorders and attention deficit hyperactivity disorder. Am J Psychiatry 158:1067–1074, 2001

Silva RR, Munoz DM, Alpert M, et al: Neuroleptic malignant syndrome in children and adolescents. J Am Acad Child Adolesc Psychiatry 38:187–194, 1999

Snyder R, Turgay A, Aman M, et al: Effects of risperidone on conduct and disruptive behavior disorders in children with subaverage IQs. J Am Acad Child Adolesc Psychiatry 41:1026–1036, 2002

Spencer EK, Alpert M, Pouget ER: Scales for the assessment of neuroleptic response in schizophrenic children: specific measures derived from the CPRS. Psychopharmacol Bull 30:199–202, 1994

Spencer T, Biederman J, Steingard R, et al: Bupropion exacerbates tics in children with attention-deficit hyperactivity disorder and Tourette's syndrome. J Am Acad Child Adolesc Psychiatry 32:211–214, 1993

Spencer T, Biederman J, Coffey B, et al: A double-blind comparison of desipramine and placebo in children and adolescents with chronic tic disorder and comorbid attention-deficit/hyperactivity disorder. Arch Gen Psychiatry 59:649–656, 2002

Strober M, Morrell W, Lampert C, et al: A family study of bipolar I illness in adolescence: early onset of symptoms linked to increased familial loading and lithium resistance. J Affect Disord 15:255–268, 1988

Strober M, Morrell W, Lampert C, et al: Relapse following discontinuation of lithium maintenance therapy in adolescents with bipolar I illness: a naturalistic study. Am J Psychiatry 147:457–461, 1990

Teicher MH, Glod CA: Neuroleptic drugs: indications and guidelines for their rational use in children and adolescents. Journal of Child and Adolescent Psychopharmacology 1:33–56, 1990

Tourette's Syndrome Study Group: Treatment of ADHD in children with tics: a randomized controlled trial. Neurology 58:527–536, 2002

Towbin KE, Dykens EM, Pugliese RG: Clozapine for early developmental delays with childhood-onset schizophrenia: protocol and 15-month outcome. J Am Acad Child Adolesc Psychiatry 33:651–657, 1994

Turgay A, Binder C, Snyder R, et al: Long-term safety and efficacy of risperidone for the treatment of disruptive behavior disorders in children with subaverage IQs. Pediatrics 110:1–12, 2002

Varley CK, McClellan J: Case study: two additional sudden deaths with tricyclic antidepressants. J Am Acad Child Adolesc Psychiatry 36:390–394, 1997

Walkup J, Labellarte M: Complications of SSRI treatment. J Child Adolesc Psychopharmacol 11:1–4, 2001

Walkup JT, Labellarte MJ, Riddle MA, et al: Fluvoxamine for the treatment of anxiety disorders in children and adolescents. N Engl J Med 344:1279–1285, 2001

Weller EB, Weller RA, Fristad MA: Lithium dosage guide for prepubertal children: a preliminary report. J Am Acad Child Adolesc Psychiatry 25:92–95, 1986

Wilens TE, Spencer TJ: Combining methylphenidate and clonidine: a clinically sound medication option. J Am Acad Child Adolesc Psychiatry 38:614–616, 1999

Wilens TE, Biederman J, Baldessarini RJ, et al: Cardiovascular effects of therapeutic doses of tricyclic antidepressants in children and adolescents. J Am Acad Child Adolesc Psychiatry 35:1491–1501, 1996

Williams DT, Mehl R, Yudofsky S, et al: The effect of propranolol on uncontrolled rage outbursts in children and adolescents with organic brain dysfunction. J Am Acad Child Adolesc Psychiatry 21:129–135, 1982

Winsberg BG, Perel JM, Hurwic MJ, et al: Imipramine protein binding and pharmacokinetics in children, in The Phenothiazines and Structurally Related Drugs. Edited by Forrest IS, Carr CJ, Usdin E. New York, Raven, 1974, pp 425–431

Yudofsky SC, Silver JM, Schneider SE: Pharmacologic treatment of aggression. Psychiatric Annals 17:397–407, 1987

Zametkin AJ, Linnoila M, Karoum F, et al: Pemoline and urinary excretion of catecholamines and indoleamines in children with attention deficit disorder. Am J Psychiatry 143:359–362, 1986

■ ADDITIONAL READING

American Academy of Child and Adolescent Psychiatry: Practice parameters for the assessment and treatment of children and adolescents with schizophrenia. J Am Acad Child Adolesc Psychiatry 40 (suppl):4S–23S, 2001

American Academy of Child and Adolescent Psychiatry: Practice parameters for the use of stimulant medications in the treatment of children, adolescents, and adults. J Am Acad Child Adolesc Psychiatry 41 (suppl): 26S–49S, 2002

Green WH: Child and Adolescent Clinical Psychopharmacology, 3rd Edition. Philadelphia, PA, Lippincott Williams & Wilkins, 2001

Kutcher SP: Child and Adolescent Psychopharmacology. Philadelphia, PA, WB Saunders, 1997

Kutcher S (ed): Practical Child and Adolescent Psychopharmacology. Cambridge, UK, Cambridge University Press, 2002

Kutcher S (ed): Child and Adolescent Psychopharmacology News (newsletter). New York, Guilford

Leonard H (ed): The Brown University Child and Adolescent Psychopharmacology Update (newsletter). Providence, RI, Manisses

Martin A, Scahill L (guest eds): Psychopharmacology. Child and Adolescent Psychiatric Clinics of North America 9(1), January 2000

Wagner MW, Markowitz JS, Patrick KS: Methylphenidate ER tablet lodging in esophagus. J Am Acad Child Adolesc Psychiatry 409:1244–1245, 2001

Werry JS, Aman MG: Practitioner's Guide to Psychoactive Drugs for Children and Adolescents, 2nd Edition. New York, Plenum Medical Book Co., 1999

9

PSYCHOSOCIAL TREATMENTS

The ideal mental health service delivery system provides a continuum of care (i.e., integrated programs at all levels of intensity). The child and family can move easily from one service to another as the clinical situation warrants.

Child and adolescent psychiatric disorders cannot be successfully treated unless the family dynamics and the school environment are considered. The parents are always involved, at a minimum to ensure coordinated treatment and to remove any secondary gain caused by the child's symptoms. For many disorders, therapeutic work with the parents or the family is just as important, or even more important, than direct therapy with the child. Often, the therapist coordinates with the school, the pediatrician, a social welfare agency, juvenile court personnel, and/or a community recreation leader. Whatever the modalities of therapy used, the therapist must be aware of the patient's level of physical, cognitive, and emotional development in order to understand the symptoms, set appropriate goals, and tailor effective interventions. A focus on the skills necessary for successful development and adaptation, with attention to improving those at which the child and parent are not sufficiently competent, may facilitate successful therapy (see Strayhorn 1988 in "Additional Reading").

In the outpatient setting, treatment by a single therapist is generally most efficient and effective. Indications for collaborative treatment (two or more therapists working as a team) include an adolescent who is unusually concerned about confidentiality, the need for different types of skills that one therapist does not have, or a clear need of the patient and parent(s) for different qualities in a therapist (e.g., the child would benefit from a male role model, but the mother has great difficulty relating to men). In collaborative treatment, the therapists must maintain free and open communication, to discuss and agree on treatment plans and to avoid aligning into competitive "teams." Unresolved conflicts over relative power and authority of the therapists will lead to difficulties in treatment.

Therapists must maintain clear guidelines for confidentiality and for relaying information between the parent and child. Adolescents are usually more sensitive to this issue than children. In general, the therapist should tell either party when and what information from his or her session will be relayed to the other. In some situations, parents and children may participate in the decision or in the communication itself. When children or adolescents are engaging in potentially dangerous activities or have serious thoughts of harming themselves or others, parents must be informed. Carefully planned joint parent–child sessions, in which the therapist coaches and supports the parent or child in sharing information, may be more useful than reports from the therapist.

■ COMMUNICATION WITH CHILDREN AND ADOLESCENTS

Children's ability to use language is limited by their cognitive immaturity. Young children often use play to express feelings, to narrate past events, and to work through trauma. In play therapy, the therapist uses the metaphor of the child's symbolic play and bases questions and comments on characters in the play rather than focusing directly on the child's own feelings and experiences (even if the connection is clear to the therapist). The skilled therapist tailors communication to the child's stage of language and cognitive development and must be aware that the vocabulary of some bright and precocious children exceeds their emotional understanding of events and concepts. Dramatic play with dolls or puppets; drawing and other art techniques; and questions about dreams, wishes, or favorite stories or television shows can provide access to children's fantasies, emotions, and concerns.

■ THE RESISTANT CHILD OR ADOLESCENT

It is not surprising that many children and adolescents do not cooperate in therapy. Most are brought to treatment by adults and often do not perceive a reason for change; they view it as "giving in" to parents or teachers. In addition, a child or an adolescent may refuse to participate in or attempt to sabotage therapy for various dynamic reasons. Strategies to reduce resistance are more effective if tailored to the cause. A child who is anxious or having difficulty separating from a parent may be helped by having the parent initially present in therapy. The therapist may address, either directly or through play, the patient's reluctance to participate and may suggest possible causes that the child is unwilling or unable to verbalize. Long silences are generally not helpful and tend to lead to increased anxiety or struggle for control. Attractive play materials help to make the therapy situation less threatening and to encourage participation while the therapist builds an alliance. Even adolescents often appreciate the availability of paper and markers. Play can be combined with therapy in techniques such as storytelling, drama, and specially designed games. The therapist must guard, however, against the danger of the sessions becoming mere play or recreation instead of therapy. Use of a token economy in the therapy situation may improve motivation, especially for materially deprived or oppositional children.

■ TYPES OF INDIVIDUAL PSYCHOTHERAPY

The common themes of individual therapies are listed in Table 9–1.

Supportive Therapy

Supportive therapy may be especially useful for children and adolescents who do not have satisfying relationships with adults because their symptoms make it very difficult to establish a positive relationship or their parents are emotionally or physically unavailable, or even hostile. For the patient in crisis, the therapist provides

TABLE 9–1.	**Common themes of individual therapies**

A relationship with a therapist who is identified as a helping person and who has some degree of control and influence over the patient

Instillation of hope, pride, and improved morale

Use of attention, encouragement, and suggestion

Goals of helping the patient to achieve greater control, competence, mastery, autonomy, and coping skills

Goals to abandon or modify unrealistic expectations of self, others, and the environment

Source. Adapted from Strupp 1973.

support until a stressor resolves, a developmental crisis has passed, or the patient or environment changes sufficiently that other adults can take on the supportive role. The patient has a real relationship with the therapist, who facilitates catharsis and provides understanding and judicious advice.

Psychodynamically Oriented Therapy

Psychodynamically oriented therapy is grounded in psychoanalytic theory but is more flexible and emphasizes the real relationship with the therapist, the provision of a corrective emotional experience, and the experience of transference. Goals include resolution of symptoms, change in behavior, and resumption of the normal developmental process. Mechanisms of change include understanding and working with transference feelings, catharsis, development of insight, strengthening of ego skills and adaptive defenses, and improvement in reality testing. The therapist forms an alliance with the child or adolescent, promotes controlled regression, identifies feelings, clarifies thoughts and events, makes interpretations, judiciously gives information and advice, and acts as an advocate for the patient. Sessions are held once or twice a week.

Possible candidates for psychodynamically oriented individual therapy include verbal youngsters (or those who can use symbolic play) who are in significant emotional distress or who are struggling to deal with a stressor or traumatic event (e.g., parental death, divorce, or abandonment; physical illness). Patients with attention-deficit/hyperactivity disorder (ADHD) or disruptive behavior disorders are unlikely to benefit. Youngsters with ADHD have little insight into their behavior and its effect on others and may be genuinely unable to report their problems or to reflect on them. Patients with oppositional defiant and conduct disorders refuse to acknowledge problem behavior and are better treated in family or group therapy or in a structured milieu.

Psychoanalysis

Psychoanalysis is infrequently used in children and adolescents, due to lack of empirical evidence of efficacy and the extreme demands on the family to sustain a process that is expensive, lasts for years, and requires four to five sessions per week. Psychoanalysis is contraindicated in psychotic children or those with cognitive deficiencies or fragile coping skills, or when the child's environment is unstable or unsupportive.

Time-Limited Therapy

All the models of time-limited therapy have in common a planned relatively brief duration (several sessions to 6 months), a predominant focus on the present, and a high degree of structure and attention to specific, limited goals. Theoretical foundations of various models include psychodynamic, crisis, family systems, cognitive, behavioral or social learning, and guidance or educational. Both the therapist and the patient must take active roles. The short duration is used to increase patient motivation and participation and limit nonadaptive dependency and regression. A great deal of attention is paid to the process of termination and to how the patient will continue to make progress after therapy stops. Psychodynamic models emphasize a firm termination of therapy, while cognitive, behavioral, and supportive may include periodic booster sessions.

Time-limited treatment appears to be at least as effective as longer-term therapy for some patients. Time-limited methods have been recommended for multiproblem, crisis-oriented families who are unlikely to persist in longer-term treatment and for well-functioning children and families with circumscribed problems of recent onset. Brief treatment is relatively contraindicated for long-standing severe problems and for children and adolescents who have endured serious losses and/or deprivation.

Other Models of Therapy

Diagnosis-specific, manualized cognitive, cognitive-behavioral, and interpersonal therapy techniques are being developed and tested for children and adolescents with depression, obsessive-compulsive disorder, posttraumatic stress disorder, anxiety disorders, or eating disorders (see "Additional Reading"). These techniques may be used individually or in diagnosis-specific groups. When parents or primary caregivers participate in these interventions, treatment adherence improves. Attention to family coping style and environment should be part of the treatment plan. Parents learn that they can make a difference for their child and that they can apply many of the skills acquired by the patient in therapy, such as emotional control, problem solving, and challenging the negative attitudes and misconceptions that reinforce emotional disorders.

■ PARENT COUNSELING AND PSYCHOEDUCATION

Parent counseling or guidance is primarily an educational intervention, conducted with individual parents or couples in groups. Parents learn about normal child development. The therapist helps parents to understand their child and his or her problems and to modify parental attitudes and behaviors that seem to be contributing to the difficulties. The therapist must try to understand the parents' point of view and to be sympathetic to the hardships of living with a disturbed child or adolescent. For parents who have serious difficulties of their own, parent counseling may merge into or pave the way for marital therapy or individual treatment of the adult.

Virtually all parents of children with psychiatric or learning problems need and deserve education on the nature of their child's disorder and how to select among treatments and manage difficult behavior. Parents spend far more time with their children than the therapist does and can powerfully assist or impede treatment. Parents of children with chronic problems must become skilled advocates, to ensure that their children receive the treatment and schooling that they need. Carefully selected reading material ("bibliotherapy") may be extremely useful to parents (see Appendix).

■ BEHAVIOR THERAPY

Behavioral therapists view symptoms as resulting from habits, faulty learning, inappropriate environmental responses to behavior, or neurodevelopmental deficits, rather than from unconscious or intrapsychic motivation. Behavior therapy is characterized by detailed assessment of problematic behaviors and the environmental conditions that elicit and maintain them, the development of strategies to produce change in the environment and therefore in the patient's behavior, and repeated assessment to evaluate the success of the intervention.

In an operant approach, positive and negative environmental contingencies (responses to the child's behavior) are identified and then modified in an attempt to decrease problem behaviors and increase adaptive ones. A *token economy* is one type of operant approach, in which points, star-shaped stickers, or tokens can be earned for desirable behaviors (and lost for problem behaviors) and then exchanged for backup reinforcers (e.g., money, food, toys, privileges, or time with an adult in a pleasant activity). Token economies can be used successfully by parents, teachers, therapists (with groups or individuals), and staff of inpatient or day treatment programs.

Social learning theory integrates operant conditioning theory with an understanding of cognitive processes and emphasizes the importance of learning new behaviors by observing or imitating others. For example, modeling is used in the treatment of children's anxiety and fears to decrease social withdrawal and teach adaptive skills.

Indications and Efficacy

Behavior therapy is by far the most thoroughly evaluated psychological treatment for children. It is the most effective treatment for simple phobias (using systematic desensitization), for enuresis and encopresis, and for a wide range of noncompliant behaviors. Maximally effective programs require home and school cooperation, focus on specific target behaviors, and implement contingencies quickly and consistently following behavior. Potential problems in the use of behavior therapy are the lack of maintenance of improvement over time and the failure to generalize the new behaviors to situations other than the ones in which training occurred. Generalization can be maximized by conducting training at varied times and places in the settings in which behavior change is desired, facilitating transfer to naturally occurring reinforcers, developing new reinforcers in the child's environment, and gradually fading reinforcement on an intermittent schedule.

Parent Management Training

Empirically tested effective training packages are available to teach parents to use behavior modification techniques to manage noncompliant, oppositional, and aggressive children (for example, see Forehand and McMahon 1981 and Webster-Stratton and Herbert 1994 in "Additional Reading"). Parents are taught to give clear instructions, to positively reinforce good behavior, and to use punishment effectively. Teaching techniques include written and verbal instruction in social learning principles and the use of behavior modification programs; modeling by the therapist; behavioral rehearsal of skills to be used; and homework assignments with subsequent review, feedback, and repetition. One frequently used negative contingency is the time-out, so called because it puts the child in a quiet, boring area where he or she experiences a "time-out" from accidental or naturally occurring positive reinforcement.

Treatment is most effective for young children and those with less severe and persistent behavior problems. Characteristics that have been associated with less positive outcome in parent training include low socioeconomic status, parental psychiatric problems, marital conflict, lack of a social support network, harsh punishment practices, and parent history of antisocial behavior (Kazdin 1997). Families with these characteristics should receive maximally potent interventions, with attention to the parents' individual or marital problems as necessary. Additional topics may need to be addressed, such as skills for resolving marital conflict or managing parental anger. More highly functioning families may be able to succeed with written materials only or by using manuals or videotapes supplemented by group discussion. The therapist must be aware of ethnic and cultural beliefs and customs regarding child development and parenting.

Behavioral intervention can be done in the context of family therapy, including techniques such as parent–child contingency contracting. A social contract is written that specifies the behaviors that the parent and child will change, with contingencies. The family is trained to negotiate and problem-solve. These techniques may be particularly useful for adolescents.

Classroom Behavior Modification

Techniques for use in schools include class rules, attention to positive behavior, token economies, and response-cost programs (reinforcers are withdrawn in response to undesirable behavior). One successful program for children with attention and conduct problems required only that the teacher observe the child for off-task behavior and give verbal feedback every 30 minutes (Pelham and Murphy 1986). The teacher may dispense simple reinforcers such as praise, stars on a chart, or classroom privileges, or parents may provide positive reinforcement and/or response cost based on a "daily report card" the teacher sends home that rates the child's performance that day on selected target behaviors. Detailed instructions and forms developed by Pelham for implementing the daily

report card are available on the Internet at http://ctadd.com/ctadd/
PDFs_CTADD/How_To_Establish_DRC.pdf.

■ FAMILY TREATMENT

Role of the Family in Treatment

Attempts to treat disorders in children or adolescents without considering the persons with whom they live or have significant relationships are doomed to failure. Any change in one family member,
whether a result of a psychiatric disorder, psychiatric treatment,
normal developmental process, or life events, will affect other family members and their relationships. Family constellations vary im-
mensely, from the traditional nuclear family to grandparents
functioning as parents, a single-parent family (with or without contact with a second parent), a step or blended family, an adoptive or
foster family, or a group home. Potential variations in sibling constellations are too numerous to count. The term *parents* refers here
to adults filling the parenting role regardless of their biological or
legal relationship to the patient.

Supportive therapy with families includes counseling in methods of changing behavior; encouraging more positive and realistic
parental feelings and attitudes toward children; helping family
members to manage their emotional reactions to the child's psychiatric disorder; detecting and obtaining treatment for psychiatric disorders in parents and siblings; and advising parents about schools,
treatment modalities, community or leisure activities, and sometimes complex custody and placement decisions.

Family Therapy

Indications

There is consistent support for the efficacy of family-based interventions for externalizing problems (including adolescent substance abuse), and there is emerging evidence for anxiety and
depression as well.

Family therapy may be particularly useful when dysfunctional interactions or impaired communication within the family appear to be related to the presenting problem or when symptoms begin or worsen with a new developmental stage or a change in the family such as divorce, remarriage, adoption, or foster placement. If more than one family member has symptoms, family therapy may be more efficient and effective than multiple individual treatments. It should be considered when one family member improves with treatment but another, not in treatment, worsens. Cases in which the identified patient is relatively unmotivated to participate or to change are likely to be more successful in family therapy than in individual therapy. Attention to family systems issues may be useful when progress is stalled in individual therapy or in behavior therapy. Often family therapy is part of a multimodal treatment plan.

If patients have clearly organic physical or mental illness or if the family equilibrium is precarious and one or more family members are at serious risk for decompensation, family therapy may be useful in combination with other treatments, such as medication or hospitalization. A patient who is acutely psychotic, violent, or delusional regarding the family should not be included in family therapy sessions. Family sessions may not be helpful when a parent has severe but unworkable or minimally relevant psychiatric disturbance or when the child or adolescent strongly prefers individual treatment. Children should not be included in family sessions when parents continue (despite redirection) to criticize them or to share inappropriate information, when the most critical issues are marital, or when parents primarily need specific concrete help with practical affairs or parent training. Cultural sensitivity and competence are even more important when working with families than with individuals.

Types of Family Therapy

Structural family therapy. Structural family therapy (developed by Minuchin) has been the model most used and studied in families in which a child or an adolescent is the identified patient. Its focus is on the present; the identified patient's symptoms are seen as serving a function for the family. The assessment process includes mapping the structure of the family, including the location and permeability of boundaries between family members and around the family and its subsystems. Other important variables are the character and flexibility of alignments of family members, including alliances (joining two or more members in a common interest or task) and coalitions (joint actions directed against one or more family members). Data are gathered on communication patterns and the distribution of power within the family and on the family's sources of stress and support in the environment.

The therapist uses assigned tasks and his or her own interactions with family members to influence the family to change its structure and thereby its functioning, resulting in resolution of the presenting symptoms. Relabeling (i.e., redefining a behavior or symptom to give it a different, usually less negative, meaning for the family) opens alternative pathways for family interactions.

Multigenerational family therapy.   Multigenerational family therapy (pioneered by Murray Bowen) emphasizes how current patterns in families repeat the past. Change results from exploring parents' families of origin and the relationships of the nuclear family to the extended family. Grandparents are often involved indirectly or even brought into the sessions.

Strategic family therapy.   Strategic family therapy (developed by Haley and elaborated by Palazolli and her colleagues) uses a complex and indirect plan of action (which is not fully shared with the family) to produce change. Seemingly paradoxical instructions are devised to upset the family equilibrium and permit change, especially in families resistant to more straightforward techniques. It can be extremely powerful but should be used only by those experienced in family therapy.

Other types.   There are other types of family therapy programs used for specific circumstances such as *family grief therapy, in-home family preservation services, family play therapy, infant or toddler–parent psychotherapy,* and *biobehavioral family approach for chronic physical illness.* Models that have been used to treat conduct disorders include Patterson's *behavioral family therapy;* Alexander's *functional family therapy,* which combines behavioral and family systems theories and techniques with attention to cognitive processes; and *multisystemic therapy,* developed by Henggeler and Borduin, which uses various home-based therapeutic techniques (strategic and structural family therapy, parent training, and cognitive-behavior therapy) along with direct practical assistance to the family in the context of the adolescent's natural environment of home, school, and neighborhood. For eating disorders, additional approaches such as Palazzoli's *Milan family systems therapy, transgenerational family therapy* developed by White, and *Maudsley family therapy* (developed in London) have been used.

Psychoeducational family therapy.   Psychoeducational family therapy has been most extensively used in families of adult schizophrenic patients but has been extended to childhood disorders, such as eating disorders, ADHD, and anxiety and mood disorders. Detailed didactic presentations about the disorder are designed to enhance the family's support networks and to improve the family's coping skills through increased understanding of the illness, its treatment, and home behavior management techniques. Ongoing treatment uses family systems interventions when educational and behavioral techniques are blocked by dysfunctional family structures or processes. Multiple family group interventions are also used in various treatment programs, including eating disorders, inpatient, or partial hospitalization programs.

■ GROUP THERAPY

Indications

Group therapy may be particularly useful for children and adolescents, who are often more willing to reveal their thoughts and feelings to peers than to adults. Forming rewarding peer relationships is one of the most crucial developmental tasks, which is often difficult for youngsters with psychiatric disorders. Group therapy offers unparalleled opportunities for the clinician to evaluate behavior with peers and for young people to observe and practice important social skills and to benefit from companionship and mutual support. Observations by peers may have a far more acute and powerful effect than those by an adult therapist. Often target symptoms such as aggression, withdrawal, shyness, and/or deficient social skills with peers are not apparent or accessible to intervention in individual therapy. Group therapy may be used as the sole treatment modality, but it is often combined with another treatment. Groups may be helpful as part of the evaluation, particularly for preschool-age children. Structured treatment such as cognitive-behavioral therapy for adolescents may be efficiently provided in groups.

Group psychotherapy is contraindicated for extremely fragile youngsters and those who are acutely depressed or anxious, psychotic, and/or paranoid. Adolescents with sociopathic traits or behaviors should not be included in groups with others who might be victimized or intimidated. Severely aggressive or hyperactive children should probably not be included in outpatient groups because of the difficulty in controlling their behavior, the risk of their modeling of problem behaviors for other children, and their intimidation of less assertive children.

All of the theoretical models used in individual therapy may be used in group therapy. Therapy may be exclusively verbal or may include expressive arts techniques (such as psychodrama, dance, or arts and crafts), sports activities, or behavioral techniques (such as anger management skills, modeling and practicing social skills, cooperation, and negotiation). Whatever the type of group, the therapist must understand the dynamics of group process. Psychoeducation and supportive treatment can be provided efficiently in groups. Multifamily groups are often used on inpatient units or partial hospitalization programs.

Technical Considerations

Composition

Patients are included in support groups because they share a single stressor (e.g., sexual abuse, parental divorce, a chronic physical illness, loss of a loved one). Other groups are specifically targeted to a single psychiatric disorder. Groups that focus on social skills work best with a mixture of patients.

Groups conducted in special schools, inpatient units, or day hospitals are typically open ended and often include all children enrolled in the program, but the patients may be divided by age. Special topic groups focusing on anger management and problem-solving skills, cognitive behavior techniques, substance use, social skills, abuse-related issues, or preparation for discharge from the program also may be offered.

The outpatient group therapist should interview prospective group members individually to assess suitability for the group, to orient the patient to the goals and methods of the group, to learn more about the patient, and to begin to develop a therapeutic alliance between the patient and the leader. Interviewing the parent(s) is also helpful for similar reasons. The younger the child, the more important is parental cooperation.

Group members should be in the same or adjacent developmental stages. Children and adolescents change so dramatically as they develop that an age span broader than 2 or 3 years is unlikely to result in a therapeutic group process. Developmental stage is often more important than chronological age in forming groups for pre- and early adolescents because girls may be more mature than boys in physical and social development related to pubertal onset, and development varies greatly even within the same gender.

Opinions differ on including boys and girls in the same group. Some issues might be better handled in single-sex groups, although children and adolescents may need more focus on getting along with opposite-sex siblings and peers. Combining boys and girls, although initially more difficult, may ultimately be more productive, depending on the setting.

Duration and Goals

Some groups have a defined, limited duration, from 6 weeks to an academic year; others are long term. Short-term groups focus on "current and explicit behavior, adaptation, coping, competency, strengths and growth.... [With] emphasis on the dynamics of the here-and-now corrective emotional experience, [and] on the patients' active participation in the change effort" (Scheidlinger 1984, p. 581). Long-term groups are more likely to aim for the promotion of insight, the resolution of unconscious conflicts, and the removal of developmental arrests.

Leadership

Of all modalities of therapy, the need for co-therapists is most clear in group treatment. Groups are complex, with many events occurring simultaneously, and a second observer is valuable. In groups of younger children, an extra pair of hands is needed. Co-leaders who differ from each other in age, sex, race, or culture may expand the opportunities for different types of patient–therapist relationships.

Rules

The group structure should fit the nature of the group and the patients. A psychodynamically oriented discussion group for depressed or anxious adolescents will need far fewer rules than a group that aims to teach social skills to school-age boys with conduct problems. The leaders are responsible for maintaining structure and control of behavior within the group. At times, strategies such as the time-out may even be required. The leaders must be explicit about the rules of confidentiality for the group because the group setting increases the risk of breach of confidentiality.

Family Contact

Involving parents is especially important for preschool- and school-age children in order to identify important events in the child's environment and to monitor progress. Adolescents are more willing and able to report and are also more sensitive to confidentiality issues. For children of all ages, the therapist should inform parents of the general goals of the group and their child's progress toward specific goals. Parent education in development and behavior management is often provided most efficiently in a coordinated parent group session. Parents may also appreciate the opportunity to meet with other parents whose children have similar problems.

Developmental Issues

Groups for Preschool-Age Children

Young children are less able to verbalize and require more structure and planned activities than older children. A group can provide a powerful context to teach social skills and language, especially for children who have pervasive developmental disorder or developmental delays.

Groups for School-Age Children

Because school-age children have great difficulty bringing in outside material for discussion or engaging in introspection, verbal portions of the group can focus on events that occur in the group itself. Games and craft activities can provide a useful structure, but the leader(s) must ensure that recreation does not become the only function of the group. Behavior modification, cognitive problem-solving techniques, and anger management skills may be efficacious. Many child patients will not spontaneously attempt to relate to other children. Others have been rejected or scapegoated by peers. If the group is successful, the children will be able to generalize the skills learned to form relationships with peers at school and in their neighborhoods.

Children with ADHD are often referred to group therapy because of their difficulty with peer relationships and their lack of insight into their difficulties. Children who are taking stimulant medication may need to receive a dose before the group meets to help them benefit from the group therapy and not disrupt it for others.

Groups for Adolescents

Cognitive-behavioral group treatment for adolescents and parents has been shown to be an effective treatment of depression (Lewinsohn et al. 1990; Brent et al. 1997). Such groups have been adapted for teens with anxiety disorders as well. Similar groups may help prevent depression in teenagers at risk. Twelve-step groups are used for adolescents who have problems with drug or alcohol abuse.

Many adolescent groups can be conducted as exclusively verbal discussion groups, although some activities may help to break the ice. If both boys and girls are included in the same group, the leaders should attempt to equalize the gender ratio as much as possible and be alert to sexual undercurrents and acting out, while facilitating the discussion of sexual concerns and the practicing of social skills.

■ WRAPAROUND SERVICES

Innovative community services, often called "wraparound" programs, are increasingly being used to avoid hospitalization or placement in residential treatment. Such services attempt to address complex needs (psychological, school, family, peer, spiritual) in a strength-based community model. Wraparound services involve a variety of interventions with individualized programming and therapy, active involvement of family and community members, integration with social services (such as child welfare, financial support, and housing), and use of interventions in the home, neighborhood, community, and school rather than in the traditional office or hospital setting. Crisis intervention teams, brief respite placement, and in-home therapy/supervision are typically included. Funding sources vary depending on the specific community or state.

■ HOSPITALIZATION AND RESIDENTIAL TREATMENT

Indications

Because children and adolescents should be treated in the setting that is least restrictive and disruptive to their lives, hospital or residential treatment is reserved for youngsters who have not responded to outpatient treatment because of severity of symptoms, lack of motivation, outright resistance, or severe disorganization of the patient or family. If there is concomitant physical illness requiring skilled medical/nursing care, hospitalization may also be necessary. In cases where seeking of psychiatric services has been delayed, more complex and severe symptoms may demand more intensive treatment from the onset, even before outpatient services are attempted.

Hospitalization is usually an acute event that is precipitated by immediate physical danger to self or others, acute psychosis, a crisis in the environment that reduces the ability of the caregiving adults to cope with the child or adolescent, or failure of less intensive forms of treatment. Some hospitalizations are needed for a more intensive, systematic, and detailed evaluation and observation of the patient and family than is possible in an outpatient or a day treatment program or if the patient is resistant to outpatient or day treatment. Over the past decades, hospital lengths of stay have become much shorter. With exceptions only for the most severely ill youngsters, hospitalization is now typically used only to stabilize the acute clinical situation and to arrange for treatment in a less restrictive setting. Placement in a residential treatment center may be indicated for children and adolescents with chronic behavior problems such as aggression, running away, truancy, substance abuse, school refusal, or self-destructive acts that the family, foster home, and/or community cannot manage.

Components of Treatment

Pharmacotherapy

Hospitalization offers an ideal opportunity for systematic trials of medications in children or adolescents whose conditions have not responded to conventional treatment, who have complicated or unclear diagnoses, who have medical problems complicating pharmacotherapy, or whose parents are not able to reliably administer medication and report on efficacy and side effects.

Individual Psychotherapy

As newer treatment methods have evolved and hospital stays have become shorter, individual psychotherapy is less often used as an inpatient primary treatment modality. Regularly scheduled individual sessions with a therapist with whom the child or adolescent can develop a trusting relationship continue to be important in developing a more complete understanding of the patient's intrapsychic, familial, and social dynamics and assisting him or her in developing more adaptive methods of coping with strong emotions. The therapist may be able to help the patient address past traumas and losses, better understand his or her own difficulties, and make use of the other treatments offered.

Milieu Therapy

Milieu therapy includes the total environment, in the context of a structured schedule for daily life. It presents a valuable opportunity to observe the patient over an extended period during meals, sleep, self-care, and play. Goals of the milieu include using clear rules and a regular routine to promote a sense of security and predictability and teaching of specific skills to increase self-esteem and competence. Many settings include a behavioral program that uses a token economy or privilege level system to manage behavior and to modify specific symptoms.

Group Therapy

In addition to general or special topic groups, many programs include community meetings in which therapists set privileges and rules, patients practice social skills, and patients learn to observe their own and others' behavior and to recognize the effect of their behavior on others.

Education

Virtually all children and adolescents who require out-of-home placement have had problems in school. The small classes and highly trained teachers of a hospital unit or residential center school can provide a detailed evaluation of a youngster's academic strengths and weaknesses. One of the most important parts of discharge planning is arranging for an appropriate educational placement and working with the teacher to set appropriate target goals. Youngsters in residential treatment centers are gradually integrated into a special education or mainstream program in the local public or private schools, although some larger residential centers have self-contained classrooms within their facility.

Family Treatment

Work with families is an essential part of hospital treatment. Interventions may include family therapy, parent counseling in behavior management, and education about the nature of the child's disorder and treatment plan. Parents may require marital therapy; individual assessment and treatment; or help with housing, finances, day care, or medical care.

■ DAY TREATMENT

A day hospital or day treatment program, often called partial hospitalization, may be best for children or adolescents who require more intensive intervention than can be provided in outpatient visits but who are able to live at home, in foster care, or in a group home. Compared with hospitalization or residential placement, day treatment is less disruptive to the patient and the family and can offer an opportunity for intensive work with parents, who typically attend the program on a regular basis. Daily planning and review of home management strategies enhance generalization and maintenance of gains made in treatment. A day program may be used to avoid the necessity of inpatient hospitalization, to aggressively address school refusal problems, or as a transition for a patient who has been hospitalized.

Day treatment programs vary in the design, the treatment techniques, and the patient populations, although all treat moderately to severely ill children and adolescents. Some programs provide a full 8-hour day, 5 days a week, and include a school program. When the patients are younger than 6 years, the program may be called a *therapeutic nursery*. Other programs may meet in the late afternoon and evening hours (typically for 3 hours), after patients attend community schools, and on weekends, which facilitates parental attendance. Some agencies offer intensive summer day treatment programs or a therapeutic day camp. The modalities of treatment are variable but tend similar to those described for inpatient units; however, the staff-to-patient ratio is often lower. Lengths of stay are decreasing in many day treatment programs, as in inpatient hospitalization.

■ ADJUNCTIVE TREATMENTS

At times, an intervention that is not, strictly speaking, a psychiatric treatment may be recommended as part of a treatment plan. These could include spiritual, recreational, or extracurricular activities. These programs may be crucial to the child's or adolescent's well-being and the treatment of the psychiatric disorder, or they may encourage progress or improve level of functioning.

Special Education Placements

Modified school programs are indicated for children and adolescents who cannot perform satisfactorily in regular classrooms or who need special structure or teaching techniques to reach their academic potential. These programs range in intensity from tutoring or resource classrooms several hours a week, to special classrooms in mainstream schools, to public or private schools that serve only children and adolescents with special educational needs. Resources differ from community to community, but most have programs for mentally retarded youth, for those with learning disabilities (specific developmental disorders), and for those whose emotional and/ or behavior problems require a special setting for learning. Classes are small, with a high teacher-to-student ratio and specially trained teachers. Vocational evaluation and education may be crucial, especially for adolescents.

Before being placed in a special class, youngsters must have an individually administered battery of psychological tests to evaluate for learning disabilities, including an intelligence test and achievement tests. Federal law 94–142 mandates that all children who need special services receive them and that service be provided in the least restrictive environment, as much in the mainstream with other children and adolescents as possible.

Child and adolescent psychiatrists are being added to the interdisciplinary team as consultants or in school-based health and mental health clinics. These programs efficiently provide coordinated medical and mental health care, although funding can be difficult to maintain.

A boarding school may be useful when a parent–child problem is unresponsive to treatment or an appropriate placement is not available in the home community. Some boarding schools have special programs for children with learning disabilities or psychiatric disorders.

Recreation

Learning to perform a sport or skill competently may be an especially important adjunct to treatment in children and adolescents who lack positive relationships with peers or adults because of social isolation, withdrawal, or being ignored or actively rejected. Trained recreation therapists work in various psychiatric and community settings and focus on teaching adaptive leisure skills and improving interactions with peers. A relationship with an adult such as a Big Brother or Sister or a YMCA counselor or sports coach offers an opportunity to interact with a peer group under supervision and may provide support and build self-esteem until the child or adolescent improves enough to establish relationships independently. Some families have employed a high school or college student one or more afternoons a week to teach the child social and play skills, develop a relationship with the child, and provide structured time. This method also gives parents a respite and an opportunity to spend time with their other children.

Day or overnight summer camps are potentially a very helpful experience. Some youngsters can attend regular camp, whereas others need a therapeutic camp program geared toward children and adolescents with psychiatric or medical problems.

Foster Care

Placement in a foster home may be needed when parents are unwilling or unable to care for their child. Indications are clearest in cases of physical or medical neglect or physical or sexual abuse. Some families may not be able to provide the appropriate emotional nurturance and supervision. Court intervention is required for placement. Foster care should be short term, until parents are rehabilitated or the courts decide that more permanent placement is needed. Unfortunately, child welfare agencies in many communities are overwhelmed, and children and adolescents may require advocacy with the appointment of a *guardian ad litem* attorney to facilitate return to parents, placement in a foster home or group home, or termination of parental rights to free the child for adoption, according to the conditions of the child and family.

Children with severe behavior or physical problems or older adolescents who are difficult to place or maintain in foster or adoptive homes may be placed in group homes with trained staff. These programs vary in staffing and intensity of the treatment offered. Some resemble residential treatment, whereas others simply provide a supervised residence.

Parent Support Groups

Various groups that provide education and support for parents, as well as conduct fund-raising and advocacy for services, have been organized by parents with professional support. Examples are listed in the Appendix. Numerous local groups (many of which are affiliated with national organizations) focus on specific medical or psychiatric disorders or on more generic psychological problems of childhood. They provide a powerful adjunct to more traditional professional services.

■ REFERENCES

Brent DA, Holder D, Kolko D, et al: A clinical psychotherapy trial for adolescent depression comparing cognitive, family, and supportive therapy. Arch Gen Psychiatry 54:877–885, 1997

Kazdin AE: Parent management training: evidence, outcomes, and issues. J Am Acad Child Adolesc Psychiatry 36:1349–1356, 1997

Lewinsohn PM, Clarke GN, Hops H, et al: Cognitive-behavioral treatment for depressed adolescents. Behavior Therapy 21:385–401, 1990

Pelham WE, Murphy HA: Attention deficit and conduct disorders, in Pharmacological and Behavioral Treatment: An Integrative Approach. Edited by Herson M. New York, Wiley, 1986, pp 108–148

Scheidlinger S: Short-term group psychotherapy for children: an overview. Int J Group Psychother 34:573–585, 1984

Strupp HH: Psychotherapy: Clinical Research, and Theoretical Issues. New York, Jason Aronson, 1973

■ ADDITIONAL READING

Adams PL: A Primer of Child Psychotherapy, 2nd Edition. Boston, MA, Little, Brown, 1982

Barker P: Basic Family Therapy, 4th Edition. New York, Oxford University Press, 1998

Barkley RA: Defiant Children: A Clinician's Manual for Assessment and Parent Training, 2nd Edition. New York, Guilford, 1997

Forehand R, Long N: Parenting the Strong-Willed Child: The Clinically Proven Five-Week Program for Parents of Two- to Six-Year-Olds. Chicago, IL, Contemporary Books, 1996

Forehand R, McMahon RJ: Helping the Non-Compliant Child: A Clinician's Guide to Parent Training. New York, Guilford, 1981

Friedberg RD, McClure JM: Clinical Practice of Cognitive Therapy With Children and Adolescents: The Nuts and Bolts. New York, Guilford, 2001

Henggeler SW, Schoenwald SK, Borduin CM, et al: Multisystemic Approach Treatment of Antisocial Behavior in Children and Adolescents. New York, Guilford, 1998

Hibbs ED, Jensen PS (eds): Psychosocial Treatments for Child and Adolescent Disorders: Empirically Based Strategies for Clinical Practice. Washington, DC, American Psychological Association, 1996

Mufson L, Moreau D, Weissman MM, et al: Interpersonal Psychotherapy for Depressed Adolescents. New York, Guilford, 1993

Patterson GR: Families: Applications of Social Learning to Family Life, Revised. Champaign, IL, Research Press, 1975

Strayhorn JM: The Competent Child: An Approach to Psychotherapy and Preventive Mental Health. New York, Guilford, 1988

Webster-Stratton C, Herbert M: Troubled Families—Problem Children. New York, Wiley, 1994

Wilkes TCR, Belsher G, Rush AJ, et al: Cognitive Therapy for Depressed Adolescents. New York, Guilford, 1994

Appendix

RESOURCES FOR PARENTS

■ INFORMATION ON THE INTERNET

American Academy of Child and Adolescent Psychiatry
Distributes Facts for Families—information sheets written for the general public on development, problem behaviors, stressors, and psychiatric disorders. Available also in Spanish and Polish.
http://www.aacap.org

Autism Society of America
7910 Woodmont Avenue, Suite 300
Bethesda, MD 20814-3067
800-3-AUTISM
http://www.autism-society.org

Bright Futures
Publications to promote and improve the health and well-being of children and adolescents.
http://www.brightfutures.org

Child and Adolescent Bipolar Foundation
http://www.bpkids.org

Note. As scientific research advances, information and advice change. Some areas are controversial, even among experts. Parents should be encouraged to discuss questions with their child's pediatrician, child and adolescent psychiatrist, psychologist, or counselor.

Children and Adults With Attention-Deficit/Hyperactivity Disorder (CHADD)
8181 Professional Place, Suite 201
Landover, MD 20785
301-306-7070
http://www.chadd.org

Federation of Families for Children's Mental Health
1021 Prince Street
Alexandria, VA 22314-2971
703-684-7710
http://www.ffcmh.org

Learning Disabilities Association of America
http://www.ldanatl.org

National Alliance for the Mentally Ill
200 North Glebe Road, Suite 1015
Arlington, VA 22203-3754
800-950-NAMI or 703-524-7600
http://www.nami.org

National Institute of Mental Health
http://www.nimh.nih.gov

Online Asperger Syndrome Information and Support (OASIS)
http://www.aspergersyndrome.org

Tourette Syndrome Association
42-40 Bell Boulevard
Bayside, NY 11361
http://www.tsa-usa.org

Zero to Three
Developmental information for parents of children ages 4 years and younger, including how to enhance children's learning and social–emotional growth.
http://www.zerotothree.org

■ BOOKS

Child Development

American Academy of Child and Adolescent Psychiatry: Your Child: What Every Parent Needs to Know. New York, Harper Collins, 1998

American Academy of Child and Adolescent Psychiatry: Your Adolescent: Emotional, Behavioral and Cognitive Development From Early Adolescence Through the Teen Years. New York, Harper Collins, 1999

Managing Child Behavior

Clark L: SOS! Help for Parents: A Practical Guide for Handling Common Everyday Behavior Problems, 2nd Edition. Bowling Green, KY, Parents Press, 1985

Faber A, Mazlish E: Siblings Without Rivalry: How to Help Your Children Live Together So You Can Live Too. New York, Avon Books, 1998

Forehand R, Long N: Parenting the Strong-Willed Child: The Clinically Proven Five-Week Program for Parents of Two- to Six-Year-Olds. Chicago, IL, Contemporary Books, 1996

Greene RW: The Explosive Child. New York, Harper Collins, 1998

Anger Management for Parents

Clark L: SOS! Help for Emotions: Managing Anxiety, Anger, and Depression, 2nd Edition. Bowling Green, KY, Parents Press, 2002

Psychiatric Disorders

Koplewicz H: It's Nobody's Fault—New Hope and Help for Difficult Children and Their Parents. New York, Random House, 1996

Anxiety

Manassis K: Keys to Parenting Your Anxious Child. Hauppage, NY, Barrons Educational Services, 1996

Shaw M: Your Anxious Child: Raising a Healthy Child in a Frightening World. New York, Tapestry Press, 1995

Attention-Deficit/Hyperactivity Disorder

Barkley R: Taking Charge of ADHD: The Complete, Authoritative Guide for Parents. New York, Guilford, 2000

Dendy C: Teenagers With ADD: A Parent's Guide. Bethesda, MD, Woodbine House, 1995

Fowler MC: Maybe You Know My Kid: A Parents' Guide to Identifying, Understanding and Helping Your Child With Attention Deficit Hyperactivity Disorder. New York, Carol Publishing Group, 1990

Ingersoll B, Goldstein S: Attention Deficit Disorder and Learning Disabilities: Realities, Myths, and Controversial Treatments. New York, Doubleday, 1993

Autism and Asperger Syndrome

Gerdtz J, Bregman J: Autism: A Practical Guide for Those Who Help Others. New York, Continuum, 1990

Bashe PR, Kirby BL: The OASIS Guide to Asperger Syndrome: Advice, Support, Insights, and Inspiration. New York, Crown, 2001

Depression

Fassler DG, Dumas LS: Help Me, I'm Sad: Recognizing, Treating and Preventing Childhood and Adolescent Depression. New York, Viking, 1997

Koplewicz HS: More Than Moody: Recognizing and Treatment Adolescent Depression. New York, Putnam, 2002

Psychiatric Medication

Dulcan MK, Lizarralde C (eds): Helping Parents, Youth, and Teachers Understand Medications for Behavioral and Emotional Problems: A Resource Book of Medication Information Handouts. Washington, DC, American Psychiatric Publishing, 2002

Wilens TE: Straight Talk About Psychiatric Medications for Kids. New York, Guilford, 1999

INDEX

*Page numbers printed in **boldface** type refer to tables or figures.*

360